THE ULTIMATE HOME APOTHECARY COLLECTION

30 BOOKS IN 1

Herbal Remedies and Natural Recipes to Enhance Your Well-Being with Holistic Healing

MEGAN MORREN

© 2024 The Ultimate Home Apothecary Collection

All rights reserved.
This document serves purely informational purposes in relation to
"The Ultimate Home Apothecary Collection"
All trademarks and brand names mentioned herein are the property of their respective owners.

GET YOUR BONUS NOW!

THE BONUS IS 100% FREE

1500 NATURAL REMEDIES

**TO GET IT SCAN
THE QR CODE BELOW OR GO TO**

skybonusbook.com/megan-morren-ha

TABLE OF CONTENTS

BOOK 1: THE FOUNDATIONS OF HERBAL MEDICINE 16
Chapter 1: The Origins of Herbal Healing 17
Ancient Civilizations' Herbal Practices 17
Herbs as Sacred Tools 17
From Ancient to Modern Herbalism 18

Chapter 2: Getting Started with Medicinal Herbs 20
Essential Tools for a Home Apothecary 20
Herbal Preparation Techniques 20
Key Herb Categories for Beginners 21

Chapter 3: Safety, Dosage, and Guidelines 23
Understanding Dosage and Potency 23
Identifying and Avoiding Toxic Plants 23
Proper Storage and Labeling for Potency 24

BOOK 2: BUILDING YOUR HOME APOTHECARY 26
Chapter 1: Growing Medicinal Herbs at Home 27
Choosing Herbs for Your Space 27
Soil Prep and Organic Pest Control 28
Seasonal Planting and Harvesting Calendar 29

Chapter 2: Harvesting and Storing Medicinal Herbs 31
Optimal Plant Harvesting Times 31
Drying and Storing Herbs 31
Preventing Contamination and Spoilage 32

Chapter 3: Organizing Your Apothecary Space 34
Designing Your Herbal Workspace 34
Essential Equipment & Storage Solutions 35
Tracking Your Herbal Inventory 35

BOOK 3: HERBAL REMEDIES FOR COMMON AILMENTS 37
Chapter 1: Herbs for Digestive Health 38
Healing the Gut with Herbal Carminatives 39
Herbs for Digestive Support 39
Liver Detox and Gallbladder Support 40

- Digestive Health Recipe 41
- Ginger and Turmeric Digestive Tonic 41

Chapter 2: Herbal Respiratory Support 43
- Herbs for Respiratory Relief 43
- Syrups and Teas for Coughs 43
- Lung Health with Mullein and Nettle 44
- Respiratory Support Recipe 45
- Eucalyptus and Honey Cough Syrup 45

Chapter 3: Natural Skin and Hair Care 47
- Herbal Salves for Skin Conditions Provides recipes for calendula and comfrey-based salves to soothe eczema, psoriasis, and minor wounds. 47
- Acne Treatments with Anti-Inflammatory Herbs 48
- Herbal Rinses and Oils for Hair Health 49
- Aloe Vera and Lavender Soothing Gel 49
- Rosemary and Peppermint Scalp Tonic 51

BOOK 4: ADVANCED HERBAL PREPARATION TECHNIQUES 53

Chapter 1: Tinctures, Infusions, and Decoctions 54
- Tinctures for Potency and Longevity 54
- Infusions and Decoctions Guide 54
- Adapting Techniques for Specific Needs 55
- Chamomile and Lemon Balm Sleep Tincture 56

Chapter 2: Crafting Herbal Ointments and Salves 58
- Infusing Carrier Oils with Herbs 58
- Balms for Pain Relief and Skin Healing 59
- Customizing Salves with Essential Oils 60
- Calendula and Comfrey Healing Salve 61

Chapter 3: Herbal Fermentation & Preservation 63
- Herbal Kombucha and Infused Ferments 63
- Herbal Vinegars and Tonics 64
- Preserving Active Compounds in Syrups 65
- Fermented Garlic Honey 66

BOOK 5: COMMON HERBS AND THEIR APPLICATIONS 68

Chapter 1: Everyday Medicinal Herbs 69
- Chamomile for Relaxation and Digestion 69
- Peppermint for Energy and Stomach Relief 69
- Lavender for Calming and Skin Health 70

Elderflower and Lemon Immune Boosting Elixir 71

Chapter 2: Healing Properties of Roots 73
Ginger: Anti-Inflammation & Digestive Aid 73
Turmeric for Joint Health and Antioxidant Power 74
Dandelion Root for Detoxification 74
Ashwagandha Root Stress Relief Tonic 75

Chapter 3: Leaves as Healing Tools 77
Nettle for Energy and Detoxification 77
Sage: Cognitive Support & Antimicrobial Uses 78
Bay Leaf: Digestion and Flavor Uses 79
Mint and Basil Breath Freshener 79

BOOK 6: RARE AND EXOTIC HERBS FOR HEALING 81

Chapter 1: Adaptogens for Stress and Energy 82
Ashwagandha: Stress Relief and Sleep Aid 82
Rhodiola Rosea: Boosting Clarity and Stamina 82
Holy Basil: A Sacred Herb for Inner Harmony 83
Rhodiola Rosea Energy Elixir 84

Chapter 2: Herbal Tonics for Longevity 86
Gotu Kola: The Brain Tonic 86
Schisandra: Five-Flavor Herb for Vitality 86
Astragalus: Immune Support & Cellular Repair 87
Ginseng and Lemon Vitality Tonic 88

Chapter 3: Exotic Herbs and Common Remedies 90
Blending Rare Herbs with Adaptogens 90
Layering Herbs for Synergistic Benefits 91
Personalized Exotic Blends for Wellness 92
Golden Milk with Ashwagandha 93

BOOK 7: HERBAL REMEDIES FOR DIGESTIVE HEALTH 95

Chapter 1: Carminatives for Digestive Relief 96
Peppermint and Fennel for Digestion 96
Ginger as a Digestive Stimulant 97
Cinnamon for Blood Sugar and Digestion 98
Fennel and Ginger Digestive Tea 99

Chapter 2: Healing the Gut Lining 101
Slippery Elm Bark: Gut Soother 101
Marshmallow Root for Digestive Health 101

Calendula for Gut Inflammation 102

Slippery Elm and Marshmallow Root Gut Soothing Tea 103

Chapter 3: Liver and Gallbladder Support 105

Milk Thistle: Liver Detox and Regeneration 105

Dandelion Root and Bile Production 105

Artichoke for Cholesterol and Digestion 106

Dandelion and Milk Thistle Liver Detox Tea 107

BOOK 8: RESPIRATORY HEALTH WITH HERBS 109

Chapter 1: Natural Decongestants and Mucolytics 110

Eucalyptus for Respiratory Relief 110

Thyme for Clearing Mucus 111

Licorice Root for Respiratory Healing 111

Eucalyptus and Peppermint Chest Rub 112

Chapter 2: Herbs for Respiratory Health 114

Mullein for Chronic Bronchitis and Asthma 114

Nettle for Seasonal Allergy Relief 115

Plantain for Coughs and Lung Healing 116

Chapter 3: Immune-Boosting Respiratory Support 117

Elderberry for Colds and Flu 117

Garlic as a Natural Antimicrobial 118

Oregano Oil for Stubborn Infections 119

Elderberry and Echinacea Immune Support Syrup 119

BOOK 9: EMOTIONAL HEALING WITH HERBS 122

Chapter 1: Adaptogens for Stress Relief 123

Ashwagandha for Cortisol Balance 123

Holy Basil for Emotional Balance 123

Rhodiola Rosea for Stress and Focus 124

Ashwagandha and Holy Basil Stress Relief Tea 125

Chapter 2: Nervines for Calmness 127

Chamomile for Restful Sleep and Anxiety 127

Valerian Root for Deep Relaxation 127

Passionflower for Anxiety Relief 128

Lavender and Valerian Root Relaxation Tea 129

Chapter 3: Uplifting Herbs for Emotional Wellbeing 131

St. John's Wort for Depression 131

Lemon Balm for Mood and Clarity 131

Saffron for Mood Regulation 133

Lemon Balm and St. John's Wort Mood Lifting Tea 133

BOOK 10: HERBAL REMEDIES FOR ATHLETES 135

Chapter 1: Pre-Workout Herbs for Energy 136

Ginseng for Sustained Energy 136

Beetroot for Athletic Performance 136

Cordyceps for Enhanced Physical Stamina 137

Ginseng and Maca Pre-Workout Elixir 138

Chapter 2: Herbal Post-Workout Recovery 140

Turmeric for Reducing Inflammation 140

Arnica for Sore Muscles 141

Ashwagandha for Post-Exercise Energy 141

Arnica and Ginger Muscle Recovery Balm 142

Chapter 3: Long-Term Athletic Health Support 144

Nettle for Mineral Replenishment 144

Horsetail for Joint and Bone Health 144

Ginger for Circulation and Flexibility 145

Beetroot and Tart Cherry Recovery Smoothie 146

BOOK 11: WOMEN'S HEALTH AND HERBAL SUPPORT 149

Chapter 1: Hormonal Balance & Reproductive Health 150

Vitex for PMS and Menstrual Regulation 150

Black Cohosh for Menopause Relief 150

Shatavari for Fertility and Hormonal Balance 151

Chasteberry and Red Clover Hormone Balancing Tea 152

Chapter 2: Herbs for Pregnancy & Postpartum 154

Red Raspberry Leaf for Uterine Health 154

Nettle for Postpartum Recovery 154

Calendula for Postpartum Healing 155

Nettle and Raspberry Leaf Pregnancy Tea 156

Chapter 3: Common Women's Health Concerns 158

Cranberry for Urinary Tract Health 158

Dong Quai for Circulation & Reproductive Health 159

Evening Primrose Oil for Skin Health 160

Red Clover and Dong Quai Hormone Balance Tincture 161

BOOK 12: HERBAL REMEDIES FOR CHILDREN 163

Chapter 1: Gentle Herbs for Common Ailments 164

  Chamomile for Colic and Restless Sleep 164
  Elderberry Syrup for Immune Support 164
  Ginger for Digestive Relief 165
  Lemon and Ginger Sore Throat Soother 166
 Chapter 2: Topical Remedies for Cuts and Rashes 168
  Calendula Cream for Diaper Rash and Minor Wounds Provides recipes for making gentle salves suitable for children's delicate skin. 168
  Aloe Vera for Burns and Scrapes 169
  Lavender Oil for Calming Skin 170
  Calendula and Chamomile Skin Soothing Balm 171
 Chapter 3: Building Immunity Naturally 173
  Echinacea for Children's Immunity 173
  Rosehip Syrup for Vitamin C 173
  Licorice Root for Respiratory Health 174
  Elderberry and Ginger Immune Boosting Tea 175

BOOK 13: HERBAL PET CARE 177
 Chapter 1: Safe Herbs for Dogs and Cats 178
  Chamomile for Calming Anxiety 178
  Slippery Elm for Digestive Relief 178
  Dandelion Root for Detoxification 179
  Chamomile and Oatmeal Calming Pet Shampoo 180
 Chapter 2: Topical and Oral Remedies 182
  Calendula for Minor Wounds 182
  Lavender for Flea Control and Relaxation 183
  Marshmallow Root for Pet Respiratory Health 183
  Arnica and Calendula Bruise Balm 184
 Chapter 3: Emergency Herbal Remedies for Pets 186
  Aloe Vera for Pet Injuries 186
  Oregon Grape Root for Infections 186
  Nettle for Seasonal Allergies 187
  Chamomile and Lavender Calming Pet Spray 188

BOOK 14: HERBAL REMEDIES FOR CARDIOVASCULAR HEALTH 190
 Chapter 1: Herbs for Blood Pressure 191
  Hawthorn for Heart Health 191
  Garlic for Lowering Blood Pressure 191
  Olive Leaf for Circulatory Support 192

Chapter 2: Cholesterol Management with Herbs 194
Fenugreek for Lowering LDL Cholesterol 194
Artichoke for Healthy Cholesterol 195
Psyllium for Cholesterol Reduction 195
Hawthorn Berry and Garlic Cholesterol Support Tonic 196

Chapter 3: Herbs for Heart Health 198
Ginkgo Biloba for Improved Circulation 198
Motherwort for Heart Rhythm Support 198
Cayenne Pepper for Circulatory Health 199
Hawthorn and Hibiscus Heart Tonic 200

BOOK 15: IMMUNE-BOOSTING HERBAL MEDICINE 202

Chapter 1: Herbs for Immune Support 203
Echinacea for Infections 203
Elderberry for Reducing Viral Load 203
Goldenseal for Immune Support 204
Elderberry and Astragalus Immune Tonic 205
Olive Leaf and Oregano Oil Immune Booster 206
Reishi Mushroom and Licorice Root Immune Elixir 208

Chapter 2: Building Long-Term Immunity 210
Astragalus for Immune Strengthening 210
Reishi Mushroom for Immune Support 210
Rosehip for Vitamin C Supplementation 211
Three Healing Recipes 212
Elderberry and Rosehip Immune Boosting Jam 212
Astragalus and Reishi Mushroom Immune Support Soup 213
Garlic and Ginger Immune Strengthening Broth 215

Chapter 3: Herbal Blends for Immune Protection 217
Cold and Flu Tea Blends Provides recipes combining elderberry, echinacea, and ginger for seasonal illness prevention. 217
Immune-Boosting Tinctures 218
Herbal Syrups for Daily Use 219
Three Ancient Healing Recipes 220
Elderberry and Ginger Immune Boosting Syrup 220
Astragalus and Elderflower Immune Tea 222
Reishi Mushroom and Echinacea Immune Support Tincture 223

BOOK 16: HERBS FOR SKIN AND WOUND HEALING 225

Chapter 1: Topical Herbs for Skin Health 226
- Calendula for Wound Healing and Eczema 226
- Plantain for Skin Irritation 226
- Comfrey for Tissue Repair 227
- Three DIY Healing Recipes 228
- Calendula and Aloe Vera Skin Repair Cream 228
- Lavender and Chamomile Facial Mist 229
- Tea Tree and Witch Hazel Acne Spot Treatment 230

Chapter 2: Herbs for Acne and Skin Conditions 232
- Tea Tree Oil for Blemish Control 232
- Witch Hazel for Oily Skin 232
- Neem for Psoriasis and Skin Issues 233
- Tea Tree and Aloe Vera Acne Gel 234
- Calendula and Witch Hazel Skin Toner 235
- Neem and Turmeric Face Mask 236

Chapter 3: Anti-Aging and Skin Rejuvenation 238
- Rosehip Oil for Skin Elasticity 238
- Aloe Vera for Hydration and Healing 238
- Ginseng for Skin Vitality 239
- Rosehip and Hibiscus Anti-Aging Serum 240
- Pomegranate and Green Tea Rejuvenating Face Mask 241
- Sea Buckthorn and Frankincense Youthful Glow Elixir 242

BOOK 17: HERBS FOR THE NERVOUS SYSTEM 244

Chapter 1: Herbs for Calming and Relaxation 245
- Valerian Root for Sleep and Anxiety 245
- Lemon Balm for Daytime Calm 245
- Skullcap for Nervous System Repair 246
- Lavender and Lemon Balm Relaxation Tea 247
- Passionflower and Chamomile Calming Elixir 248
- Hops and Valerian Root Sleep Aid 249

Chapter 2: Herbs for Mental Focus 251
- Ginkgo Biloba for Cognitive Enhancement 251
- Rosemary for Mental Alertness 251
- Gotu Kola for Brain Health 252
- Ginkgo and Rosemary Memory Elixir 253
- Bacopa and Lemon Balm Concentration Tea 254

  Gotu Kola and Peppermint Focus Tonic 256

Chapter 3: Nervous System Tonics 258
  Oat Straw for Nervous System Health 258
  Ashwagandha for Stress Resilience 259
  Passionflower for Relaxation 260
  Lemon Balm and Passionflower Nerve Tonic 260
  Skullcap and Oat Straw Calming Elixir 261
  Blue Vervain and Hops Relaxation Tonic 263

BOOK 18: HERBAL FIRST AID ESSENTIALS 265

Chapter 1: Quick-Action Remedies 266
  Arnica for Bruising and Swelling 266
  Yarrow for Cuts and Bleeding 266
  Plantain for Bug Bites 267
  Arnica and Comfrey Bruise Cream 268
  Plantain and Yarrow Wound Poultice 269
  Cayenne and Ginger Pain Relief Balm 270

Chapter 2: Antiseptics and Anti-Inflammatories 273
  Calendula for Wound Care..273
  Goldenseal as a Natural Antiseptic 274
  Witch Hazel for Swelling and Irritation 275
  Tea Tree and Lavender Antiseptic Spray 275
  Calendula and Turmeric Anti-Inflammatory Cream 277
  Witch Hazel and Chamomile Soothing Antiseptic Gel 278

Chapter 3: Herbal Emergency Kit Essentials 280
  Portable Herbal Kit Essentials 280
  Combining Herbs for First-Aid Blends... 280
  Herbal Kits: Storage and Maintenance 281

BOOK 19: GROWING MEDICINAL HERBS 283

Chapter 1: Starting a Medicinal Herb Garden 284
  Beginner-Friendly Herbs Selection 284
  Understanding Soil and Climate Needs... 284
  Container Gardening for Limited Space 285

Chapter 2: Herb Garden Planting and Care 287
  Seed Planting vs. Transplanting 287
  Seasonal Herb Care and Pest Management 288
  Pruning and Harvesting for Growth... 288

Chapter 3: Preserving and Storing Your Harvest 290
Drying Herbs for Storage 290
Herbal Powders and Infusions 290
Freezing and Storing Fresh Herbs 291

BOOK 20: SUSTAINABLE HERBAL PRACTICES 293

Chapter 1: Ethical Wildcrafting and Foraging 294

Chapter 2: Composting and Recycling in Herbalism 295
Building Nutrient-Rich Compost 296
Recycling Herbal Byproducts 296
Herbal Mulches and Fertilizers 297

Chapter 3: Creating a Sustainable Apothecary 299
Eco-Friendly Packaging Choices 299
Sustainable Herbal Practices 300

BOOK 21: ADVANCED HERBAL EXTRACTION TECHNIQUES 302

Chapter 1: Essential Oil Distillation at Home 303
Essential Oil Extraction Tools 303
Essential Oil Distillation Process 303
Essential Oil Safety and Storage 304

Chapter 2: Alcohol-Free Tinctures and Extracts 306
Glycerites: Alcohol-Free Herbal Extracts 306
Vinegar Infusions for Health 307
Honey-Based Herbal Syrups 307

Chapter 3: Advanced Preservation Methods 309
Solar Infusion for Herbal Oils 309
Encapsulation of Herbal Powders 310
Freezing Tinctures and Infusions 311

BOOK 22: HERBS FOR RARE AND CHRONIC CONDITIONS 312

Chapter 1: Herbal Management of Autoimmune Diseases 313
Turmeric for Reducing Inflammation 313
Ashwagandha for Adrenal Support 314
Astragalus for Immune Modulation 314
Turmeric and Black Pepper Anti-Inflammatory Tonic 315
Licorice Root and Ginger Immune Support Tea 316
Boswellia and Ashwagandha Joint Relief Elixir 317

Chapter 2: Herbal Remedies for Chronic Pain 320
Willow Bark for Pain Relief 320

 Devil's Claw for Joint Pain Relief 320

 Boswellia for Pain Relief 321

 White Willow Bark Pain Relief Tea 322

 Turmeric and Ginger Anti-Inflammatory Smoothie 324

 Devil's Claw Joint Support Tincture 325

Chapter 3: Herbs for Recovery and Healing 327

 Comfrey for Tissue Regeneration 327

 Schisandra for Liver Support 327

 Milk Thistle for Liver Health 328

 Arnica and St. John's Wort Healing Balm 329

 Gotu Kola and Ashwagandha Recovery Tonic 330

 Turmeric and Boswellia Joint Healing Elixir 332

BOOK 23: COMBINING HERBS FOR SYNERGY 334

Chapter 1: The Science of Herbal Synergy 336

Chapter 2: Synergistic Herbal Blends 337

Chapter 3: Personalizing Herbal Remedies 338

 Adjusting Blends for Individual Needs 338

 Blending for Age and Lifestyle 338

 Creating Seasonal Herbal Formulas 339

BOOK 24: HERBAL BUSINESS BASICS 341

Chapter 1: Starting Your Herbal Business 342

 Finding Your Herbal Market Niche 342

 Setting Up a Legal Herbal Business 343

 Developing a Brand Identity 344

Chapter 2: Creating and Packaging Products 346

Chapter 3: Marketing Your Herbal Products 347

 Creating an Online Presence 347

 Engaging with Your Audience 347

BOOK 25: SPIRITUAL AND ENERGETIC HERBAL PRACTICES 349

Chapter 1: Herbs for Cleansing and Grounding 350

 Sage and Palo Santo for Energy Clearing 350

 Lavender and Rosemary for Emotional Balance 350

 Mugwort for Intuition and Psychic Energy 351

Chapter 2: Rituals and Herbal Practices 353

Chapter 3: Herbs for Spiritual Growth 354

 Frankincense and Myrrh for Meditation 354

- Holy Basil for Divine Connection 355
- Rose for Heart Chakra Healing 355

BOOK 26: PREPARING FOR HERBAL EMERGENCIES 357

Chapter 1: Herbal First Aid Kit 358
- Essential Herbs for Cuts and Bruises 358
- Herbs for Common Ailments 358
- Portable Kits for Travel 359

Chapter 2: Emergency Herbal Preparations 360

Chapter 3: Herbal Remedies for Long-Term Crises 361

BOOK 27: SEASONAL HERBAL PRACTICES 362

Chapter 1: Spring Renewal with Herbs 363

Chapter 2: Summer Cooling and Protection 364
- Cooling Teas for Heat Relief Provides recipes using peppermint and hibiscus to beat the heat. 364
- Bug Repellent Sprays and Balms 365

Chapter 3: Autumn and Winter Wellness 366
- Immune Support with Elderberry & Echinacea 366
- Warming Herbal Teas and Tonics 367

BOOK 28: HERBAL APPLICATIONS IN COOKING 369

Chapter 1: Culinary Herbs for Everyday Health 370

Chapter 2: Herbal Infusions for Beverages 371
- Teas for Digestion and Relaxation Provides recipes using chamomile, mint, and fennel. 372
- Herbal Tonics and Cordials 373
- Infused Waters for Everyday Hydration 374
- Lemon Verbena and Mint Iced Tea 374
- Hibiscus and Rosehip Refreshing Cooler 376
- Lavender and Lemon Zest Herbal Water 377

BOOK 29: HERBS FOR GLOBAL HEALING 379

Chapter 1: African and Native Herbal Wisdom 380

Chapter 2: Asian and European Herbal Practices 381

Chapter 3: Integrating Global Practices 382

BOOK 30: SUSTAINING HERBAL KNOWLEDGE 383

Chapter 1: Teaching Herbal Wisdom 384

Chapter 2: Building a Legacy of Herbal Practices 385

Chapter 3: Preserving Herbal Traditions 386

BOOK 1: THE FOUNDATIONS OF HERBAL MEDICINE

CHAPTER 1: THE ORIGINS OF HERBAL HEALING

Ancient Civilizations' Herbal Practices

Ancient civilizations across the globe have long recognized the potent healing properties of herbs, integrating them into their daily lives and wellness practices with remarkable sophistication. The Egyptians, for instance, meticulously documented herbal remedies on papyrus scrolls, such as the Ebers Papyrus, which dates back to 1550 BCE. This ancient medical document lists over 850 herbal prescriptions for a variety of ailments, indicating a deep understanding of plant-based healing. Ingredients like garlic, which was used for its broad-spectrum antimicrobial properties, and aloe vera, revered for its skin-healing benefits, were staples in their medicinal arsenal.

Similarly, in ancient China, the foundational text of Chinese medicine, the "Shennong Bencao Jing" (The Divine Farmer's Materia Medica), compiled around the 3rd century AD, categorizes hundreds of medicinal plants and their uses. This text laid the groundwork for the development of Traditional Chinese Medicine (TCM), which continues to influence modern herbal practices. For example, ginseng, recognized for its adaptogenic properties, was used to enhance vitality and balance bodily systems, while licorice was often prescribed for its soothing effect on the gastrointestinal tract and its ability to harmonize the effects of other herbs.

The Indian subcontinent's contribution to herbal medicine is encapsulated in the ancient texts of Ayurveda, which date back over 3,000 years. Ayurveda emphasizes the holistic balance between body, mind, and spirit, employing a wide array of herbs tailored to individual constitutions. Turmeric, with its potent anti-inflammatory and antioxidant properties, and Ashwagandha, known for its stress-reducing effects, are just two examples of herbs that have been used for millennia in Ayurvedic practices. In the Americas, indigenous tribes possessed extensive knowledge of the medicinal properties of their native plants, a practice deeply intertwined with spiritual beliefs. The Mayans, for example, were adept herbalists who utilized plants like cacao for its stimulating properties and chilis for their pain-relieving capsaicin. North American tribes such as the Cherokee and Navajo used herbs in both healing and ceremonial contexts, employing plants like echinacea to enhance the immune system and white sage for purification rituals.

The Greeks and Romans also made significant contributions to herbal medicine, with figures like Hippocrates and Galen emphasizing the importance of plants in treating disease. The Greek physician Dioscorides wrote "De Materia Medica," a comprehensive text that described the medicinal uses of over 600 plants. This work became a standard reference for herbal knowledge throughout the Middle Ages in Europe.

Each of these ancient civilizations understood the necessity of observing and interacting with the natural world to unlock the healing potential of plants. They relied on empirical evidence and a deep spiritual connection to the earth, carefully documenting the effects of various herbs to treat a wide range of conditions. This rich tradition of herbal medicine laid the foundation for many modern practices and continues to inspire contemporary herbalists to explore the synergistic relationships between plants and human health.

Herbs as Sacred Tools

Throughout history, herbs have been revered not only for their medicinal properties but also for their spiritual significance. In various cultures, certain herbs are considered sacred and are used in rituals, ceremonies, and spiritual practices to purify, protect, and connect with the divine. These practices underscore the belief in the intrinsic power of herbs to influence the spiritual realm and enhance human consciousness.

Sage, for instance, is widely used for **smudging**, a practice where the herb is burned, and the smoke is directed around a person or space to cleanse negative energies. This ritual, rooted in Native American traditions, is believed to promote healing, wisdom, and protection. To perform a smudging ceremony, one would typically use a dried sage bundle, light it, and gently blow out the flame, allowing the smoke to rise. The person conducting the ceremony then guides the smoke around the body or room with their hands or a feather, focusing on intention and prayer.

Frankincense, another herb with deep spiritual roots, has been used for thousands of years in religious ceremonies across Christian, Jewish, Islamic, and other spiritual traditions. Its resin, when burned as incense, is believed to elevate the soul, deepen meditation, and invite divine presence. The use of frankincense involves placing its resin on a hot charcoal disc in a heat-resistant container, allowing the aromatic smoke to fill the space and facilitate spiritual connection.

Palo Santo, known as "holy wood" from South America, is burned similarly to sage for cleansing and healing. The wood is harvested from fallen branches of the Bursera graveolens tree, respecting its sacredness and sustainability. To use Palo Santo for spiritual cleansing, one lights the end of a stick, allows it to burn for a few seconds, then blows it out, letting the smoke permeate the area or aura that needs purification.

Cedar is another herb used in purification rituals, especially in Native American and other indigenous cultures. It is believed to attract good spirits and eliminate negative energy. Cedar branches or leaves can be burned, or fresh boughs can be placed in homes or ceremonial spaces to protect and sanctify them. The process involves lighting dried cedar in a fireproof bowl and using the smoke in a similar manner to sage smudging.

Lavender, while widely recognized for its calming and therapeutic properties, also holds spiritual significance. It is often used in rituals to promote peace, purification, and love. Lavender can be added to bath water for a cleansing ritual, dried flowers can be placed in sachets for protection, or its oil can be anointed on the body to promote calm and clarity.

Incorporating these herbs into spiritual practices involves a deep respect for their power and an understanding of their traditional uses. It is essential to source these herbs ethically, acknowledging their sacredness and ensuring they are harvested sustainably. Engaging with these herbs in a mindful, intentional way can enhance spiritual practices, connect us more deeply to the natural world, and support our overall well-being.

From Ancient to Modern Herbalism

The transition from ancient practices to modern herbalism represents a fascinating evolution of knowledge, blending centuries-old wisdom with contemporary scientific understanding. This evolution has not only preserved the essence of herbal medicine but also enhanced its application, making it more accessible and relevant to today's health challenges. Modern herbalism, while deeply rooted in the traditions of ancient civilizations, has embraced advancements in technology and science to validate and expand the use of medicinal plants. One of the pivotal changes in modern herbalism is the rigorous scientific research that supports the efficacy of herbal remedies. Unlike ancient times, where empirical evidence and traditional knowledge were the primary bases for the use of herbs, today's herbalists can draw upon a wealth of clinical studies and pharmacological data. This scientific backing has led to a more nuanced understanding of how active compounds in herbs interact with the human body at a cellular level. For instance, the anti-inflammatory properties of turmeric, once attributed to its general healing power, are now understood to be due to curcumin, a compound that has been extensively studied for its role in modulating biological processes involved in inflammation and pain.

Another significant advancement in modern herbalism is the standardization of herbal extracts. This process ensures that herbal supplements contain a consistent level of active ingredients, addressing one of the challenges of using whole herbs—the variability in potency due to factors like growing conditions and harvesting methods. Standardization has made it possible to use herbs more precisely, enhancing their safety and effectiveness. For example, standardized extracts of St. John's Wort for depression or Ginkgo Biloba for cognitive enhancement provide reliable dosages that facilitate their integration into conventional healthcare settings.

The integration of technology in modern herbalism extends beyond research and standardization. Today, sophisticated techniques like CO_2 extraction and lyophilization (freeze-drying) are employed to preserve the integrity of herbal constituents, ensuring they remain potent from harvest to shelf. These methods allow for the creation of highly concentrated extracts that are free from solvents and impurities, offering a purity that was unattainable with the simpler extraction methods of the past.

Moreover, the global exchange of herbal knowledge, facilitated by the internet and digital communication, has broadened the scope of modern herbalism. Herbalists now have access to a vast array of plants from around the world, along with traditional uses documented by diverse cultures. This global perspective not only enriches the practice of herbalism but also fosters a more inclusive approach, recognizing the value of indigenous knowledge and practices. As a result, remedies like Ashwagandha from Ayurvedic medicine or Baical Skullcap from Traditional Chinese Medicine are now part of the modern herbalist's repertoire, used alongside native herbs like Echinacea and Goldenseal.

Education and regulation have also played crucial roles in the evolution of herbalism. The establishment of accredited programs in herbal medicine and naturopathy has raised the standard of practice, ensuring practitioners have a comprehensive understanding of both the science and tradition behind herbal remedies. Furthermore, regulatory frameworks in many countries have been developed to oversee the safety and marketing of herbal products, protecting consumers while allowing them to benefit from these natural remedies.

In essence, modern herbalism represents a confluence of tradition and innovation. It honors the wisdom of ancient practices while embracing the advancements that allow for a deeper understanding and more effective use of medicinal plants. This dynamic field continues to evolve, driven by ongoing research, technological advancements, and a growing interest in natural health solutions. As it does, it remains a testament to the enduring power of plants to heal and nurture human health, bridging the gap between the past and the present in the quest for wellness.

CHAPTER 2: GETTING STARTED WITH MEDICINAL HERBS

Essential Tools for a Home Apothecary

To establish a functional home apothecary, certain essential tools are indispensable for the preparation and storage of herbal remedies. Each tool serves a specific purpose in the creation of effective, natural medicines from the comfort of your home. Understanding the role and proper use of these tools will ensure that your herbal preparations are both potent and safe.

Mortar and Pestle: This timeless tool is crucial for grinding and crushing dried herbs into powders or pastes. A ceramic or stone mortar and pestle is recommended for its durability and non-reactive surface. When using, place the herbs in the mortar (bowl) and, with a firm, circular motion, press and crush them with the pestle until the desired consistency is achieved. This method allows for the release of the herbs' essential oils, maximizing their therapeutic benefits.

Strainer: A fine mesh strainer is essential for separating solids from liquids after infusing herbs in water, oil, or alcohol. Stainless steel strainers are preferred for their longevity and ease of cleaning. When straining an infusion, place the strainer over a bowl or jar and pour the mixture through, using a spoon to press out any remaining liquid from the plant material. This ensures a clear, particle-free final product.

Dark Glass Jars: Light exposure can degrade the potency of herbal preparations. Amber or cobalt blue glass jars offer protection from UV rays, preserving the integrity of tinctures, oils, and other herbal products. Ensure jars are clean and completely dry before use to prevent contamination. Label each jar with the contents and date of preparation for future reference.

Scales: Precision is key in herbalism. Digital scales allow for accurate measurement of herbs and other ingredients, ensuring consistent and safe dosages. Look for scales that measure in both grams and ounces with a tare function to account for the weight of containers. When measuring herbs, place a piece of parchment paper or a small dish on the scale, zero out the weight, and then add your herbs until the desired weight is achieved.

Sourcing quality herbs is as important as having the right tools. Opt for organically grown herbs from reputable suppliers to ensure they are free from pesticides and contaminants. Freshness is also vital; dried herbs should be vibrant in color and aroma, indicating they have been properly harvested and stored.

Maintaining a clean, organized apothecary space is crucial for the safety and efficacy of your herbal remedies. Store herbs and preparations in a cool, dark place, ideally in a cabinet or closet dedicated solely to your apothecary supplies. This not only protects the herbs from light and temperature fluctuations but also prevents accidental contamination from kitchen activities or household chemicals. Regularly check your stock for any signs of spoilage or pest infestation and clean all tools and containers thoroughly after use.

By equipping your home apothecary with these essential tools and adhering to best practices for sourcing and storage, you'll be well-prepared to craft a wide range of herbal remedies. This foundation supports the timeless art of herbal medicine, allowing you to harness the natural healing power of plants for the well-being of yourself and your loved ones.

Herbal Preparation Techniques

Embarking on the journey of creating herbal remedies at home begins with mastering three fundamental techniques: infusions, decoctions, and tinctures. These methods, each suited to extracting the healing properties of different parts of plants, form the cornerstone of a versatile home apothecary. By understanding and applying these techniques, you can unlock the medicinal benefits of herbs and create remedies tailored to your health needs.

Infusions are akin to making tea and are best used for the delicate parts of the plant, such as leaves, flowers, and sometimes thin, aromatic roots. To prepare a chamomile tea for relaxation, start with about one to two teaspoons of dried chamomile flowers per cup of boiling water. Place the chamomile in a teapot or jar, pour the boiling water over the herbs, and cover to prevent the escape of volatile oils. Let it steep for 5 to 10 minutes, depending on desired strength. Strain the tea into a cup, and it's ready to enjoy. This method can be adapted to other herbs like peppermint, which is excellent for aiding digestion. Use fresh or dried peppermint leaves and follow the same process, adjusting the amount to taste.

Decoctions are the preferred method for extracting the deeper essences from tougher plant materials such as roots, barks, and hard seeds. To make a ginger decoction, which can soothe an upset stomach, begin by coarsely chopping an inch of fresh ginger root. Add this to a pot with about a cup of water. Bring the mixture to a boil, then reduce the heat and simmer gently for 20 to 30 minutes, allowing the water to reduce by about a third. Strain the liquid, and it is ready to drink. You may add honey or lemon to taste. This technique ensures that the robust, water-soluble compounds are efficiently extracted.

Tinctures involve the use of alcohol or vinegar to extract and preserve the medicinal properties of herbs. They are particularly useful for creating concentrated remedies that are easy to store and administer in small doses. To prepare a simple tincture, fill a jar one-third to one-half full with dried herbs. Do not pack the herbs too tightly. Cover the herbs completely with a solvent like vodka or apple cider vinegar, ensuring there's about an inch of liquid above the herbs to allow for expansion. Seal the jar tightly and store it in a cool, dark place, shaking it daily. After four to six weeks, strain the liquid through a fine mesh strainer or cheesecloth into a clean, dark glass bottle. Label the bottle with the herb and date of preparation. A standard dose is typically 1-2 milliliters, taken 2-3 times daily, but this can vary depending on the herb and the individual.

When preparing herbal remedies, always use high-quality, organic herbs to ensure the purity and efficacy of your preparations. It's also important to label your creations clearly, noting the herb, date of preparation, and expiration date if applicable. Most tinctures will last for several years if stored in a cool, dark place, while decoctions and infusions are best consumed within a day or two for maximum potency.

Key Herb Categories for Beginners

Embarking on the journey of creating a home apothecary begins with understanding the key categories of herbs that form the cornerstone of herbal medicine. These categories include nervines, adaptogens, and carminatives, each playing a unique role in supporting health and wellness. By familiarizing oneself with these categories and a few starter herbs such as chamomile, peppermint, and ginger, beginners can confidently start to explore the vast world of herbal remedies.

Nervines are a class of herbs known for their ability to support the nervous system. These herbs can have a calming effect, helping to alleviate stress, anxiety, and promote a sense of calm. Chamomile is a prime example of a nervine herb. It's not only widely available but also easy to use. To prepare a chamomile tea, one would need about 1-2 teaspoons of dried chamomile flowers per cup of boiling water. Steeping the flowers for 5-10 minutes creates a soothing tea that can be enjoyed throughout the day to help calm nerves and promote relaxation. Chamomile's gentle nature makes it suitable for all ages, highlighting its versatility and ease of use for beginners.

Adaptogens, on the other hand, help the body resist stressors of all kinds, whether physical, chemical, or biological. These herbs and roots have been used for centuries in traditional Chinese and Ayurvedic healing practices. Ginseng and ashwagandha are among the most well-known adaptogens, but for those just starting their herbal journey, peppermint serves as an accessible and versatile adaptogen. Peppermint can be used to make a revitalizing tea by steeping 1 teaspoon of dried peppermint leaves in a cup of boiling water for about 7 minutes. This refreshing beverage can aid digestion, relieve stress headaches, and boost energy levels without the side effects of caffeine.

Carminatives are herbs that help improve digestion, reduce gas, and soothe the digestive tract. Ginger is a powerful carminative with a long history of use in herbal medicine for its ability to relieve nausea, improve digestion, and reduce inflammation. To harness the digestive benefits of ginger, one can prepare a simple ginger tea by slicing about one inch of fresh ginger root and steeping it in boiling water for 10 minutes. This potent tea can be consumed before meals to stimulate digestion or after meals to soothe the digestive system.

For those beginning their exploration into herbal remedies, starting with these three categories of herbs—nervines, adaptogens, and carminatives—provides a solid foundation. Chamomile, peppermint, and ginger are not only effective in their respective categories but are also readily available, easy to prepare, and offer a gentle introduction to the benefits of herbal medicine. As beginners grow more comfortable and experienced in working with these herbs, they can expand their apothecary to include a wider range of herbs, each with its own unique properties and benefits.

CHAPTER 3: SAFETY, DOSAGE, AND GUIDELINES

Understanding Dosage and Potency

Determining the correct dosage and understanding the potency of herbal remedies are critical components of safely incorporating herbs into your health regimen. The effectiveness and safety of herbal treatments depend significantly on administering the right amount, which varies based on the individual's weight, sensitivity to the herb, and any underlying health conditions. This detailed guide aims to provide clarity on calculating dosages for adults, children, and pets, ensuring that each group receives the therapeutic benefits of herbs without adverse effects.

For adults, the standard dosage of dried herbs in a tea form is generally 1-2 teaspoons (5-10 grams) per cup of water. When dealing with tinctures, a common dosage is 1-2 milliliters, taken three times daily. However, these dosages can vary depending on the herb's potency and the condition being treated. It's essential to start with the lower dosage range and gradually increase as needed, observing any reactions or side effects.

Children's dosages require more precise adjustments, primarily based on weight. A safe and commonly used method to determine the correct dose for children is the Young's Rule or the age-to-dose formula. This involves dividing the child's age by twelve plus the age, then multiplying the adult dosage by the result. For example, for a 6-year-old child, the formula would be $6/(6+12) = 6/18 = 1/3$ of the adult dosage. It's crucial to consult with a healthcare provider before administering any herbal remedy to a child, as some herbs may not be safe for young individuals.

When it comes to pets, particularly dogs and cats, the dosage must be adjusted not only for weight but also for species-specific sensitivities. A general guideline for dogs is to administer 1/4 of the adult human dose for every 20 pounds of the animal's body weight. Cats, being more sensitive to many compounds due to their unique liver metabolism, often require a more conservative approach, typically 1/10 of the adult human dose, adjusted for the cat's weight. Always consult with a veterinarian experienced in herbal medicine before treating pets, as some herbs can be toxic to animals. In addition to weight, sensitivity to specific herbs is another critical factor to consider. Individuals, including pets, may have varying reactions to the same herb, influenced by factors such as genetics, existing health conditions, and concurrent use of other medications. Start with the lowest possible dose to assess tolerance and avoid potential adverse reactions. Finally, underlying health conditions can significantly impact the appropriate dosage of herbal remedies. Herbs that may be beneficial for one condition could exacerbate another, and the presence of chronic diseases, especially those involving the liver or kidneys, can alter the body's ability to process and eliminate herbal compounds. Consulting with a healthcare professional knowledgeable in both herbal medicine and the individual's health history is essential to safely and effectively use herbal remedies.

By carefully considering these factors and starting with conservative dosages, individuals can safely explore the benefits of herbal medicine while minimizing the risk of adverse effects. Remember, the goal of using herbs is to support health and wellness, which requires a thoughtful and informed approach to dosage and potency.

Identifying and Avoiding Toxic Plants

In the realm of herbal medicine, the ability to distinguish between safe and toxic plants is paramount for ensuring the health and safety of those who seek to harness the power of herbs. This section delves into the critical skills needed to identify common toxic herbs and outlines guidelines for differentiating between safe and dangerous plants in the wild. Recognizing toxic plants involves a keen observation of specific characteristics, including leaf shape, plant structure, and the presence of unique markers such as milky sap or certain flower colors. For instance, plants like poison hemlock (Conium maculatum) can be identified by their smooth, hollow stems with purple spots, which starkly contrast with the safe and beneficial Queen Anne's lace (Daucus carota), despite their superficial similarity in flower appearance.

Toxic herbs often share common habitats with their beneficial counterparts, making it crucial for foragers and herbalists to familiarize themselves with the botanical and ecological nuances that distinguish safe plants from their toxic look-alikes. For example, while foraging for wild herbs, one must pay close attention to the environment; wetlands and shaded areas are often home to both medicinal plants and their toxic relatives. Learning to identify plants by their botanical Latin names rather than common names can significantly reduce the risk of confusion, as common names can be misleading and vary by region.

One effective method for avoiding toxic plants is to study and carry a field guide with clear photographs and descriptions of both safe and toxic plants native to the area of interest. Digital applications for smartphones that allow users to take pictures and compare them with a database can also be helpful, though they should not replace the guidance of an experienced herbalist or botanist.

When examining a plant, observe its leaves, flowers, and roots carefully. Many toxic plants, such as foxglove (Digitalis purpurea), which is poisonous despite its therapeutic use under controlled conditions, have distinctive features like bell-shaped flowers and a basal rosette of leaves. The presence of certain insects or the absence of animal grazing on a particular plant can also serve as an indicator of its toxicity.

Another critical aspect of recognizing and avoiding toxic plants is understanding the specific toxic compounds they contain and the symptoms they can cause. For instance, plants containing alkaloids, such as belladonna (Atropa belladonna), often have sedative and toxic effects on the nervous system, leading to symptoms like dilated pupils, dry mouth, and hallucinations. Glycosides, found in plants like oleander (Nerium oleander), affect the heart and can cause symptoms ranging from nausea and vomiting to cardiac arrest in severe cases.

For those new to herbal foraging, it is advisable to start with plants that have no toxic look-alikes and are widely regarded as safe. Engaging in workshops or guided walks led by experienced herbalists can provide invaluable hands-on learning opportunities. Additionally, cultivating a personal garden with medicinal herbs offers a controlled environment to learn about plant growth, characteristics, and safe harvesting practices without the risk of encountering toxic wild plants.

Proper Storage and Labeling for Potency

To ensure the longevity and efficacy of your home apothecary, proper storage and labeling of dried herbs, tinctures, and oils are paramount. The key to preserving the potency of these remedies lies in understanding the factors that can degrade their quality—light, heat, moisture, and air—and implementing strategies to mitigate these risks.

Dried Herbs: Store dried herbs in airtight containers made of dark glass or opaque materials to protect them from light, which can fade their color and diminish their therapeutic properties. Mason jars with tight-fitting lids or vacuum-sealed bags are ideal options. Place these containers in a cool, dry area, away from direct sunlight, heat sources, and significant temperature fluctuations, such as a pantry or a cabinet in a room that remains consistently cool. Ensure the herbs are completely dry before sealing them in containers to prevent mold growth. Silica gel packets can be added to absorb any residual moisture.

Tinctures: Similar to dried herbs, tinctures should be stored in dark glass bottles, preferably with a dropper for ease of use. The alcohol or glycerin base of tinctures acts as a natural preservative, allowing them to be stored at room temperature. However, they should still be kept out of direct sunlight and away from heat to maintain their potency. A cabinet or a shelf in a cool, dark room will suffice.

Oils: Herbal oils, whether infused or essential, are sensitive to light and heat. Store these in dark glass bottles in a cool, dark place. If using essential oils, consider refrigeration to extend their shelf life, but ensure the oils are brought to room temperature before use to avoid condensation inside the bottle. Infused oils, particularly those made with fresh plants, have a shorter shelf life and benefit significantly from refrigeration.

Labeling: Every container in your apothecary should be clearly labeled with the following information:

- **Name of the herb or preparation**: Include both the common name and the botanical name to avoid any confusion, especially when dealing with herbs that have multiple common names or look-alikes.

- **Date of preparation**: This is crucial for tracking the age of the remedy. Over time, even well-stored herbs, tinctures, and oils can lose their potency, so knowing when they were prepared helps you gauge their effectiveness.

- **Use or indication**: Note the intended use or specific indications for the remedy. This can be particularly helpful when you have multiple preparations that might be used for different purposes, ensuring you reach for the right remedy when needed.

- **Dosage (for tinctures and oils)**: Include the recommended dosage, especially for tinctures, to avoid the need to look it up each time you use it.

For added organization, consider keeping a logbook or a digital document with detailed records of all the items in your apothecary, including recipes, sources of herbs, dates of harvest or purchase, and any observations on the efficacy of the remedies. This practice not only aids in the efficient management of your apothecary but also enriches your understanding and experience of working with herbal remedies.

By adhering to these guidelines for storage and labeling, you can significantly extend the shelf life of your herbal remedies, ensuring they retain their therapeutic benefits for as long as possible. This careful attention to detail underscores the respect and reverence for the plants and their healing properties, a cornerstone of herbal medicine practice.

BOOK 2: BUILDING YOUR HOME APOTHECARY

CHAPTER 1: GROWING MEDICINAL HERBS AT HOME

When selecting the right herbs for your space, consider the climate you live in and whether you have a garden or need to opt for container gardening. For those new to growing medicinal herbs, starting with plants that are known for their resilience and minimal care requirements can make the process more manageable and rewarding. Herbs such as basil, thyme, and lavender are excellent choices for beginners due to their versatile uses and relatively easy care.

Basil thrives in warm environments and requires at least six to eight hours of sunlight daily. It's best to plant basil in well-draining soil with a neutral pH. If you're growing basil in containers, ensure they are at least 8 inches deep to accommodate the roots comfortably. Water the plant regularly, allowing the soil to dry out slightly between watering sessions to prevent root rot. Basil can be harvested as soon as it starts to leaf out. Pinching off the tips can encourage a bushier growth and prevent early flowering, which can cause the leaves to taste bitter.

Thyme is a hardy perennial that prefers full sun and well-draining soil. It's particularly drought-tolerant, making it a great option for gardeners in dryer climates or those who might not be able to water their plants as frequently. When planting thyme, space the plants about 9 inches apart to allow for proper air circulation and reduce the risk of fungal diseases. Thyme can be harvested at any time, but the flavors are most potent just before the plant flowers. To ensure the plant continues to produce, only harvest up to one-third of the plant at a time.

Lavender, known for its calming aroma, requires full sun, good air circulation, and well-draining soil with a slightly alkaline pH. Lavender is particularly sensitive to overwatering and wet conditions, so it's crucial to let the soil dry out between watering. If you're using containers, choose ones with plenty of drainage holes. Lavender can be harvested once the buds are formed but before they fully open. Cutting the stems in the morning after the dew has dried but before the sun is at its strongest will help preserve the oils and fragrance.

For those with limited outdoor space, container gardening can be a viable alternative. When choosing containers, ensure they are large enough to accommodate the plant's root system and have adequate drainage holes. Use a high-quality potting mix specifically designed for container gardening to ensure your herbs receive the right nutrients and moisture level. Regularly check the soil moisture, as containers can dry out more quickly than garden beds, especially during warmer months. Additionally, consider the placement of your containers; herbs grown on balconies or patios may need more frequent watering due to increased exposure to wind and sun.

Regardless of the method you choose, growing medicinal herbs at home can be a rewarding way to enhance your apothecary and deepen your connection to herbal medicine. By starting with these beginner-friendly herbs and paying close attention to their specific needs, you can create a thriving herbal garden that supports your health and wellness journey.

Choosing Herbs for Your Space

When selecting herbs for your home apothecary, understanding the specific needs of each plant is crucial to ensure they thrive in your space. **Basil**, **thyme**, and **lavender** are excellent starting points due to their adaptability and the minimal care they require, making them perfect for beginners.

Basil thrives in warm environments and requires six to eight hours of sunlight daily. For optimal growth, choose a south-facing window if growing indoors or a spot in your garden that receives ample sunlight. Basil prefers moist, well-drained soil. When watering, aim for the soil to be damp to the touch but not waterlogged. Use a pot with sufficient drainage holes and consider a well-draining potting mix to prevent root rot.

Thyme, on the other hand, is known for its drought tolerance, making it a forgiving choice for those new to gardening. It requires a similar amount of sunlight as basil but is less demanding regarding watering. Allow the soil to dry out completely between waterings to mimic the Mediterranean conditions it naturally thrives in. Thyme is an excellent candidate for container gardening due to its compact growth habit. When planting thyme, mix in some sand or gravel with your potting soil to improve drainage and replicate its native growing conditions.

Lavender demands full sun and well-drained soil, much like thyme. It prefers alkaline conditions, so consider adding a small amount of lime to the soil if your pH levels are too low. Lavender is particularly well-suited for container gardening because it allows for better control over soil conditions. Ensure your container is large enough to accommodate growth and has plenty of drainage holes. Water sparingly, as lavender's primary requirement is good air circulation around the roots and dry soil conditions.

For those with limited outdoor space, **container gardening** offers a versatile solution. Select containers that provide adequate drainage and are large enough to accommodate the mature size of the herbs. Terracotta pots are ideal for herbs due to their porous nature, allowing the soil to breathe and preventing moisture buildup.

When considering **climate**, it's important to remember that basil is sensitive to cold, so it should be brought indoors or protected on chilly nights. Thyme and lavender, however, are more tolerant of varying temperatures but should be shielded from extreme cold. In regions with harsh winters, consider growing these herbs in pots that can be moved indoors or to a sheltered area during the colder months.

Soil Prep and Organic Pest Control

To ensure your medicinal herbs thrive, **soil preparation** and **organic pest control** are fundamental steps that cannot be overlooked. Starting with soil preparation, the goal is to create a fertile, well-draining environment that supports robust plant growth. Begin by assessing your soil type; sandy soil drains too quickly, while clay soil retains moisture for too long. To amend either condition, incorporate **organic compost** into the top 6-8 inches of soil. Compost improves drainage in clay soils and increases water retention in sandy soils, creating an ideal growing medium. For an added nutrient boost, consider mixing in aged manure or a balanced organic fertilizer, following the manufacturer's guidelines for quantities.

The pH level of your soil also plays a critical role in plant health. Most medicinal herbs prefer a pH between 6.0 and 7.0. Use a soil pH tester, available at garden centers, to determine your soil's current state. To raise the pH, add garden lime; to lower it, incorporate sulfur or aluminum sulfate, adhering to package instructions for application rates based on your soil's current pH and the desired level.

Moving on to **organic pest control**, the first line of defense is selecting disease-resistant herb varieties and ensuring they are planted in their preferred conditions, as stressed plants are more susceptible to disease and pest infestations. Implement **crop rotation** to prevent soil-borne diseases from becoming established. Avoid planting the same herb or its family members in the same spot more than once every three years.

For **insect pests**, encourage natural predators like ladybugs, lacewings, and predatory mites by planting a diversity of plants that provide them with nectar, pollen, and shelter. **Physical barriers**, such as floating row covers, can protect young plants from flying insects and rabbits without the need for chemical interventions.

When pests are detected, **neem oil** serves as a powerful organic option. It's effective against a wide range of pests, including aphids, mites, and whiteflies, and it also has some fungicidal properties. Apply according to the label directions, typically at dusk or dawn to avoid harming beneficial insects and to minimize leaf burn.

Diatomaceous earth is another versatile tool in organic pest control. Made from the fossilized remains of tiny, aquatic organisms called diatoms, its sharp edges cut through the exoskeletons of insects, leading to dehydration. It's effective against slugs, snails, and other soft-bodied pests. Sprinkle it around the base of plants, reapplying after rain.

For **fungal diseases**, a homemade baking soda spray can offer prevention and treatment. Mix 1 tablespoon of baking soda with 2.5 tablespoons of vegetable oil in a gallon of water. Add a few drops of liquid soap to help the mixture adhere to plant leaves and apply to affected areas. This solution changes the pH on the leaf surface, making it less hospitable to fungal spores.

Seasonal Planting and Harvesting Calendar

Creating a **seasonal planting and harvesting calendar** is essential for optimizing the growth and potency of your medicinal herbs. This guide will provide month-by-month instructions tailored to a temperate climate zone, which can be adjusted based on your local climate conditions. Remember, the key to a successful home apothecary garden is understanding the unique growth cycle of each herb and planning accordingly.

January & February:

- **Planning Phase**: Use these colder months to plan your garden layout and decide which herbs you want to grow. Research each herb's specific needs regarding sunlight, water, and soil pH. This is also the time to order seeds or purchase starter plants from local nurseries.
- **Indoor Starting**: Some herbs, such as **chamomile** and **lavender**, can be started indoors in these months. Use peat pots and a seed starting mix, placing them in a south-facing window or under grow lights to ensure they receive enough light.

March:

- **Soil Preparation**: As the ground thaws, begin preparing your outdoor garden beds. Incorporate organic compost or well-rotted manure to enrich the soil. Test and adjust the soil pH if necessary, aiming for a range between 6.0 and 7.0 for most herbs.
- **Indoor to Outdoor Transition**: Begin to harden off indoor-started seedlings by gradually exposing them to outdoor conditions for a few hours each day.

April:

- **Direct Sowing**: Hardy herbs like **cilantro**, **dill**, and **parsley** can be sown directly into the garden as they can withstand cooler temperatures.
- **Transplanting**: Continue to transplant seedlings started indoors to their outdoor positions, ensuring the risk of frost has passed.

May:

- **Main Planting Season**: This month is ideal for planting most of your herbs, including **basil**, **thyme**, and **oregano**. Ensure all danger of frost has passed before planting sensitive herbs outdoors.
- **Watering Regimen**: Establish a consistent watering schedule, keeping the soil moist but not waterlogged to encourage strong root development.

June:

- **Maintenance**: Keep an eye on weed growth and use mulch to suppress weeds and retain soil moisture. Continue monitoring water needs, especially during dry spells.

- **Pest and Disease Inspection**: Regularly inspect plants for signs of pests or disease and address any issues promptly to prevent spread.

July & August:
- **Harvesting Begins**: Many herbs, such as **mint** and **rosemary**, can be harvested at this time. Cut them in the morning when their oil content is highest for maximum potency.
- **Continuous Sowing**: Sow fast-growing herbs like **cilantro** and **dill** every few weeks for a continuous harvest.

September:
- **Late Season Planting**: Plant perennials like **sage** and **lavender** now so they can establish themselves before winter.
- **Harvesting**: Continue harvesting herbs, paying attention to each plant's specific harvesting guidelines to ensure the best quality.

October:
- **Final Harvests**: Complete the harvesting of tender herbs before the first frost. Hardy herbs can often withstand the first few frosts and may be harvested into late fall.
- **Preparation for Dormancy**: Begin to prepare your garden for winter. Cut back perennials to ground level, and cover them with a layer of mulch for protection.

November & December:
- **Garden Cleanup**: Remove any dead plant material to reduce the risk of disease next season.
- **Planning for Next Year**: Reflect on the year's successes and challenges to plan for improvements in the next growing season.

By following this calendar, you can ensure your home apothecary garden is both productive and rewarding. Adjustments may be necessary based on your specific climate zone and weather conditions, so always monitor local forecasts and adjust your gardening activities accordingly.

CHAPTER 2: HARVESTING AND STORING MEDICINAL HERBS

Optimal Plant Harvesting Times

Harvesting your medicinal herbs at the optimal time is crucial for maximizing their therapeutic benefits. Each part of the plant – flowers, leaves, and roots – has a specific harvest time that aligns with its peak potency. Understanding these timings ensures that you capture the plant's medicinal properties most effectively.

Flowers should be harvested when they are fully open and before they begin to wilt. This is when their essential oils and active compounds are most concentrated. For most flowering herbs, the best time to harvest is in the morning after the dew has evaporated but before the sun becomes too intense. This timing helps preserve the delicate oils and aromas. Examples include **lavender**, **chamomile**, and **calendula**. Using scissors or garden shears, cut the flower heads cleanly off the stem, taking care not to crush or damage them.

Leaves are often harvested for their medicinal oils, and the timing here varies slightly more than with flowers. Young leaves are generally more tender and aromatic, but it's the mature leaves that often contain the highest concentration of active compounds. The optimal time to harvest most leaves is in the morning, as with flowers, when their essential oils are most potent yet before the midday sun can start the evaporation process. For perennial herbs like **rosemary** or **sage**, which can be harvested throughout their growing season, choose leaves from the outside of the plant first, as this will encourage new growth. Use a sharp pair of garden scissors to snip leaves or stems, ensuring a clean cut that will heal quickly.

Roots require a bit more patience and timing for their harvest. The best time to harvest roots is in the fall of the plant's first or second year, depending on the species. By this time, the plant has had the entire growing season to develop a robust root system rich in medicinal compounds. For annuals, harvest in the late fall before the first frost. For perennials, the second year of growth is often the most potent time. Digging up roots should be done carefully to avoid damaging them. Use a garden fork to loosen the soil around the plant, then gently lift the root from the ground. Shake off excess soil, and rinse the roots with cool water to remove any remaining dirt.

To ensure the highest quality of dried medicinal parts, it's essential to process them immediately after harvest. Flowers and leaves can be dried in a dehydrator set to a low temperature, in an airy, shaded area, or tied in bunches and hung upside down in a dry, well-ventilated space. Roots should be cleaned, chopped into uniform pieces, and dried similarly to ensure even drying.

Remember, the potency of herbs is not only determined by how they are grown but also by how they are harvested and processed. By adhering to these guidelines, you can ensure that your home apothecary is stocked with high-quality, potent medicinal herbs ready for use in teas, tinctures, and other remedies.

Drying and Storing Herbs

Drying and storing herbs effectively is essential for preserving their medicinal properties and ensuring they remain potent for use in your home apothecary. Three primary methods can be employed: air-drying, oven-drying, and freezing. Each technique has its specific applications and best practices to maximize the preservation of the herbs' active compounds.

Air-drying is the most traditional method and is particularly suited for herbs with low moisture content in their leaves, such as rosemary, thyme, and oregano. To air-dry herbs, gather them in small bunches, tying the stems together with twine. Hang these bunches upside down in a warm, dry, and well-ventilated area out of direct sunlight. An attic, a shed, or a room with good airflow will suffice. The drying process can take anywhere from one to three weeks, depending on the moisture content of the herbs and the humidity levels in the drying environment. To test if the herbs are sufficiently dry, check if the leaves crumble easily between your fingers. Once dried, remove the leaves from the stems and store them in airtight containers, labeling each with the herb name and the date of drying. Glass jars with tight-fitting lids or vacuum-sealed bags are ideal for storage, protecting the herbs from light and moisture, which can diminish their potency.

Oven-drying is a faster method that is suitable for herbs with higher moisture content, such as basil, mint, and lemon balm, which might mold if not dried quickly. Preheat your oven to the lowest possible setting, ideally below 180°F (82°C), as higher temperatures can lead to the loss of the herbs' volatile oils and, consequently, their therapeutic benefits. Spread the herbs in a single layer on a baking sheet lined with parchment paper to prevent sticking. Place the baking sheet in the oven, leaving the door slightly ajar to allow moisture to escape. Check the herbs every 30 minutes, turning them occasionally to ensure even drying. Depending on the herb and oven temperature, this process can take 1 to 4 hours. Once the herbs are brittle and crumble easily, remove them from the oven and allow them to cool before storing in airtight containers.

Freezing is an excellent option for preserving the freshness and color of herbs that do not dry well, such as cilantro, parsley, and dill. To freeze herbs, wash and pat them dry with paper towels. Chop the herbs finely and pack them into ice cube trays, filling each compartment halfway. Top up with water or olive oil, which helps preserve the herbs' flavor and prevents freezer burn. Once frozen, transfer the herb cubes to a freezer bag, label it with the herb name and date, and store it in the freezer. These herb cubes can be directly added to soups, stews, or sauces, offering a convenient way to incorporate fresh herbs into your cooking year-round.

Creating herbal powders and infusions from dried herbs further extends their shelf life and potency. To make a powder, grind the dried herbs using a coffee grinder or mortar and pestle until they reach a fine consistency. Store the powdered herbs in small, airtight jars, keeping them in a cool, dark place to maintain their medicinal qualities. For infusions, steep the dried herbs in a carrier oil or alcohol to extract their active compounds, creating potent tinctures and oil infusions for therapeutic use.

By meticulously following these drying and storing techniques, you can ensure that your home apothecary is well-stocked with high-quality, potent herbs ready for creating a wide range of natural remedies and health-boosting infusions.

Preventing Contamination and Spoilage

Preventing contamination and spoilage during the preservation process of medicinal herbs is crucial to maintain their effectiveness and safety. The presence of mold or other contaminants can significantly reduce the therapeutic properties of herbs and, in some cases, render them unsafe for consumption. To ensure the longevity and potency of your home apothecary supplies, meticulous attention must be paid to the methods of drying, storing, and handling your herbs.

The first step in preventing contamination and spoilage is to harvest herbs at the correct time and under the right conditions. Herbs should be collected in dry weather, ideally after the morning dew has evaporated but before the heat of the day, which can cause essential oils to evaporate. This timing helps minimize the moisture content in the herbs, reducing the risk of mold growth during the drying process.

Once harvested, herbs should be cleaned gently to remove any dirt, insects, or other foreign matter. Avoid washing herbs with water unless absolutely necessary, as this can introduce additional moisture. If washing is required, do so lightly and ensure the herbs are thoroughly dried immediately afterward using a salad spinner or patting dry with clean towels.

Drying herbs effectively is paramount to preventing spoilage. Herbs can be air-dried, oven-dried, or dehydrator-dried, depending on the specific herb and available resources. For air-drying, herbs should be tied in small bundles and hung upside down in a well-ventilated, dry, and dark space. This method is suitable for most leafy herbs and flowers. Oven drying should be done at the lowest possible temperature, with the oven door slightly open to allow moisture to escape. A dehydrator provides the most controlled environment for drying herbs, with adjustable temperature settings that can accommodate different types of herbs.

Proper storage is equally important in preventing contamination and spoilage. Once dried, herbs should be stored in airtight containers made of glass, ceramic, or metal, which can protect the herbs from moisture and air, both of which can lead to spoilage. Plastic containers are not recommended as they can leach chemicals into the herbs over time. Containers should be labeled clearly with the herb name and date of storage and placed in a cool, dark location. Exposure to light, heat, or humidity can degrade the quality of the herbs and encourage the growth of mold or bacteria.

Monitoring your stored herbs regularly for signs of spoilage or contamination is a critical ongoing step. Any signs of mold, unusual odors, or changes in color indicate that the herbs have been compromised and should be discarded. It's also essential to use clean, dry utensils when handling herbs to prevent introducing moisture or contaminants.

For herbs that are particularly prone to moisture, such as roots or thicker leaves, silica gel packets or a small amount of uncooked rice can be added to the storage containers to absorb any excess moisture. However, these should not come into direct contact with the herbs to avoid contamination.

By adhering to these detailed steps for harvesting, drying, and storing medicinal herbs, you can significantly reduce the risk of contamination and spoilage. This careful attention to detail ensures that your home apothecary remains a safe, effective source of natural remedies for health and wellness.

CHAPTER 3: ORGANIZING YOUR APOTHECARY SPACE

Designing Your Herbal Workspace

When designing your herbal workspace in a small space, the key is to maximize efficiency and organization while maintaining a clean and accessible area for your apothecary practices. Here are detailed strategies and specific recommendations to create an effective herbal workspace even in limited spaces.

Utilize Vertical Space: In small areas, vertical space is your best friend. Consider installing **hanging herb racks** on unused wall spaces or over doors. Use S-hooks and lightweight, durable materials like bamboo or wire mesh to construct the racks. Ensure they are securely anchored to wall studs to safely hold glass jars and dried herb bundles. This not only saves valuable counter space but also keeps your herbs within easy reach.

Opt for Modular Shelving: Modular shelving units allow you to customize your storage solutions according to your space and needs. Look for units that can be adjusted vertically and horizontally, with options for add-on components like hooks for hanging tools (scissors, strainers, etc.) and under-shelf baskets for additional small items. Materials such as powder-coated steel or solid pine provide durability and resistance against moisture, which is crucial in storing herbs.

Magnetic Spice Containers: Transform your refrigerator door or any metal surface into a storage space using magnetic spice containers. These containers can be used to store small quantities of dried herbs or blends. Opt for clear lids to easily identify contents and ensure they have an airtight seal to preserve the herbs' potency.

Label Everything Clearly: Use waterproof, easy-to-remove labels on all jars, containers, and shelves. This not only helps in quickly identifying your herbs but also keeps your workspace organized and efficient. Consider a label maker for uniformity and legibility.

Incorporate a Fold-Down Worktable: If space is at a premium, a fold-down worktable can be a game-changer. Install a wall-mounted drop-leaf table that can be folded away when not in use. Look for a table with a durable surface that's easy to clean, such as laminated wood or stainless steel. This provides a temporary workspace for preparing your herbal remedies without permanently occupying floor space.

Use Clear Storage Jars: Opt for clear, airtight glass jars for storing dried herbs. This allows you to see what's inside without opening the jar, maintaining the herbs' freshness. Choose jars of various sizes to accommodate different quantities and label them with both the common and botanical names of the herbs.

Implement Drawer Dividers: For smaller tools and supplies, use drawer dividers to keep everything organized and in its place. Adjustable dividers allow you to customize the layout of each drawer according to the items you're storing, such as measuring spoons, pipettes, and labels.

Dedicate a Space for Drying Herbs: Even in a small space, you can create an area for drying herbs. Use a retractable clothesline or a small, foldable drying rack that can be easily set up when needed and stored away when not in use. Ensure this area has good air circulation and is away from direct sunlight to optimize the drying process.

By implementing these specific strategies and utilizing recommended materials and tools, you can design an efficient, organized, and functional herbal workspace, even within the constraints of a small space. This approach not only maximizes your available area but also enhances the overall productivity and enjoyment of your herbal apothecary practices.

Essential Equipment & Storage Solutions

In building a home apothecary, the selection of essential equipment and storage solutions is foundational to maintaining a clean, organized, and efficient workspace. This involves choosing the right tools and containers that not only preserve the potency of herbs and preparations but also facilitate ease of use and accessibility. Here, we delve into the specifics of such equipment and storage solutions, emphasizing their importance and offering guidance on optimal utilization.

Tincture bottles, pivotal for any home apothecary, are available in various sizes, typically ranging from 1 ounce to 4 ounces, and are best chosen in amber or cobalt blue glass. These colored glasses are not merely aesthetic; they serve a critical function by filtering out harmful UV rays, thus preserving the integrity of the tincture. When selecting tincture bottles, ensure they come with dropper caps or spray tops depending on your application needs. Dropper caps facilitate precise dosage, crucial for internal use, while spray tops are ideal for topical applications.

Mason jars, another indispensable item, offer versatile storage solutions for dried herbs, teas, and larger batches of infusions or decoctions. Ranging in capacity from 4 ounces to 32 ounces, these glass jars are preferred for their airtight seals, which are vital in preventing moisture and air from compromising the quality of the contents. For dried herbs, opt for wide-mouth jars for easier access and packing. It's also beneficial to select jars with measurement markings, providing convenience in tracking quantities for recipes or when preparing remedies.

Airtight containers, though similar in function to mason jars, are typically used for powders, seeds, or very finely chopped herbs that may lose their potency to oxidation. Materials can vary, but food-grade stainless steel or high-quality BPA-free plastic with locking lids are recommended for their durability and seal integrity. These containers come in various sizes, so choosing a range that suits the volume of materials you work with regularly is wise.

Maintaining a clean, organized setup is not merely about aesthetics but is crucial for the efficacy and safety of herbal preparations. Labeling is an essential practice in organization, where each bottle, jar, or container should be clearly marked with the contents and date of storage. Waterproof, removable labels are ideal as they can be updated without leaving residue that could obscure visibility or contribute to clutter.

To ensure efficiency, organize your apothecary space by categorizing tools and herbs according to their use or properties. For instance, keeping all materials needed for tincture making in one designated area, including alcohol, bottles, and herbs, streamlines the process. Similarly, dedicating a specific shelf or cabinet for dried herbs, categorized alphabetically or by their purpose (e.g., digestive aids, nervines), enhances accessibility and minimizes time spent searching for ingredients.

Regular cleaning and maintenance of equipment are also paramount. Glassware should be sterilized between uses, especially when switching between different types of preparations to prevent cross-contamination. Stainless steel tools like funnels, spoons, or measuring cups should be washed and dried thoroughly to prevent rust or residue buildup.

Tracking Your Herbal Inventory

To maintain an efficient and functional home apothecary, tracking your herbal inventory is crucial. This involves a systematic approach to **labeling**, **dating**, and **categorizing** your herbs and remedies. Implementing a clear system not only helps in quickly identifying and accessing your supplies but also ensures the potency and safety of your herbal preparations. Here's how to effectively manage your herbal inventory:

Labeling: Every container, whether it's a jar of dried herbs, a bottle of tincture, or a tin of salve, should have a clear, durable label. Use waterproof labels to withstand moisture and handling. The label should include the **common name** and **botanical name** of the herb, to avoid any confusion, especially when dealing with multiple species. For added clarity, include the **part of the plant** used (e.g., root, leaf, flower).

Dating: Alongside the name, each label should display the **date of processing** or **purchase**. For dried herbs, note the date they were dried or acquired. For tinctures, salves, and other preparations, mark the date they were made. This is vital for tracking the shelf life and ensuring you're using your herbs and remedies while they're most potent. Most dried herbs maintain their potency for 1-2 years, while tinctures can last up to 5 years if stored properly.

Categorizing: Organize your apothecary space by categorizing herbs and remedies by their **purpose** or **type**. For example, keep all digestive aids together, separate from herbs used for respiratory health. Alternatively, you can categorize by the **form** of the herb (dried, tincture, oil, etc.). Use separate shelves, drawers, or boxes for each category, and clearly mark the category on the storage unit.

Inventory Tracking System: Consider creating a digital or physical inventory log. This can be as simple as a notebook or spreadsheet where you record each herb's name, quantity, location, and expiration date. Update this log whenever you add to or use items from your inventory. This system not only helps in keeping track of what you have and what you might need to restock but also in planning your herb harvesting or purchasing schedule.

Storage Solutions: Use clear, airtight containers for storing dried herbs and ensure tinctures are in amber or cobalt bottles to protect from light. Assigning a specific place for each category and labeling the shelves or drawers can further streamline your inventory management. For larger collections, consider using a bin or box system where each bin represents a category, and individual containers within are labeled with specifics.

Regular Audits: Schedule regular checks of your inventory to assess the condition and potency of your herbs and remedies. This is the time to remove any items that are past their prime or to note which supplies are running low. It's also an opportunity to update your inventory log with any changes.

Visibility and Accessibility: Ensure that your most frequently used herbs and remedies are the most accessible. This might mean keeping a small, separate area or container for your daily or weekly needs, distinct from your main inventory. This approach minimizes the disruption to the rest of your apothecary and keeps your primary inventory organized.

By implementing these detailed strategies for tracking your herbal inventory, you can maintain a well-organized, efficient, and safe home apothecary. This system not only ensures the optimal use of your herbal remedies but also enhances your overall experience in practicing home herbalism.

BOOK 3: HERBAL REMEDIES FOR COMMON AILMENTS

CHAPTER 1: HERBS FOR DIGESTIVE HEALTH

Ginger and Turmeric Digestive Tonic is a potent remedy designed to soothe the digestive system, reduce inflammation, and enhance overall gut health. This tonic leverages the powerful anti-inflammatory properties of turmeric and the gastrointestinal soothing effects of ginger, making it an excellent choice for those seeking natural relief from digestive discomforts such as bloating, gas, and indigestion. Here's how to prepare this beneficial tonic:

Ingredients:

- 1 tablespoon of freshly grated ginger root
- 1 tablespoon of freshly grated turmeric root (or 1 teaspoon of turmeric powder if fresh is not available)
- 4 cups of filtered water
- Juice of 1 lemon
- 2 tablespoons of raw honey (adjust to taste)
- A pinch of black pepper (to enhance the absorption of turmeric)

Preparation Steps:

1. **Prepare the Roots:** Begin by thoroughly washing the ginger and turmeric roots. Grate them finely to maximize the surface area, which will help extract their beneficial compounds during the boiling process.

2. **Boil the Roots:** In a medium-sized pot, combine the grated ginger and turmeric with 4 cups of filtered water. Bring the mixture to a boil over high heat, then reduce to a simmer.

3. **Simmer:** Allow the mixture to simmer gently for about 20 minutes. This slow cooking process helps to extract the active compounds from the ginger and turmeric, infusing the water with their potent properties.

4. **Strain:** After simmering, remove the pot from the heat. Pour the mixture through a fine mesh strainer into a large pitcher or jar, discarding the solid remnants. This step ensures a smooth tonic free from gritty particles.

5. **Add Lemon and Honey:** While the mixture is still warm, stir in the fresh lemon juice and raw honey. Lemon adds a refreshing tang and vitamin C, while honey provides a natural sweetness that balances the spicy flavors of ginger and turmeric. Adjust the honey according to your taste preference.

6. **Incorporate Black Pepper:** Sprinkle a pinch of black pepper into the tonic and stir well. Black pepper contains piperine, a compound that significantly boosts the bioavailability of curcumin, the active ingredient in turmeric, making it more effective.

7. **Cool and Serve:** Allow the tonic to cool to room temperature. For an extra refreshing experience, you can chill it in the refrigerator before serving. Serve the tonic over ice if desired.

8. **Storage:** Any leftover tonic can be stored in a sealed container in the refrigerator for up to 5 days. Shake well before each use as natural separation may occur.

Serving Suggestion: For optimal digestive support, consume a glass of this tonic about 20 minutes before meals. This timing allows the ginger and turmeric to prime the digestive system, promoting smoother digestion and absorption of nutrients from your food.

Note: While this tonic is generally safe for most individuals, those on medication or with specific health conditions should consult with a healthcare provider before incorporating it regularly into their diet, especially due to the potent effects of ginger and turmeric on blood thinning and blood sugar levels.

By following these detailed steps, you can create a Ginger and Turmeric Digestive Tonic that not only offers relief from digestive issues but also serves as a refreshing and healthful beverage option for everyday wellness.

Healing the Gut with Herbal Carminatives

Herbal carminatives play a pivotal role in soothing and improving digestive health by relaxing the digestive tract and reducing symptoms such as bloating, gas, and cramping. Among the most effective of these herbs are **peppermint**, **fennel**, and **ginger**. Each of these herbs contains specific compounds that aid in the digestion process, offering relief and comfort. Here's a detailed look at how to incorporate these carminative herbs into your daily regimen for optimal digestive health.

Peppermint (Mentha piperita) is renowned for its menthol content, which provides a cooling sensation and helps to relax the muscles of the digestive tract. This relaxation can alleviate spasms and gas, making peppermint a go-to remedy for IBS (Irritable Bowel Syndrome) symptoms. To harness peppermint's benefits, prepare a **peppermint tea** by steeping 1 teaspoon of dried peppermint leaves in 1 cup of boiling water for 10 minutes. Strain and drink this tea 2-3 times daily, preferably between meals, to ease digestive discomfort.

Fennel (Foeniculum vulgare) seeds contain anethole, a compound that can reduce inflammation and help relax the muscles in the gastrointestinal tract, thus reducing gas and bloating. A simple way to use fennel is to chew on half a teaspoon of the seeds after meals. Alternatively, you can make a **fennel seed tea** by crushing 1 teaspoon of fennel seeds and steeping them in 1 cup of boiling water for 10 minutes. Strain and enjoy the tea after meals to aid digestion.

Ginger (Zingiber officinale) is another powerful carminative that can help stimulate saliva, bile, and gastric enzymes that aid digestion, thereby reducing nausea and abdominal discomfort. To prepare a **ginger digestive aid**, peel and grate a 1-inch piece of fresh ginger. Boil the grated ginger in 2 cups of water for about 15 minutes. Strain the liquid, add honey to taste, and sip the tea slowly before or after meals to relieve digestive symptoms.

For individuals looking to combine the benefits of these herbs, a **blended digestive tea** can be made by mixing equal parts of dried peppermint leaves, fennel seeds, and sliced ginger root. Use 1 teaspoon of this blend per cup of boiling water, steep for 10 minutes, and strain. This tea combines the soothing effects of all three herbs and can be consumed 2-3 times daily to support digestive health.

When incorporating these herbs into your diet, it's essential to consider any potential interactions with medications or underlying health conditions. Peppermint, for example, may not be suitable for individuals with GERD (Gastroesophageal Reflux Disease) as it can relax the sphincter between the stomach and esophagus, potentially worsening symptoms. Always consult with a healthcare provider before adding new herbal remedies to your regimen, especially if you are pregnant, nursing, or have existing health concerns.

Herbs for Digestive Support

Marshmallow root and slippery elm are two powerful herbs that have been used for centuries to provide relief and healing for a variety of digestive issues, including irritable bowel syndrome (IBS) and acid reflux. These herbs work by forming a protective layer over the mucous membranes of the digestive tract, soothing irritation, and promoting healing. This detailed guide will explain how to use marshmallow root and slippery elm effectively for long-term digestive support.

Marshmallow root, derived from Althaea officinalis, contains a high mucilage content that becomes gel-like when mixed with water. This mucilage coats the lining of the stomach and intestines, providing a protective barrier against acidity and irritation. To prepare a marshmallow root infusion, measure out 1 to 2 tablespoons of dried marshmallow root into a jar and cover with about 16 ounces of cold water. Allow this mixture to steep overnight, or for at least 8 hours, to fully extract the mucilage. Strain the mixture and drink on an empty stomach first thing in the morning to maximize its soothing effect on the digestive tract. For ongoing support, consume up to 3 cups throughout the day, especially before meals.

Slippery elm, sourced from the inner bark of the Ulmus rubra tree, also boasts a high mucilage content, which similarly coats and soothes the digestive tract. To create a slippery elm porridge, which is particularly beneficial for those with IBS or acid reflux, mix 1 tablespoon of slippery elm powder with 2 cups of hot water. Stir continuously until the mixture thickens. Once cooled, the porridge can be consumed directly or mixed with a bit of honey or yogurt to enhance the flavor. This porridge forms a soothing, protective layer in the gut, alleviating discomfort and inflammation. It's recommended to consume this porridge 2-3 times daily, particularly before meals or at bedtime, to aid in digestion and provide relief from acid reflux.

Both marshmallow root and slippery elm can be integrated into your daily regimen for digestive health. However, it's important to ensure that these herbs do not interfere with any medications you may be taking, as their mucilaginous properties can affect absorption. Always consult with a healthcare professional before introducing new herbal remedies into your routine, especially if you are pregnant, nursing, or have existing health concerns. For individuals seeking to enhance the effectiveness of these herbs, consider incorporating lifestyle changes that support digestive health, such as maintaining a balanced diet rich in fiber, staying hydrated, and managing stress through mindfulness or yoga.

Liver Detox and Gallbladder Support

Dandelion and milk thistle stand out as powerful herbs that support liver function and bile production, essential processes for optimal digestion and detoxification. These plants offer a wealth of benefits, particularly in their ability to cleanse the liver and enhance gallbladder health. Here, we delve into the specifics of how each herb contributes to digestive wellness and the practical ways to incorporate them into your daily regimen for natural health support.

Dandelion (Taraxacum officinale) is not just a common yard weed; it's a potent medicinal plant with deep roots in herbal medicine for liver support. The leaves and roots of dandelion are rich in vitamins and minerals, particularly potassium, which is crucial for maintaining electrolyte balance and blood pressure. For liver detoxification, dandelion root plays a pivotal role by stimulating bile production. Bile, produced by the liver and stored in the gallbladder, is vital for breaking down fats and aiding in the absorption of fat-soluble vitamins (A, D, E, and K). Increasing bile flow helps to remove waste products from the liver, facilitating a natural detox process.

To harness the benefits of dandelion for liver health, consider preparing a **dandelion root tea**. Use about 1 to 2 teaspoons of dried dandelion root per cup of boiling water. Steep for 10 to 15 minutes before straining. This tea can be consumed two to three times a day. Not only does this support liver function, but it also promotes hydration, which is essential for flushing toxins from the body.

Milk Thistle (Silybum marianum) contains silymarin, a group of compounds said to have antioxidant and anti-inflammatory properties that protect liver cells from damage. Silymarin encourages liver cell regeneration and has been shown to improve liver function in people with liver diseases. Milk thistle is particularly beneficial for those exposed to toxins or who consume high amounts of alcohol, as it can help cleanse and repair the liver.

For incorporating milk thistle into your diet, **milk thistle supplements** are widely available and can be an effective way to ensure you're getting a concentrated dose of silymarin. Look for supplements standardized to contain 70 to 80% silymarin. The recommended dosage can vary, but a general guideline is 140 to 210 milligrams of silymarin three times a day. Always consult with a healthcare provider before starting any new supplement, especially if you have a pre-existing liver condition or are taking medications that the liver processes.

Combining **dandelion and milk thistle** can amplify their liver-supporting effects. Both herbs work synergistically to enhance bile production and facilitate the liver's detoxifying role. This combination can be particularly beneficial during seasonal changes or after periods of heavy indulgence when the liver may benefit from additional support.

Digestive Health Recipe

Ginger and Turmeric Digestive Tonic

Beneficial effects

Ginger and Turmeric Digestive Tonic is designed to support digestive health by reducing inflammation, stimulating digestion, and alleviating symptoms of bloating and gas. Ginger contains gingerol, which helps to speed up stomach emptying and reduce nausea. Turmeric, on the other hand, contains curcumin, a compound known for its anti-inflammatory properties that can help soothe the digestive tract. Together, they create a powerful tonic for enhancing digestive wellness.

Portions

Makes about 4 servings

Preparation time

10 minutes

Cooking time

5 minutes

Ingredients

- 4 cups of filtered water
- 2 inches of fresh ginger root, thinly sliced
- 2 inches of fresh turmeric root, thinly sliced (or 1 teaspoon of turmeric powder if fresh is unavailable)
- 1 tablespoon of honey, or to taste (optional)
- Juice of 1/2 lemon
- A pinch of black pepper (to enhance curcumin absorption)

Instructions

1. In a medium saucepan, bring the 4 cups of filtered water to a gentle boil.
2. Add the thinly sliced ginger and turmeric root to the boiling water. If using turmeric powder, ensure it's thoroughly dissolved.
3. Reduce the heat and simmer for about 5 minutes. The water will start to take on a rich, golden color as the roots release their beneficial compounds.
4. After simmering, remove the saucepan from the heat and let it cool for a few minutes.
5. Strain the tonic through a fine mesh strainer into a large pitcher or jar, removing the ginger and turmeric pieces.
6. Stir in the honey until it's fully dissolved for a touch of sweetness. This step is optional and can be adjusted based on personal preference.
7. Add the juice of 1/2 lemon, mixing well. The lemon not only adds vitamin C but also enhances the flavor of the tonic.

8. Finish with a pinch of black pepper. This might seem like a small addition, but it significantly increases the bioavailability of curcumin from turmeric.

9. Serve the tonic warm, or allow it to cool completely and enjoy it chilled.

Variations

- For an extra digestive boost, add a cinnamon stick during the simmering process.
- If you prefer a spicier tonic, include a small slice of fresh cayenne pepper or a dash of cayenne powder.
- Substitute lemon with lime for a different citrus twist.

Storage tips

Store any leftover tonic in an airtight container in the refrigerator for up to 5 days. Gently reheat on the stove or enjoy cold.

Tips for allergens

For those with honey allergies or vegan preferences, substitute honey with maple syrup or agave nectar as a sweetener.

Scientific references

- "Ginger in gastrointestinal disorders: A systematic review of clinical trials," published in Food Science & Nutrition, highlights ginger's effectiveness in enhancing gastrointestinal function.

CHAPTER 2: HERBAL RESPIRATORY SUPPORT

Herbs for Respiratory Relief

Eucalyptus, thyme, and peppermint stand as natural decongestants with a long history of use in herbal medicine for alleviating symptoms associated with upper respiratory conditions. These herbs work by opening airways, clearing sinus blockages, and providing relief from coughs and colds. Their effectiveness lies in their unique compounds that exhibit anti-inflammatory, antibacterial, and expectorant properties, making them invaluable for respiratory support.

Eucalyptus (Eucalyptus globulus) is renowned for its potent eucalyptol content, a compound known for its ability to break up mucus and reduce inflammation. To harness the benefits of eucalyptus for respiratory relief, one can inhale steam infused with eucalyptus oil. This involves adding a few drops of eucalyptus essential oil to a bowl of hot water, covering the head with a towel, and deeply inhaling the steam. The warmth of the steam combined with the therapeutic properties of eucalyptus helps to loosen mucus, allowing for easier breathing. Eucalyptus oil can also be diluted with a carrier oil and applied topically to the chest and throat to ease congestion.

Thyme (Thymus vulgaris) contains thymol, an essential oil with powerful expectorant and antibacterial qualities. Thyme is particularly effective in treating bronchitis and coughs. A simple way to utilize thyme for respiratory issues is by preparing a thyme tea. This involves steeping 1-2 teaspoons of dried thyme leaves in boiling water for about 10 minutes, then straining and drinking the tea. The warmth of the tea soothes the throat, while the thyme works to expel mucus and combat infection. For added benefit, honey, a natural cough suppressant, can be stirred into the tea.

Peppermint (Mentha piperita) is another herb that significantly benefits respiratory health, primarily due to its menthol content. Menthol helps relax the muscles of the respiratory tract, making breathing easier. Peppermint can be used in several ways for respiratory relief. Drinking peppermint tea is a soothing way to benefit from its decongestant properties. Alternatively, inhaling peppermint steam or using a peppermint essential oil diffuser can provide immediate relief for congested sinuses and chests. Peppermint essential oil can also be applied topically in a diluted form to the chest, back, and soles of the feet to help clear congestion.

When using these herbs, especially essential oils, it is crucial to ensure they are of high quality and purity. Always perform a patch test before applying oils to the skin to rule out any allergic reactions. Pregnant women, nursing mothers, and individuals with specific health conditions should consult a healthcare professional before using these remedies.

Syrups and Teas for Coughs

Creating soothing syrups and teas for coughs and sore throats involves a careful selection of ingredients known for their therapeutic properties. Honey, elderberry, and slippery elm bark stand out for their ability to offer relief from both dry and productive coughs, soothing the throat and easing discomfort. Here, we delve into the methodology of crafting these remedies, ensuring each step is detailed for clarity and effectiveness.

To begin with, honey is recognized for its antimicrobial and soothing effects, making it an ideal base for cough syrups. When selecting honey, opt for raw, unprocessed varieties to maximize its medicinal benefits. Elderberry, rich in antioxidants and vitamins, has been traditionally used to boost the immune system and fight off respiratory infections. Slippery elm bark contains mucilage, a gel-like substance that coats and soothes the throat, providing relief from irritation.

Elderberry and Honey Cough Syrup:

Ingredients:

- 1 cup fresh or 1/2 cup dried elderberries
- 3 cups water
- 1 cup raw honey
- A small piece of ginger root (optional for additional anti-inflammatory benefits)

Instructions:

1. Combine the elderberries and water in a saucepan. If using, add the ginger root. Bring the mixture to a boil, then reduce heat and simmer for about 45 minutes to an hour, or until the liquid has reduced by about half.

2. Remove from heat and let cool until it is safe to handle. Mash the berries carefully using a spoon or masher.

3. Strain the mixture through a fine mesh strainer or cheesecloth into a bowl, pressing on the berry mixture to extract all the liquid.

4. Once the liquid is at room temperature, stir in the honey until well combined. The reason for waiting is to ensure the raw honey doesn't lose its medicinal properties through exposure to high heat.

5. Transfer the syrup to a clean, airtight glass jar. Store in the refrigerator for up to two months.

Slippery Elm Bark Tea:

Ingredients:

- 1 tablespoon slippery elm bark powder
- 1 cup boiling water
- Honey or lemon to taste (optional)

Instructions:

1. Place the slippery elm bark powder in a heat-safe mug or bowl.

2. Pour the boiling water over the powder, stirring continuously to prevent clumping. Ensure the powder is fully dissolved.

3. Allow the tea to steep for 3-5 minutes. The mixture will thicken slightly due to the mucilage in the slippery elm.

4. Add honey or lemon to taste, if desired. Honey will provide additional soothing effects, while lemon can offer a refreshing flavor and vitamin C boost.

When preparing these remedies, it's crucial to source high-quality, organic ingredients to ensure the purity and potency of your concoctions. Always label your syrup or tea with the date it was made to keep track of its freshness. For adults, the recommended dosage for the elderberry syrup is one tablespoon taken 3-4 times a day during a cough or cold. For the slippery elm tea, sipping on one cup 2-3 times a day can provide throat relief.

It's important to note that while these remedies can offer relief from symptoms, they are not a substitute for professional medical advice or treatment. Always consult with a healthcare provider if symptoms persist or worsen. These natural syrups and teas can be a comforting addition to your wellness routine, harnessing the power of nature to support respiratory health.

Lung Health with Mullein and Nettle

Mullein (Verbascum thapsus) and nettle (Urtica dioica) are two potent herbs that have been traditionally used to support respiratory health, particularly for strengthening the lungs and reducing inflammation. These herbs are beneficial for individuals suffering from chronic respiratory conditions such as asthma, providing a natural approach to improving lung function and overall respiratory wellness.

Mullein is renowned for its soothing properties on the bronchial tubes and lungs. It acts as an expectorant, facilitating the expulsion of excess mucus and reducing congestion. This herb's leaves and flowers contain saponins, mucilage, and flavonoids, which contribute to its anti-inflammatory and antispasmodic effects, making it an excellent choice for easing coughs and soothing irritated respiratory tracts. To harness the benefits of mullein, a tea can be prepared by steeping 1 to 2 teaspoons of dried mullein leaves or flowers in boiling water for 10 to 15 minutes. This allows the therapeutic compounds to be released. Strain the tea to remove any fine hairs from the plant material, as these can be irritating if ingested. Drinking mullein tea 2 to 3 times a day can significantly improve respiratory symptoms and enhance lung health.

Nettle, on the other hand, is packed with vitamins and minerals, including vitamin C, potassium, and iron, which support the body's immune response and overall health. Its anti-inflammatory properties make it an effective remedy for reducing allergic reactions and inflammation in the respiratory system, which is particularly beneficial for asthma sufferers. Nettle can be consumed as a tea, made by steeping dried nettle leaves in boiling water for about 10 minutes. This method extracts the beneficial compounds from the leaves, offering a simple yet effective way to incorporate nettle into your respiratory health regimen. Drinking nettle tea daily can help to alleviate symptoms of respiratory conditions and support lung function.

For those dealing with chronic respiratory issues, incorporating both mullein and nettle into a daily wellness routine can offer significant benefits. Combining the two herbs can enhance their individual effects, providing a comprehensive approach to lung health. A blend can be created by mixing equal parts of dried mullein and nettle leaves, which can then be used to prepare tea. This combination leverages mullein's soothing and expectorant properties alongside nettle's anti-inflammatory benefits, offering a powerful herbal remedy for respiratory support.

When preparing and using mullein and nettle, it's crucial to source high-quality, organic herbs to ensure the purity and effectiveness of your remedies. Always consult with a healthcare provider before incorporating new herbs into your regimen, especially if you are pregnant, nursing, or taking prescription medications. While these herbs offer a natural way to support respiratory health, they should complement, not replace, conventional treatments prescribed by your healthcare provider.

By integrating mullein and nettle into your health care practices, you can take advantage of their powerful properties to support lung strengthening and long-term respiratory wellness. These herbs provide a natural and accessible means to improve respiratory function and alleviate symptoms associated with chronic respiratory conditions, enhancing your overall quality of life.

Respiratory Support Recipe

Eucalyptus and Honey Cough Syrup

Beneficial effects

Eucalyptus and Honey Cough Syrup harnesses the power of eucalyptus to relieve coughs and respiratory congestion, combined with the soothing properties of honey to coat and calm irritated throats. Eucalyptus is known for its cineole content, a compound that can help break up mucus, making it easier to expel and thus easing coughs. Honey, on the other hand, has been studied for its effectiveness in soothing sore throats and reducing cough frequency, making it an ideal natural sweetener for cough syrups.

Portions

Makes approximately 10 servings

Preparation time
5 minutes
Cooking time
10 minutes
Ingredients
- 1 cup of water
- 1/4 cup of dried eucalyptus leaves
- 1 cup of raw honey
- 1 tablespoon of lemon juice
- 1/2 teaspoon of ground ginger (optional)

Instructions
1. Pour 1 cup of water into a small saucepan and bring it to a boil over medium heat.
2. Add 1/4 cup of dried eucalyptus leaves to the boiling water. Reduce the heat to low, allowing the mixture to simmer gently for 10 minutes. This process extracts the beneficial compounds from the eucalyptus leaves.
3. After simmering, remove the saucepan from the heat. Strain the eucalyptus infusion using a fine mesh strainer into a heat-resistant bowl or measuring cup, discarding the eucalyptus leaves.
4. While the eucalyptus infusion is still warm (but not too hot to touch), add 1 cup of raw honey to the bowl. Stir the mixture thoroughly until the honey is completely dissolved into the eucalyptus infusion.
5. Incorporate 1 tablespoon of lemon juice into the syrup, adding a touch of vitamin C and enhancing its flavor. If desired, stir in 1/2 teaspoon of ground ginger for its additional anti-inflammatory and anti-nausea benefits.
6. Transfer the finished cough syrup into a clean, dry bottle or jar with a tight-fitting lid. Label the container with the date and contents.

Variations
- For an extra immune boost, add 1 teaspoon of cinnamon powder or a cinnamon stick during the simmering process.
- Substitute lemon juice with orange juice for a different citrus twist and additional vitamin C.

Storage tips
Store the eucalyptus and honey cough syrup in the refrigerator for up to 2 weeks. Ensure the container is sealed properly to maintain freshness and potency.

Tips for allergens
For those with allergies to honey, substitute it with maple syrup or agave nectar, though be mindful that the texture and soothing properties may vary.

Scientific references
- "Honey for acute cough in children," published in the Cochrane Database of Systematic Reviews, highlights honey's effectiveness in cough management.
- "The effects of cineole in the treatment of acute bronchitis in children," featured in Phytomedicine, discusses the benefits of cineole, found in eucalyptus, for respiratory conditions.

CHAPTER 3: NATURAL SKIN AND HAIR CARE

Herbal Salves for Skin Conditions Provides recipes for calendula and comfrey-based salves to soothe eczema, psoriasis, and minor wounds.

Beneficial effects

This herbal salve combines the healing properties of calendula and comfrey to soothe and repair skin affected by eczema, psoriasis, and minor wounds. Calendula is renowned for its anti-inflammatory and antimicrobial benefits, which promote skin healing and cell regeneration. Comfrey, with its allantoin content, aids in the growth of new skin cells and reduces inflammation. Together, these herbs create a powerful salve that can accelerate the healing process, soothe irritated skin, and provide a protective barrier against environmental irritants.

Portions

Makes approximately 8 ounces (240 ml) of salve

Preparation time

15 minutes

Cooking time

1 hour to infuse oil + 20 minutes to prepare the salve

Ingredients

- 1 cup of calendula-infused oil (see instructions below for infusion)
- 1 cup of comfrey-infused oil (see instructions below for infusion)
- 1/4 cup of beeswax pellets
- 2 tablespoons of shea butter
- 1 teaspoon of vitamin E oil
- 10-15 drops of lavender essential oil (optional for added antimicrobial and soothing properties)

Instructions

1. **To prepare the infused oils:** Place dried calendula and comfrey leaves in separate jars, covering each with a carrier oil such as olive or almond oil. Seal the jars and place them in a warm, sunny spot for 4-6 weeks, shaking daily. Alternatively, for a quicker method, gently heat the herbs and oil in a double boiler for 2-3 hours on low heat, ensuring the oil does not boil. Strain the herbs from the oil using cheesecloth or a fine mesh strainer.

2. In a double boiler, combine the calendula and comfrey-infused oils with beeswax pellets. Heat gently until the beeswax is completely melted, stirring occasionally.

3. Once the beeswax is melted, add shea butter to the mixture, stirring until it is fully incorporated and melted.

4. Remove the mixture from the heat and stir in the vitamin E oil and lavender essential oil, if using. The vitamin E acts as a natural preservative and skin healer, while the lavender adds a soothing fragrance and additional antimicrobial properties.

5. Carefully pour the hot salve mixture into clean, dry tins or jars. Allow the salve to cool and solidify at room temperature, which may take several hours.

6. Once cooled, seal the containers with lids to prevent contamination.

Variations
- For extra healing properties, add a few drops of tea tree oil for its antiseptic qualities.
- If allergic to beeswax, substitute with an equal amount of candelilla wax or soy wax for a vegan-friendly version.
- For a softer salve, especially in colder climates, reduce the amount of beeswax by a few grams.

Storage tips
Store the salve in a cool, dark place. If stored properly, the salve can last for up to 1 year. Avoid exposing the salve to extreme temperatures, which can cause it to melt or become too hard.

Tips for allergens
For those with sensitivities to shea butter, substitute with mango butter or cocoa butter for similar consistency and skin benefits. Always patch test before applying to affected areas, especially for sensitive skin or known allergies.

Scientific references
- "Anti-inflammatory and skin barrier repair effects of topical application of some plant oils," published in the International Journal of Molecular Sciences, discusses the benefits of plant oils, including calendula, for skin health.
- "The effect of lavender oil on stress, bispectral index values, and needle insertion pain in volunteers," found in the Journal of Alternative and Complementary Medicine, highlights the soothing properties of lavender essential oil.

Acne Treatments with Anti-Inflammatory Herbs

Witch hazel, tea tree oil, and lavender stand out as natural allies in the fight against acne, primarily due to their potent anti-inflammatory and antibacterial properties. These herbs work synergistically to reduce redness, control bacterial growth, and soothe irritated skin, making them invaluable components of any acne treatment regimen.

Witch hazel, derived from the bark and leaves of the Hamamelis virginiana plant, acts as a natural astringent. Its high tannin content effectively reduces inflammation and minimizes the appearance of pores. For application, soak a cotton ball with witch hazel extract and gently dab onto the affected areas. Its calming effect on the skin reduces redness and swelling, providing a cooling sensation that soothes irritation.

Tea tree oil, extracted from the leaves of Melaleuca alternifolia, is renowned for its antimicrobial and antiseptic qualities. Its ability to combat a wide range of bacteria, including those responsible for acne, makes it a powerful tool in acne treatment. To use, mix a few drops of tea tree oil with a carrier oil, such as jojoba or almond oil, to prevent irritation, and apply directly to blemishes using a clean cotton swab. This method targets acne-causing bacteria, reducing inflammation and preventing future outbreaks.

Lavender, known for its aromatic and therapeutic properties, also possesses anti-inflammatory and antibacterial effects that benefit acne-prone skin. Its gentle action soothes the skin, reduces stress-related breakouts, and promotes healing. Create a lavender-infused oil by steeping dried lavender in a carrier oil for several weeks. Strain and apply the oil lightly to the skin, focusing on areas prone to acne. Lavender's calming scent additionally offers a relaxing effect, which indirectly benefits skin health by mitigating stress, a known acne trigger.

Incorporating witch hazel, tea tree oil, and lavender into your skincare routine can provide a natural, effective way to manage acne. These herbs offer a holistic approach to skin care, addressing not only the symptoms but also the underlying causes of acne, such as bacteria proliferation and inflammation, without the harsh side effects associated with chemical treatments.

Herbal Rinses and Oils for Hair Health

Harnessing the power of rosemary and nettle for hair health begins with understanding their unique properties and how to effectively incorporate them into your hair care routine. Rosemary, scientifically known as Rosmarinus officinalis, is renowned for its ability to stimulate hair follicles, encouraging growth and resulting in thicker, more lustrous hair. Nettle, or Urtica dioica, is packed with vitamins and minerals essential for hair health, such as vitamins A, C, and K, along with amino acids and iron, which can combat hair loss and aid in the regeneration of hair strands.

To create a rosemary rinse that can enhance hair growth and impart a natural shine, start by boiling 2 cups of water. Once boiling, remove from heat and add 1/2 cup of dried rosemary leaves. Cover and allow the mixture to steep for at least 30 minutes, ensuring that the essential oils and properties of the rosemary are fully infused into the water. After steeping, strain the mixture to remove the leaves, and allow the liquid to cool to room temperature. For application, after shampooing, pour the rosemary rinse through your hair as a final rinse, gently massaging into the scalp and hair strands. Do not rinse out; the solution is designed to be left in the hair to maximize its beneficial effects. This process can be repeated 2-3 times a week.

For addressing issues such as dandruff and scalp irritation, a nettle rinse can provide soothing relief and promote a healthy scalp environment. Begin by preparing a nettle infusion similar to the rosemary rinse. Boil 2 cups of water and add 1/2 cup of dried nettle leaves. Allow the mixture to steep, covered, for 30 minutes to an hour, which will create a potent infusion rich in the nutrients nettle is celebrated for. After steeping, strain the liquid and let it cool. This nettle rinse can be applied to the scalp and hair after shampooing, massaging gently to ensure full coverage. Like the rosemary rinse, it should be left in the hair to dry naturally. Regular use can significantly reduce dandruff and scalp irritation.

For those interested in an oil treatment that combines the benefits of both rosemary and nettle for a more intensive approach, creating an infused oil is an excellent method. Start with a base oil, such as jojoba or coconut oil, known for their compatibility with hair and scalp health. In a clean jar, combine 1 cup of your chosen base oil with 1/4 cup dried rosemary leaves and 1/4 cup dried nettle leaves. Seal the jar and place it in a sunny spot for 2-4 weeks, shaking it every few days to ensure the herbs are fully infused into the oil. After the infusion period, strain the oil to remove the herbs, and store the oil in a clean, airtight container. To use, apply a small amount of the oil to the scalp and hair, massaging thoroughly. For best results, leave the oil in for at least an hour or overnight before washing out with a gentle shampoo. This treatment can be done once a week to nourish the scalp, promote hair growth, and add a healthy shine to the hair.

Aloe Vera and Lavender Soothing Gel

Beneficial effects

Aloe Vera and Lavender Soothing Gel combines the cooling, hydrating properties of aloe vera with the calming, anti-inflammatory benefits of lavender. Aloe vera, known for its ability to soothe burns, hydrate skin, and accelerate wound healing, pairs perfectly with lavender, which can reduce redness, calm irritation, and promote relaxation. This gel is ideal for sunburns, minor cuts, and daily skin hydration, offering a natural, gentle remedy for skin care.

Portions

Makes about 8 ounces (240 ml)

Preparation time

15 minutes

Ingredients
- 1 cup pure aloe vera gel
- 2 tablespoons lavender hydrosol
- 1 teaspoon vitamin E oil
- 10 drops lavender essential oil
- 1 tablespoon witch hazel extract (optional for added skin healing benefits)

Instructions
1. Start by ensuring all your utensils and containers are clean and sterilized to prevent contamination.
2. In a mixing bowl, combine 1 cup of pure aloe vera gel with 2 tablespoons of lavender hydrosol. Stir gently to maintain the gel's consistency.
3. Add 1 teaspoon of vitamin E oil to the mixture. Vitamin E acts as a natural preservative and helps nourish and protect the skin.
4. Incorporate 10 drops of lavender essential oil into the bowl. This not only adds a calming scent but also enhances the gel's soothing properties.
5. For additional skin healing benefits, mix in 1 tablespoon of witch hazel extract. This step is optional but recommended for its astringent and anti-inflammatory effects.
6. Using a whisk or a fork, mix all the ingredients thoroughly until you achieve a uniform consistency.
7. Carefully transfer the gel into a clean, airtight glass jar or bottle. Use a funnel if necessary to avoid spills.
8. Label your container with the date and contents for future reference.

Variations
- For a cooling after-sun gel, add a few drops of peppermint essential oil for its refreshing and cooling properties.
- Incorporate chamomile hydrosol instead of lavender for sensitive skin, offering similar soothing effects with a gentler touch.
- Add aloe vera juice in place of part of the gel for a thinner consistency, suitable for use as a spray.

Storage tips
Store the Aloe Vera and Lavender Soothing Gel in the refrigerator for an enhanced cooling effect upon application. The gel should remain fresh for up to 1 month when stored properly. Always use clean hands or a spatula to scoop out the gel to maintain its purity.

Tips for allergens
For those with sensitivities to lavender, simply omit the lavender essential oil and hydrosol. The base of aloe vera and vitamin E alone still provides excellent skin-soothing benefits. Alternatively, substitute with hypoallergenic essential oils like chamomile or rose for fragrance and additional skin care benefits.

Scientific references
- "Aloe vera: a short review," published in the Indian Journal of Dermatology, highlights the moisturizing, healing, and anti-inflammatory properties of aloe vera.
- "Lavender and the Nervous System," published in Evidence-Based Complementary and Alternative Medicine, discusses the calming, anti-inflammatory, and antimicrobial effects of lavender on the skin.

Rosemary and Peppermint Scalp Tonic

Beneficial effects

Rosemary and peppermint are not only refreshing but also packed with properties beneficial for scalp health and hair growth. Rosemary oil is known for its ability to improve circulation, which can stimulate hair follicles and promote growth. Peppermint oil offers a cooling effect that soothes an itchy scalp and can help to dandruff control. Together, they create a tonic that revitalizes the scalp, encourages healthy hair growth, and leaves a pleasant, invigorating scent.

Portions

Makes about 8 ounces

Preparation time

10 minutes

Cooking time

No cooking required

Ingredients

- 1/2 cup of distilled water
- 1/4 cup of witch hazel
- 2 tablespoons of fresh rosemary leaves, finely chopped
- 10 drops of peppermint essential oil
- 5 drops of rosemary essential oil
- 1 tablespoon of aloe vera gel
- 1 teaspoon of apple cider vinegar

Instructions

1. Begin by combining the distilled water and witch hazel in a clean spray bottle. Witch hazel acts as a natural astringent, which can help to cleanse the scalp and regulate oil production.

2. Add the finely chopped fresh rosemary leaves to the mixture. The fresh leaves will infuse the tonic with potent botanical compounds beneficial for scalp health.

3. Incorporate 10 drops of peppermint essential oil into the bottle. Peppermint oil is known for its cooling and soothing properties, which can help to relieve scalp irritation.

4. Add 5 drops of rosemary essential oil to the mix. Rosemary essential oil is reputed for its ability to stimulate hair growth and improve scalp circulation.

5. Include 1 tablespoon of aloe vera gel to the tonic. Aloe vera gel is a natural moisturizer that can hydrate the scalp and hair, reducing dryness and flakiness.

6. Pour in 1 teaspoon of apple cider vinegar. Apple cider vinegar helps to balance the pH of the scalp, enhancing overall scalp health and adding shine to the hair.

7. Secure the lid on the spray bottle and shake vigorously to ensure all ingredients are well combined. The shaking process helps to evenly distribute the essential oils and aloe vera gel throughout the tonic.

8. To use, spray the tonic directly onto the scalp and hair roots after shampooing and conditioning. Massage gently with your fingertips for a few minutes to enhance absorption and stimulate circulation. There's no need to rinse out the tonic; let your hair air dry or style as usual.

Variations

- For an extra nourishing boost, add 1 teaspoon of jojoba oil to the mixture. Jojoba oil closely mimics the scalp's natural oils, providing moisture without weighing hair down.

- If you have sensitive skin, reduce the amount of essential oils by half to prevent potential irritation.

Storage tips

Store the rosemary and peppermint scalp tonic in a cool, dark place. The tonic should remain effective for up to 1 month when stored properly. If the tonic appears cloudy or has an off smell, it's time to make a fresh batch.

Tips for allergens

For those with sensitivities to witch hazel, you can substitute it with more distilled water or a floral water such as rose water for its soothing properties. Always perform a patch test on a small area of your skin before applying the tonic to your scalp to ensure there's no allergic reaction.

Scientific references

- "Peppermint Oil Promotes Hair Growth without Toxic Signs," published in Toxicological Research, highlights the hair growth-promoting effects of peppermint oil.

- "Rosemary oil vs minoxidil 2% for the treatment of androgenetic alopecia: a randomized comparative trial," found in Skinmed Journal, discusses the effectiveness of rosemary oil in treating hair loss compared to conventional treatments.

BOOK 4: ADVANCED HERBAL PREPARATION TECHNIQUES

CHAPTER 1: TINCTURES, INFUSIONS, AND DECOCTIONS

Tinctures for Potency and Longevity

Tinctures are concentrated herbal extracts made by soaking herbs in alcohol or glycerin. They are valued for their ability to preserve the active compounds of herbs, ensuring potency and longevity. The process of making a tincture involves several detailed steps, each critical to achieving a high-quality product.

To start, choose high-proof alcohol for alcohol-based tinctures as it effectively extracts a wide range of water-soluble and alcohol-soluble compounds. For those avoiding alcohol, vegetable glycerin, a sweet, syrupy liquid derived from plant oils, offers an alternative solvent, though it may not extract as wide a range of compounds.

Selecting the right herb is crucial. Fresh or dried herbs can be used, but ensure they are of the highest quality, organically grown or wildcrafted, and free from pesticides and contaminants. The herb-to-solvent ratio is pivotal and varies depending on the herb's form and the desired strength of the tincture. A common starting point is 1:2 for fresh herbs (one part herb to two parts solvent by weight) and 1:4 for dried herbs.

For alcohol-based tinctures, a solvent with 40-60% alcohol content is generally effective. Vodka, with its neutral flavor, is a popular choice, but brandy or rum can also be used for their distinct flavors. When using glycerin, a typical ratio is 3:1, glycerin to water, to ensure proper preservation and extraction.

The maceration process begins with finely chopping or grinding the herbs to increase the surface area for extraction. Place the herbs in a clean, dry jar, then pour the solvent over the herbs, completely covering them. Seal the jar tightly to prevent evaporation and store it in a cool, dark place. Shake the jar daily to mix the herbs and solvent.

Maceration time varies from two weeks to a month, depending on the herb and desired strength. After maceration, strain the mixture through a fine mesh strainer or cheesecloth, squeezing out as much liquid as possible. For a clearer tincture, filter the liquid again through a coffee filter.

Bottle the tincture in dark glass dropper bottles to protect it from light, which can degrade its potency. Label each bottle with the herb name, date of production, and type of solvent used. Store the bottles in a cool, dark place. Properly made and stored, alcohol-based tinctures can last several years, while glycerin-based tinctures have a shorter shelf life of approximately 1-2 years.

To use, tinctures are typically administered by the dropperful, diluted in a small amount of water or tea. The dosage varies depending on the herb, the condition being treated, and the individual's body weight and sensitivity. It is essential to research or consult a healthcare professional for guidance on appropriate dosages.

Creating tinctures is both an art and a science, allowing for the preservation of herbal remedies in a potent and convenient form. By following these detailed steps and recommendations, individuals can harness the therapeutic benefits of herbs for use in natural health and wellness practices.

Infusions and Decoctions Guide

Infusions and decoctions are foundational techniques in herbal medicine, each serving a specific purpose based on the parts of the plant being used and the desired therapeutic benefits.

Understanding these differences is crucial for anyone looking to harness the full potential of medicinal herbs.

Infusions are best suited for the more delicate parts of the plant, such as leaves, flowers, and some thin barks. This method involves pouring boiling water over the plant material and allowing it to steep for a specified period, usually 15 to 20 minutes for leaves and flowers, and up to 8 hours for roots in a cold infusion. The goal is to extract the volatile oils and other soluble compounds into the water.

To prepare an infusion:

1. Measure 1-2 teaspoons of dried herb or 2-4 teaspoons of fresh herb per cup of water.

2. Boil water in a kettle and pour it over the herb in a heat-proof container.

3. Cover the container to prevent the escape of volatile oils.

4. Steep for the recommended time, then strain the plant material from the liquid.

5. The resulting infusion can be consumed immediately or stored in a refrigerator for up to 24 hours for best flavor and efficacy.

Decoctions are used for the tougher parts of the plant, like roots, seeds, and some hard barks, which require more processing to break down cell walls and release their active compounds. This method involves simmering the plant material in water over a period, typically 20 minutes to several hours, depending on the hardness of the material.

To prepare a decoction:

1. Begin with cold water, using approximately 1 teaspoon of dried herb or 2 teaspoons of fresh herb per cup of water.

2. Add the plant material to the water and bring to a boil in a covered pot to minimize the loss of any volatile substances.

3. Reduce the heat and simmer for the recommended time, checking periodically to ensure the mixture does not boil dry.

4. After simmering, remove from heat and strain the decoction, pressing the plant material to extract as much liquid as possible.

5. Consume the decoction while warm, or store it in the refrigerator for up to 48 hours.

Both infusions and decoctions can be made **stronger or weaker**, depending on personal preference or therapeutic need, by adjusting the amount of herb used or the steeping time. For those new to herbal preparations, starting with the lower recommended amounts and gradually increasing can help gauge personal tolerance and effectiveness.

Adapting Techniques for Specific Needs

When adapting herbal preparation techniques to meet specific needs, it's essential to consider the unique properties of each herb, as well as the intended use of the final product. This approach ensures that the active compounds of the herbs are efficiently extracted, and their therapeutic benefits are maximized. Here's how to tailor the preparation methods of tinctures, infusions, and decoctions to specific herbs and health conditions.

Tinctures: The concentration of a tincture can be adjusted by varying the ratio of herb to solvent or altering the maceration time. For herbs with robust, hardy constituents, such as **dandelion root** or **milk thistle seeds**, a higher alcohol percentage (about 60-70%) may be necessary to effectively extract the active compounds. Conversely, for delicate herbs like **chamomile** or **lavender**, a lower alcohol content (around 40-50%) is sufficient and preserves the herb's volatile oils. If creating a tincture for someone sensitive to alcohol, consider using a glycerin base, keeping in mind that glycerin may not extract all compounds as effectively as alcohol. The maceration period can also be extended from the standard two to four weeks to six weeks or longer for tougher materials, ensuring a potent and therapeutic extract.

Infusions: The temperature and steeping time are critical factors in preparing herbal infusions. For heat-sensitive herbs, such as **lemon balm** or **peppermint**, water should be heated to just below boiling before pouring over the herbs to preserve their delicate essential oils. Steeping time can be adjusted based on the desired strength; however, a general guideline is 15-20 minutes for leaves and flowers, and up to 12 hours (overnight) for a cold infusion of roots or barks. For a stronger medicinal effect, increase the amount of herb per cup of water, using up to 2 tablespoons of dried herb or 4 tablespoons of fresh herb.

Decoctions: When preparing decoctions for hard, woody herbs or roots, such as **astragalus** or **burdock root**, it's beneficial to simmer the herbs for an extended period, often 20 minutes to an hour, to fully extract the tougher constituents. The water level should be monitored closely, adding more as necessary to prevent the decoction from becoming too concentrated or burning. For herbs that are particularly bitter or strong-tasting, reducing the simmering time and adding complementary flavoring herbs can make the decoction more palatable without significantly compromising its therapeutic value.

Adjusting for Specific Needs: When crafting herbal remedies for specific health conditions, consider the herb's affinity for the condition. For instance, **ginger** and **turmeric** are excellent for inflammatory conditions and can be prepared in both tincture and decoction forms to enhance their bioavailability and effectiveness. For sleep or anxiety, a tincture of **valerian root** and **passionflower**, adjusted for a higher herb-to-solvent ratio, creates a potent remedy that can be easily dosed before bedtime.

Materials and Tools: Use high-quality, organic herbs to ensure the purity and potency of your preparations. Glass jars with tight-fitting lids are ideal for macerating tinctures, while stainless steel or enamel-coated pots are best for decoctions to prevent interaction with the herbs. For infusions, a French press or a simple glass jar covered with a lid can be used to steep the herbs, allowing for easy straining.

Chamomile and Lemon Balm Sleep Tincture

Beneficial effects

Chamomile and Lemon Balm Sleep Tincture combines the soothing properties of chamomile with the calming effects of lemon balm, creating a powerful ally for those struggling with sleeplessness or anxiety. Chamomile is widely recognized for its mild sedative effects, which can help to ease the mind into a peaceful state, conducive to sleep. Lemon balm complements chamomile by promoting relaxation and reducing stress, thanks to its ability to increase GABA levels in the brain, a neurotransmitter that helps control the nervous system's response to stress. Together, these herbs offer a natural remedy to encourage deeper, more restful sleep.

Portions

Makes approximately 2 cups

Preparation time

24 hours for maceration

Cooking time

N/A

Ingredients

- 1/2 cup dried chamomile flowers
- 1/2 cup dried lemon balm leaves

- 1 quart (4 cups) vodka or brandy (80-100 proof)
- 1 large glass jar with a tight-fitting lid

Instructions

1. Begin by sterilizing the glass jar and lid to ensure it's free from bacteria and other contaminants. You can do this by boiling them in water for 10 minutes and then allowing them to air dry completely.

2. Place the dried chamomile flowers and lemon balm leaves into the sterilized jar. Try to break the leaves into smaller pieces to increase the surface area for extraction.

3. Pour the vodka or brandy over the herbs, ensuring they are completely submerged. The alcohol should be at least 80-100 proof to effectively extract the active compounds from the herbs and preserve the tincture.

4. Seal the jar tightly with the lid. Shake the jar gently to mix the herbs with the alcohol.

5. Store the jar in a cool, dark place away from direct sunlight. Shake the jar once daily to agitate the herbs and aid in the extraction process.

6. After 4-6 weeks, strain the tincture through a fine mesh strainer or cheesecloth into another sterilized jar or bottles. Press or squeeze the herbs to extract as much liquid as possible.

7. Label the bottles with the name of the tincture and the date of preparation.

Variations

- For a non-alcoholic version, replace the vodka or brandy with glycerin and water. Use 3 parts glycerin to 1 part water as the solvent.
- Add a cinnamon stick or vanilla bean to the jar during the maceration process for additional flavor and potential blood sugar regulation benefits.

Storage tips

Store the chamomile and lemon balm sleep tincture in a cool, dark place. The tincture will remain potent for up to 3 years if stored properly. Ensure the bottles are tightly sealed to prevent evaporation of the alcohol.

Tips for allergens

For those with allergies to chamomile or lemon balm, consider substituting with lavender or valerian root, which also possess calming and sleep-inducing properties. Always perform a patch test or consult with a healthcare provider before trying a new herbal remedy.

Scientific references

- "A review of the bioactivity and potential health benefits of chamomile tea (Matricaria recutita L.)," published in Phytotherapy Research, outlines the sedative and anti-anxiety effects of chamomile.
- "Melissa officinalis L. – A review of its traditional uses, phytochemistry, and pharmacology," in the Journal of Ethnopharmacology, discusses lemon balm's role in improving sleep quality and reducing anxiety.

CHAPTER 2: CRAFTING HERBAL OINTMENTS AND SALVES

Infusing Carrier Oils with Herbs

Infusing carrier oils with medicinal herbs is a foundational skill for anyone looking to delve into the world of herbal ointments and salves. This process, when done correctly, extracts the active compounds from herbs and transfers their healing properties into oils, creating a potent medium for a variety of topical applications. To achieve this, two primary methods can be employed: slow heat infusion and solar infusion. Each method has its unique benefits and requirements, and understanding the nuances of both will enable you to choose the most effective technique for your specific needs.

For the slow heat method, you will need a double boiler, a heat source, your chosen carrier oil (such as olive oil, coconut oil, or almond oil), and dried medicinal herbs. The choice of carrier oil depends on the intended use of the final product, as each oil has its own therapeutic properties. Begin by placing your dried herbs in the top section of the double boiler and covering them with the carrier oil. It's crucial to ensure that the herbs are completely submerged to facilitate optimal extraction. Set the double boiler over a low heat source, allowing the mixture to gently warm. The key here is to maintain a low temperature (ideally between 100°F to 120°F) to prevent the destruction of the herbs' delicate compounds and the oil from overheating. This process should be sustained for 2 to 4 hours, stirring occasionally, to allow the active ingredients of the herbs to infuse into the oil.

Alternatively, the solar infusion method harnesses the power of the sun to naturally infuse the oil with herbal properties. This method requires a clean, dry glass jar, your chosen carrier oil, and dried herbs. Fill the jar one-third to one-half full with dried herbs, then pour the carrier oil over the herbs, ensuring they are completely covered. Seal the jar tightly and place it in a location where it will receive direct sunlight, such as a windowsill facing south. The infusion should be left in the sun for 2 to 4 weeks, shaking the jar gently every few days to mix the contents. The warmth from the sun facilitates a gentle infusion process, slowly coaxing the medicinal properties out of the herbs and into the oil without the risk of overheating.

Regardless of the method chosen, after the infusion period, the next step involves straining the oil to remove the herbal material. A fine mesh strainer or cheesecloth can be used for this purpose. It's important to press or squeeze the herbs to extract as much oil as possible. The final product should be stored in a clean, dry glass bottle or jar, ideally amber or dark blue to protect the oil from light, which can degrade its quality over time. Label the container with the date of production and the ingredients used for future reference.

Creating herb-infused oils is both an art and a science, requiring patience and attention to detail. Whether you opt for the slow heat or solar method, the key to success lies in using quality ingredients, maintaining the correct temperature, and allowing sufficient time for the herbs to impart their healing virtues to the oil. These infused oils can serve as the base for a myriad of homemade herbal remedies, including salves, balms, and ointments, each tailored to address specific health concerns or to nourish the skin and body.

Balms for Pain Relief and Skin Healing

Beneficial effects
This balm harnesses the natural anti-inflammatory and pain-relieving properties of herbs infused in oils, combined with beeswax to create a protective, soothing salve. It's designed for pain relief, inflammation reduction, and wound care, making it a versatile addition to any home apothecary. The beeswax forms a barrier that helps protect wounds while retaining moisture, aiding in the skin's natural healing process. The infused oils carry the therapeutic properties of the herbs deep into the skin, offering natural relief for sore muscles, joint pain, and various skin conditions.

Portions
Makes approximately 8 ounces (240 ml) of balm

Preparation time
30 minutes (plus 2-3 hours for infusing oils if not pre-prepared)

Cooking time
10 minutes

Ingredients
- 1/2 cup of coconut oil
- 1/2 cup of olive oil
- 1/4 cup of dried calendula petals
- 1/4 cup of dried arnica flowers
- 1/4 cup of beeswax pellets
- 20 drops of lavender essential oil
- 20 drops of peppermint essential oil
- 10 drops of eucalyptus essential oil
- A double boiler
- Cheesecloth or fine mesh strainer
- Clean, dry jars or tins for storage

Instructions
1. Begin by infusing the coconut and olive oils with calendula and arnica. Combine the oils and dried herbs in the top part of a double boiler, ensuring the water in the bottom part is simmering, not boiling. Allow the herbs to infuse in the oils over low heat for 2-3 hours. Stir occasionally to ensure even heat distribution.

2. After infusion, remove the oil mixture from heat and let it cool slightly. Strain the infused oil through cheesecloth or a fine mesh strainer into a clean bowl, discarding the used herbs.

3. Clean the top part of the double boiler and return the strained infused oil to it. Add the beeswax pellets to the infused oil and melt them together over low heat, stirring constantly to ensure they combine thoroughly.

4. Once the beeswax is completely melted and mixed with the infused oil, remove from heat. Allow the mixture to cool for a few minutes but not solidify.

5. Stir in the lavender, peppermint, and eucalyptus essential oils into the slightly cooled mixture. Each of these essential oils adds additional pain-relieving and anti-inflammatory benefits to the balm, as well as a pleasant scent.

6. Carefully pour the final mixture into clean, dry jars or tins. Allow the balm to cool and solidify at room temperature. This process may take a few hours.

7. Once solidified, close the containers with lids to prevent contamination and preserve the balm's properties.

Variations
- For a vegan version, substitute beeswax pellets with an equal amount of candelilla wax.
- Add vitamin E oil to the balm as an antioxidant and to extend shelf life.
- Customize the essential oils based on preferences or specific therapeutic needs. For example, rosemary essential oil can be used for its muscle pain relief properties.

Storage tips
Store the balm in a cool, dark place to maintain its consistency and therapeutic properties. If stored properly, the balm can last for up to 1 year.

Tips for allergens
For those with sensitivities to coconut or olive oil, substitute with another carrier oil like almond oil or jojoba oil. Always conduct a patch test before applying the balm extensively, especially if you have sensitive skin or known allergies to any of the ingredients.

Scientific references
- "Anti-inflammatory and wound healing activity of a growth substance in Aloe vera," published in the Journal of the American Podiatric Medical Association, highlights the healing properties of aloe vera, which can be infused in the oils for additional benefits.
- "Effect of aromatherapy on symptoms of dysmenorrhea in college students: A randomized placebo-controlled clinical trial," found in the Journal of Alternative and Complementary Medicine, discusses the pain-relieving effects of lavender essential oil.

Customizing Salves with Essential Oils

Once you have your base salve prepared from infused oils, customizing it with essential oils can significantly enhance its therapeutic properties. Essential oils, concentrated plant extracts, bring potent medicinal qualities to your salves. This section will guide you through selecting and incorporating essential oils like **lavender**, **peppermint**, and **tea tree** into your herbal salves for added benefits.

Selecting Essential Oils:
- **Lavender Essential Oil**: Known for its calming and relaxing properties, lavender is ideal for salves aimed at soothing skin irritations, promoting wound healing, and reducing anxiety when applied topically.
- **Peppermint Essential Oil**: With its cooling effect, peppermint is excellent for relieving muscle pain, headaches, and itching. It also offers digestive benefits when used in abdominal salves.
- **Tea Tree Essential Oil**: Recognized for its antimicrobial and antiseptic qualities, tea tree oil is a powerful addition to salves intended for treating acne, fungal infections, and other skin conditions.

Incorporating Essential Oils into Salves:
1. **Calculate the Proper Dilution**: For topical applications, a safe dilution rate is typically 1-2% of the total salve volume. This equates to 6-12 drops of essential oil per ounce (30ml) of carrier oil or salve base. It's crucial to adhere to this dilution to prevent skin irritation or sensitization.
2. **Mixing Essential Oils**: In a clean, sterilized container, start by adding your prepared salve base. Gently heat the salve if solid to achieve a slightly liquid consistency for easier mixing. Then, carefully measure and add the essential oils using a dropper, aiming for the calculated dilution rate based on the volume of your salve.

3. **Homogenize the Mixture**: Using a clean stir stick or spatula, thoroughly mix the essential oils into the salve base. Ensure the mixture is uniform to distribute the essential oils evenly throughout the salve.
4. **Test for Sensitivity**: Before applying broadly, it's wise to conduct a patch test on a small skin area to check for any adverse reactions, especially when using potent oils like tea tree or peppermint.
5. **Storage**: Transfer the finalized salve into dark glass jars to protect the essential oils from light degradation. Label your containers with the ingredients, date of production, and intended use. Properly stored, your custom salve can last up to a year, depending on the shelf life of the base oils and essential oils used.

Tips for Customization:

- For **skin healing** salves, combine lavender with chamomile essential oil for enhanced anti-inflammatory effects.
- For **pain relief** salves, blend peppermint with eucalyptus essential oil to amplify the cooling sensation and analgesic properties.
- For **antifungal** salves, tea tree can be paired with lavender to improve efficacy and add a soothing scent.

Remember, the key to successful salve customization lies in understanding the properties of each essential oil and how they can complement the base salve to address specific health concerns. Experimenting with different combinations within safe dilution guidelines allows you to create personalized, effective herbal remedies.

Calendula and Comfrey Healing Salve

Beneficial effects

This Calendula and Comfrey Healing Salve is a potent blend designed to soothe, repair, and protect the skin. Calendula, known for its anti-inflammatory and antimicrobial properties, works to promote wound healing and skin regeneration. Comfrey, rich in allantoin, aids in the healing of cuts, bruises, and sprains by stimulating cell growth. Together, these herbs create a powerful salve that can help heal minor wounds, soothe irritated skin, and provide a barrier against environmental damage.

Portions

Makes approximately 10 ounces (300 ml) of salve

Preparation time

30 minutes

Cooking time

1 hour

Ingredients

- 1/2 cup dried calendula flowers
- 1/2 cup dried comfrey leaves
- 1 cup olive oil or almond oil
- 1/4 cup beeswax pellets
- 2 tablespoons coconut oil
- 1 teaspoon vitamin E oil
- 10 drops lavender essential oil (optional for fragrance and additional antimicrobial properties)

Instructions

1. Begin by infusing the olive or almond oil with dried calendula flowers and comfrey leaves. Combine the herbs and oil in a double boiler, heating gently over low heat for 1 hour to allow the herbs to infuse. Stir occasionally to ensure even heat distribution.

2. After the infusion process, strain the oil through a cheesecloth or fine mesh strainer into a clean bowl, pressing the herbs to extract as much oil as possible. Discard the used herbs.

3. Return the infused oil to the double boiler, and add the beeswax pellets. Heat gently, stirring constantly, until the beeswax is completely melted and combined with the oil.

4. Remove the mixture from heat and stir in the coconut oil until it is fully melted and integrated into the mixture.

5. While the mixture is still warm, stir in the vitamin E oil and lavender essential oil, if using. Vitamin E oil acts as a natural antioxidant that can extend the shelf life of the salve and support skin healing, while lavender oil can provide a calming scent and additional antimicrobial benefits.

6. Carefully pour the warm salve mixture into clean, dry jars or tins. Allow the salve to cool and solidify at room temperature, which may take several hours depending on the size of the containers.

7. Once solidified, secure the lids on the containers to prevent contamination.

Variations

- For a vegan version, substitute beeswax pellets with an equal amount of candelilla wax or soy wax.
- Add a few drops of tea tree oil for its powerful antiseptic properties, especially beneficial for treating acne-prone or oily skin types.
- For extra moisturizing properties, include shea butter or cocoa butter in the salve. Reduce the amount of olive or almond oil by the amount of butter added to maintain consistency.

Storage tips

Store the salve in a cool, dark place to preserve its therapeutic properties. If stored properly, the salve can last for up to 1 year. Avoid exposing the salve to direct sunlight or high temperatures, which can cause it to melt.

Tips for allergens

For individuals with sensitivities to nuts, use olive oil instead of almond oil as the base for the salve. Always conduct a patch test on a small area of skin before widespread use, especially if you have sensitive skin or are prone to allergies.

Scientific references

- "Anti-inflammatory and wound healing activity of a growth substance in Aloe vera," published in the Journal of the American Podiatric Medical Association, highlights the healing properties of aloe vera, which can be infused in the oils for additional benefits.
- "Effect of aromatherapy on symptoms of dysmenorrhea in college students: A randomized placebo-controlled clinical trial," found in the Journal of Alternative and Complementary Medicine, discusses the pain-relieving effects of lavender essential oil.

CHAPTER 3: HERBAL FERMENTATION & PRESERVATION

Herbal Kombucha and Infused Ferments

Making herbal kombucha and infused ferments introduces an exciting dimension to traditional fermentation practices, allowing for the incorporation of various herbs such as ginger and hibiscus to enhance flavor, nutritional value, and therapeutic benefits. The process begins with the preparation of a basic kombucha, which serves as a foundation for the infusion of medicinal herbs. Kombucha itself is a fermented tea beverage cultivated with a symbiotic culture of bacteria and yeast (SCOBY). The fermentation process transforms sweet tea into a tangy, effervescent drink rich in probiotics, aiding in digestion and overall gut health.

To start, you'll need to brew a base kombucha. This requires filtered water, black or green tea, granulated sugar, and an active SCOBY with starter tea. The sugar acts not as a sweetening agent but as food for the SCOBY, which metabolizes the sugar, producing various acids, vitamins, and enzymes. For one gallon of water, use about 8 tea bags or 2 tablespoons of loose-leaf tea and 1 cup of sugar. Once the tea is steeped and the sugar dissolved, allow the mixture to cool to room temperature before adding the SCOBY and starter tea. This mixture should ferment in a glass jar covered with a breathable cloth in a warm, dark place for 7 to 14 days.

After the initial fermentation, the kombucha is ready for the infusion of herbs. Ginger and hibiscus are popular choices for their health benefits and flavor profiles. Ginger, known for its anti-inflammatory and digestive properties, adds a spicy kick to the kombucha. Hibiscus, on the other hand, imparts a tart flavor and vibrant color, along with antioxidants and vitamin C. To infuse these herbs, remove the SCOBY from the fermented kombucha and add either fresh or dried ginger slices and dried hibiscus flowers directly to the brew. The quantity of herbs depends on personal taste preferences but start with a tablespoon of dried hibiscus flowers and an equivalent amount of ginger per quart of kombucha for a balanced flavor. Allow this mixture to undergo a secondary fermentation for an additional 3 to 7 days, tasting periodically until the desired flavor intensity is achieved. This secondary fermentation can also be done in bottles to increase carbonation, but ensure to burp the bottles daily to release excess pressure.

For those interested in exploring beyond kombucha, infused ferments can also be created with other bases such as water kefir or apple cider vinegar. The infusion process remains similar, with the addition of herbs during the secondary fermentation phase to impart their flavors and medicinal properties. When using apple cider vinegar as a base, herbs can be steeped directly in the vinegar for a period of 2 to 4 weeks, creating a potent herbal tonic that can be used in culinary applications or taken as a dietary supplement.

Throughout the fermentation and infusion processes, it's crucial to maintain cleanliness and monitor the development of the brews closely. Any signs of mold or unusual odors necessitate discarding the batch to prevent the risk of contamination. Additionally, when experimenting with different herbs, it's important to research their properties and potential interactions to ensure they complement the health benefits of the fermented base without causing adverse effects.

Herbal kombucha and infused ferments not only offer a delightful sensory experience but also embody the principles of ancient herbal medicine, providing a creative and enjoyable way to incorporate these timeless remedies into modern wellness practices.

Herbal Vinegars and Tonics

Herbal vinegars and tonics are potent concoctions that harness the medicinal properties of herbs, offering a versatile way to incorporate these benefits into daily life. The process of creating these infusions involves steeping herbs in vinegar or a mixture of water and alcohol to extract their active compounds. This section outlines the detailed steps to craft your own herbal vinegars and tonics, ensuring you can create effective and flavorful remedies at home.

Selecting Your Vinegar: Choose an organic, high-quality vinegar as your base. Apple cider vinegar is a popular choice due to its health benefits, including digestive support and antimicrobial properties. White wine and red wine vinegars are also suitable and offer a different flavor profile for culinary uses. Ensure the vinegar has a 5% acidity level, ideal for extracting the medicinal qualities of the herbs.

Choosing Herbs: Focus on herbs known for their culinary and medicinal properties. Common herbs include rosemary, thyme, oregano, and dandelion. Each herb offers unique benefits, such as rosemary for memory enhancement and thyme for respiratory health. For tonics, consider herbs like echinacea for immune support and elderberry for antiviral properties.

Preparation: Begin by sterilizing a glass jar and lid in boiling water for 10 minutes. This step is crucial to prevent contamination and ensure the longevity of your herbal vinegar or tonic. Once sterilized, carefully dry the jar and lid to remove any moisture.

Herb-to-Vinegar Ratio: For a potent infusion, use a ratio of 1 part herb to 2 parts vinegar by volume. If using fresh herbs, gently bruise the leaves and stems to release their essential oils. For dried herbs, ensure they are not powdered but whole or coarsely chopped to maximize the extraction of medicinal compounds.

Infusion Process: Place the prepared herbs in the sterilized jar, and pour the vinegar over them, ensuring the herbs are completely submerged. If the herbs float to the top, consider adding a clean, sterilized weight to keep them immersed. Seal the jar tightly with the lid or, if using a metal lid, place a piece of wax paper between the jar and the lid to prevent corrosion from the vinegar.

Steeping Time: Store the jar in a cool, dark place for 3 to 6 weeks. The length of time will depend on the desired strength of the infusion. Gently shake the jar every few days to mix the herbs and vinegar.

Straining and Bottling: After the steeping period, strain the vinegar through a fine mesh sieve or cheesecloth into a clean, sterilized bottle. Press or squeeze the herbs to extract as much liquid as possible. For a clearer vinegar, strain a second time. Label the bottle with the date and ingredients used.

Storage: Store the herbal vinegar in a cool, dark place. It does not require refrigeration but should be kept away from direct sunlight to preserve its potency and flavor. Properly stored, herbal vinegars can last up to a year.

Creating Herbal Tonics: The process for creating herbal tonics is similar, with the primary difference being the inclusion of alcohol, such as vodka or brandy, to extract the herbs' properties. A common ratio is 1 part herb to 3 parts liquid (a combination of water and alcohol). The alcohol percentage should be at least 40% to preserve the tonic and extract the active compounds effectively.

Usage: Herbal vinegars can be used in salad dressings, marinades, or taken daily as a health tonic. Herbal tonics can be consumed in small doses as dietary supplements to support overall health or address specific health concerns.

By following these detailed steps, you can create your own herbal vinegars and tonics tailored to your taste preferences and health needs. These preparations not only offer a way to enjoy the flavors of various herbs but also provide a method to incorporate their healing properties into your daily routine.

Preserving Active Compounds in Syrups

Creating long-lasting herbal syrups and honeys involves a meticulous process that ensures the preservation of active compounds found in herbs, making these sweeteners not only flavorful but also beneficial for health. This section provides a step-by-step guide on how to infuse syrups and honeys with the essence and medicinal properties of herbs, using natural sweeteners as the base.

Herbal Syrups:

1. **Select Your Herbs**: Choose herbs based on the desired health benefits. For instance, ginger for digestion, echinacea for immune support, or lavender for relaxation. Use fresh or dried herbs; however, remember that dried herbs are more concentrated.

2. **Prepare the Herbal Infusion**: Combine 1 cup of water with 1 cup of your chosen herb(s) in a saucepan. If using dried herbs, reduce the amount to 1/2 cup as they are more potent than fresh herbs. Bring the mixture to a boil, then reduce the heat and simmer for 30 to 40 minutes until the volume of water is reduced by approximately half.

3. **Strain the Herbs**: After simmering, remove the saucepan from the heat. Pour the infusion through a fine mesh strainer or cheesecloth into a clean container, pressing or squeezing the herbs to extract as much liquid as possible.

4. **Add Natural Sweetener**: Measure the volume of your herbal infusion. For every cup of infusion, add 3/4 to 1 cup of a natural sweetener such as honey, maple syrup, or agave nectar. Return the mixture to the saucepan.

5. **Simmer to Combine**: Heat the mixture over low heat, stirring constantly until the sweetener is fully dissolved. Do not boil to preserve the integrity of the honey or syrup and to prevent degradation of the herbs' active compounds.

6. **Preserve with Alcohol (Optional)**: For added preservation, you can fortify the syrup with alcohol. Add 1 tablespoon of high-proof alcohol, like vodka or brandy, for every cup of syrup. This step is optional but extends the shelf life.

7. **Bottle and Store**: Pour the finished syrup into sterilized glass bottles. Label each bottle with the date and ingredients. Store in the refrigerator for up to 6 months.

Herbal Honeys:

1. **Choose Your Herbs**: Similar to syrups, select herbs based on their therapeutic properties. Lavender, rosemary, and thyme work well for their antimicrobial and soothing effects.

2. **Prepare the Herbs**: If using fresh herbs, ensure they are completely dry to prevent moisture from diluting the honey. Dried herbs are preferable for a longer shelf life.

3. **Infuse the Honey**: Fill a clean, dry jar one-third full with dried herbs. Pour raw, organic honey over the herbs, filling the jar. Stir the mixture to ensure all the herbs are coated.

4. **Seal and Store for Infusion**: Tightly seal the jar with a lid. Place the jar in a warm, sunny spot, such as a windowsill, for 1 to 2 weeks. Every few days, turn the jar upside down to mix the herbs and honey.

5. **Strain the Honey**: After the infusion period, warm the honey slightly by placing the jar in a warm water bath. This makes straining easier. Pour the honey through a fine mesh strainer or cheesecloth into a clean jar, pressing the herbs to extract infused honey.

6. **Bottle and Label**: Transfer the strained honey into sterilized jars. Label with the date and infused herbs. Store in a cool, dark place. Herbal honey can last up to a year or longer if stored properly.

By following these detailed steps, you can create herbal syrups and honeys that not only add natural sweetness but also incorporate the healthful benefits of herbs into your daily diet. These preparations offer a delightful way to enjoy the flavors and therapeutic qualities of herbs, preserved in a form that's both versatile and enjoyable.

Fermented Garlic Honey

Beneficial effects

Fermented Garlic Honey is a powerful combination that leverages the natural antibacterial and antiviral properties of both ingredients. Garlic, known for its immune-boosting effects, contains allicin, a compound that has been shown to help reduce the severity of colds and other infections. Honey, a natural antioxidant, provides soothing relief for sore throats and coughs while acting as a medium for fermenting garlic, enhancing its beneficial properties. Together, they create a potent remedy that can support immune health, aid in digestion, and offer anti-inflammatory benefits.

Portions

Makes about 1 pint

Preparation time

10 minutes

Cooking time

N/A

Ingredients

- 1 cup of raw, peeled garlic cloves
- 1 pint of raw honey

Instructions

1. Start by selecting a clean, dry jar with a tight-fitting lid. Sterilize the jar by boiling it in water for 10 minutes or washing it in a dishwasher on a high heat setting. This step is crucial to prevent any unwanted bacteria from influencing the fermentation process.

2. Peel the garlic cloves. Ensure each clove is free from blemishes or green sprouts, as these can affect the flavor and potency of your fermented honey.

3. Place the peeled garlic cloves into the sterilized jar, filling it to about ¾ full. Avoid overpacking the jar to allow space for the honey to cover the garlic and for air to circulate.

4. Slowly pour raw honey over the garlic cloves, ensuring they are completely submerged. Leave at least an inch of space at the top of the jar to allow for expansion during fermentation.

5. Using a clean spoon or stick, gently stir the mixture to release any air bubbles trapped between the garlic cloves. This step helps to ensure an even fermentation process.

6. Seal the jar with its lid, but not too tightly. Fermentation produces gases that need to escape, so a loosely fitted lid or a piece of cloth secured with a rubber band can be used to cover the jar.

7. Store the jar in a dark, room-temperature spot, away from direct sunlight. A kitchen cupboard or pantry shelf works well.

8. Check the jar every day for the first few days, opening it to release any gases that have built up and to stir the mixture gently. This also prevents mold from forming on the surface.

9. After a week, begin tasting the mixture. The fermentation process can take anywhere from one week to a month, depending on your taste preference and the room temperature. The garlic will gradually become sweeter and less pungent, while the honey will thin out slightly and take on a tangy flavor.

10. Once the fermented garlic honey reaches your desired taste, store it in the refrigerator to slow down the fermentation process. It can be consumed immediately or allowed to age for a deeper flavor.

Variations

- Add herbs such as thyme, rosemary, or oregano to the jar for additional flavor and health benefits.
- For a spicier kick, include a few dried chili peppers to the mixture.
- Incorporate a tablespoon of apple cider vinegar to introduce additional probiotic properties and to kickstart the fermentation process.

Storage tips

Keep the fermented garlic honey in the refrigerator once it has reached your desired level of fermentation. This will preserve its potency and prevent further fermentation. When stored properly, fermented garlic honey can last up to a year or longer.

Tips for allergens

For those with allergies to honey, a similar fermentation process can be applied using maple syrup, although the end product will differ in taste and health benefits. Always ensure that you are not allergic to garlic, as it is a common allergen for some individuals.

Scientific references

- "Allicin: chemistry and biological properties" in the journal Molecules highlights the antimicrobial and antiviral properties of garlic.
- "Honey: its medicinal property and antibacterial activity" published in the Asian Pacific Journal of Tropical Biomedicine discusses honey's role in immune support and wound healing.

BOOK 5: COMMON HERBS AND THEIR APPLICATIONS

CHAPTER 1: EVERYDAY MEDICINAL HERBS

Chamomile for Relaxation and Digestion

Chamomile, scientifically known as Matricaria chamomilla or Chamomilla recutita, stands out as a versatile herb renowned for its calming and digestive support properties. This herb has been utilized for centuries, offering a gentle yet effective remedy for a variety of ailments. Its applications as a tea, topical wash, and compress make it a staple in the home apothecary, providing a natural and accessible means to enhance wellness.

When preparing chamomile tea, the focus should be on extracting the maximum beneficial compounds from the flowers. Begin by boiling water and then allowing it to cool for about a minute to approximately 200°F, a temperature that ensures the delicate chamomile flowers do not get scorched, preserving their therapeutic properties. Use about one tablespoon of dried chamomile flowers per cup of water, or if using fresh chamomile, increase the quantity to two tablespoons, as fresh flowers contain more water. Steep the chamomile flowers in the hot water, covered, for 5 to 10 minutes. Covering the tea as it steeps is crucial to prevent the evaporation of essential oils into the air. The longer steeping time allows for a more potent tea, enhancing its effectiveness in promoting relaxation and aiding digestion. Strain the flowers from the liquid before drinking. For digestive support, consume chamomile tea 20 to 30 minutes before meals to prepare the digestive system or after meals to ease digestion.

Chamomile's application as a topical wash or compress offers another dimension of its healing capabilities, particularly beneficial for skin irritations, eye inflammations, and abdominal cramps. To create a chamomile wash, steep the flowers as you would for tea, but in a larger quantity of water, creating a more diluted solution. Once cooled to a comfortable temperature, the solution can be applied directly to the affected area with a clean cloth or used as a rinse. For eye applications, ensure the solution is thoroughly strained through a fine mesh to remove all flower particles, preventing any irritation to the eyes. A compress soaked in chamomile tea and applied to the abdomen can provide relief from cramps and bloating, with the warmth of the compress enhancing the herb's soothing effects.

In crafting a chamomile compress for relaxation or digestive support, soak a clean, soft cloth in freshly prepared chamomile tea. Wring out the excess liquid until the cloth is damp but not dripping. Apply the compress to the forehead, abdomen, or other affected areas, leaving it in place for 10 to 15 minutes. The compress can be reheated as needed or applied cool, depending on the desired effect. For added benefit, combine chamomile with other herbs such as peppermint for digestion or lavender for relaxation, creating a synergistic blend that enhances the therapeutic properties of each herb.

Peppermint for Energy and Stomach Relief

Peppermint, scientifically known as Mentha piperita, is a perennial herb that thrives in temperate climates worldwide. Its leaves contain several essential compounds, including menthol, which is primarily responsible for the plant's cooling sensation and therapeutic effects. When considering peppermint for energy and stomach relief, it's crucial to understand the specific ways in which this herb can be utilized to maximize its benefits effectively.

For energy enhancement, peppermint oil can be used in aromatherapy. The process involves diffusing a few drops of peppermint essential oil in a water-based diffuser. This method disperses the oil into the air, allowing for inhalation and direct absorption through the lungs. The menthol in peppermint oil stimulates the hippocampus area of the brain, which is responsible for mental clarity and focus, thus providing an energy boost. For personal use, applying one to two drops of diluted peppermint oil to the temples and back of the neck can invigorate the senses, promoting alertness. It's important to dilute the essential oil with a carrier oil, such as jojoba or coconut oil, to prevent skin irritation, using a ratio of one drop of peppermint oil to one teaspoon of carrier oil.

Peppermint's role in providing stomach relief is well-documented. Its antispasmodic properties can relax the muscles of the gastrointestinal system, helping to alleviate symptoms of nausea and indigestion. A simple way to harness these benefits is through peppermint tea. To prepare, add one tablespoon of dried peppermint leaves to one cup of boiling water. Cover and steep for 10 minutes to ensure the volatile oils are not lost to evaporation. Straining the leaves, the tea can be consumed two to three times a day, especially before meals to aid digestion or at the onset of nausea. For those on the go, peppermint capsules are an alternative, providing a measured dose that can be taken with water; however, it's essential to follow the manufacturer's dosage recommendations to avoid overconsumption, which can lead to heartburn or irritation.

In cases of headaches and congestion, peppermint oil can be applied topically in a diluted form. Mixing a few drops of peppermint essential oil with a carrier oil and massaging into the forehead, temples, and sinuses can alleviate headache symptoms. The cooling effect of menthol helps to relax muscles and ease tension headaches. Additionally, inhaling peppermint oil can provide relief from nasal congestion. This can be achieved by adding a couple of drops of the oil to a bowl of hot water and inhaling the steam, covering the head with a towel to trap the vapors. The menthol in peppermint acts as a natural expectorant, helping to break up phlegm and clear the nasal passages.

When incorporating peppermint into your wellness routine, it's crucial to note that while peppermint tea is generally safe for most people, the essential oil should be used with caution. Peppermint oil is highly concentrated and can be toxic if ingested in large quantities. Always ensure that peppermint products, especially essential oils, are kept out of reach of children and pets. Pregnant or nursing women and individuals with gallstones should consult a healthcare provider before using peppermint as a remedy.

Lavender for Calming and Skin Health

Lavender, scientifically known as Lavandula angustifolia, has been revered for centuries not only for its captivating fragrance but also for its versatile therapeutic properties. This herb plays a pivotal role in both calming the mind and enhancing skin health, making it an indispensable component of any home apothecary. When delving into the utilization of lavender in teas, oils, and topical treatments, it's essential to understand the specific methodologies to harness its full potential effectively.

For creating a calming lavender tea, the process begins with selecting high-quality, dried lavender flowers. The ideal proportion is one to two teaspoons of dried lavender per cup of boiling water. To preserve the delicate essential oils, pour the boiling water over the lavender in a teapot and cover it, allowing it to steep for about 5 to 10 minutes. This method ensures that the volatile oils, which are responsible for lavender's soothing effects, are not lost to evaporation. Straining the lavender flowers before consumption results in a fragrant tea that can reduce anxiety, promote relaxation, and aid in a restful night's sleep.

Lavender oil, renowned for its aromatic and therapeutic qualities, can be prepared through a process of infusion. Begin with a carrier oil of your choice, such as sweet almond or jojoba oil, known for their skin-nourishing properties. Add dried lavender flowers to the carrier oil in a ratio that supports the desired potency, typically a quarter cup of lavender per cup of oil. This mixture should be gently heated in a double boiler for 2 to 3 hours, keeping the temperature low to avoid degrading the oil's beneficial properties. After cooling, the oil needs to be strained through a fine mesh or cheesecloth to remove all plant material, resulting in a fragrant oil that can be used for massages, skin care, or as a stress-relieving aroma.

For topical treatments, lavender's anti-inflammatory and antibacterial properties make it an excellent choice for addressing skin conditions such as eczema, acne, and minor burns. To create a lavender salve, begin by infusing lavender into a carrier oil, as previously described. This infused oil can then be combined with beeswax at a ratio of approximately one ounce of beeswax per cup of infused oil. The mixture should be gently heated until the beeswax melts completely, then poured into clean containers to solidify. Once cooled, this salve can be applied directly to the skin to soothe irritation, promote healing, and hydrate dry areas.

Elderflower and Lemon Immune Boosting Elixir

Beneficial effects

Elderflower and lemon combine in this elixir to create a powerful immune-boosting drink. Elderflower is known for its antiviral and anti-inflammatory properties, making it excellent for fighting colds and flu. Lemon adds a high dose of vitamin C, which is crucial for the immune system's proper function. Together, they stimulate the body's defenses and provide a refreshing, soothing remedy that can help shorten the duration of illnesses and bolster overall health.

Portions

Makes about 4 cups

Preparation time

15 minutes

Cooking time

5 minutes to heat water, then allow to infuse for 24 hours

Ingredients

- 1/2 cup dried elderflowers
- 2 large lemons, organic if possible
- 4 cups boiling water
- 1/4 cup raw honey, or to taste

Instructions

1. Begin by thoroughly washing the lemons. Using a vegetable peeler or a sharp knife, carefully peel the lemons, avoiding as much of the white pith as possible to prevent bitterness. After peeling, juice the lemons and set aside.

2. Place the dried elderflowers in a large heatproof jar or a glass bowl. Add the lemon peels to the elderflowers.

3. Boil 4 cups of water. Once boiled, pour the hot water over the elderflowers and lemon peels, ensuring they are completely submerged.

4. Cover the jar or bowl with a lid or a clean cloth and let it infuse at room temperature for about 24 hours. This slow infusion process allows the water to extract the flavors and beneficial properties of the elderflowers and lemon peels fully.

5. After the infusion period, strain the mixture through a fine mesh sieve or cheesecloth into another clean jar or bottle, pressing on the solids to extract as much liquid as possible. Discard the elderflowers and lemon peels.

6. Stir in the freshly squeezed lemon juice and raw honey into the strained liquid. Mix well until the honey is completely dissolved. Adjust the sweetness according to taste by adding more honey if desired.

7. Transfer the elixir to the refrigerator to chill. Serve cold for a refreshing and immune-boosting drink.

Variations

- For an extra immune boost, add a 1-inch piece of ginger, thinly sliced, to the infusion.
- Incorporate a few sprigs of fresh mint or thyme for additional flavor complexity and health benefits.
- Replace honey with maple syrup for a vegan alternative.

Storage tips

Store the elderflower and lemon immune boosting elixir in a sealed container in the refrigerator for up to 1 week. For longer storage, the elixir can be frozen in ice cube trays and then transferred to a freezer bag, keeping it fresh for up to 3 months. Thaw in the refrigerator or add directly to hot water for a warm, soothing drink.

Tips for allergens

For those with allergies to honey, maple syrup or agave nectar are suitable substitutes that do not compromise the elixir's beneficial properties. Always ensure to use organic lemons to minimize exposure to pesticides, especially since the peel is used in the infusion.

Scientific references

- "Antiviral effect of flavonoids on human viruses" in the Journal of Medical Virology highlights the antiviral properties of compounds found in elderflowers.
- "Vitamin C and Immune Function" in Nutrients discusses the role of vitamin C, found in lemons, in supporting various cellular functions of both the innate and adaptive immune system.

CHAPTER 2: HEALING PROPERTIES OF ROOTS

Ginger: Anti-Inflammation & Digestive Aid

Ginger, scientifically known as Zingiber officinale, is a root herb cherished for its medicinal properties, particularly its anti-inflammatory effects and its role as a digestive aid. This section delves into the mechanisms by which ginger exerts its warming properties and stimulates circulation, contributing to its therapeutic benefits. Ginger contains bioactive compounds such as gingerols and shogaols, which are primarily responsible for its potent anti-inflammatory and antioxidant effects. These compounds inhibit the synthesis of pro-inflammatory cytokines, thereby reducing inflammation and providing relief from conditions such as arthritis, muscle soreness, and migraines.

To harness ginger's benefits for digestion, it's important to understand its effects on the gastrointestinal system. Ginger promotes the secretion of saliva and gastric juices, enhancing digestion and the absorption of nutrients. It also exhibits prokinetic effects, improving gastrointestinal motility and alleviating symptoms of dyspepsia, including bloating, gas, and indigestion. Furthermore, ginger's warming effect on the body is attributed to its ability to increase blood circulation, which not only aids in the distribution of nutrients but also enhances the detoxification process.

For those looking to incorporate ginger into their wellness routine, consider the following detailed recommendations:

1. **Preparation of Ginger Tea**: Start with fresh ginger root, which contains higher levels of gingerols compared to dried ginger. Peel and thinly slice approximately one inch of ginger root. Boil the slices in two cups of water for about 10 to 15 minutes, depending on the desired strength. The longer you boil the ginger, the more potent the tea will be. Strain the tea into a cup and add lemon or honey to taste. Drinking ginger tea 20 to 30 minutes before meals can stimulate digestion and prevent indigestion.

2. **Ginger Compress for Inflammation**: Grate a 2-inch piece of fresh ginger and wrap it in a thin cloth or cheesecloth. Boil water and place the wrapped ginger in it for 30 seconds to 1 minute, allowing it to warm up. Carefully remove the ginger compress from the water and check the temperature to ensure it's warm but not scalding. Apply the compress to the affected area, such as sore muscles or joints, for 15 to 20 minutes. The warmth from the ginger compress not only delivers ginger's anti-inflammatory compounds directly to the affected area but also improves circulation, aiding in the healing process.

3. **Ginger Infusion for Circulatory Support**: To create a ginger infusion that can be taken orally to support circulation, peel and finely chop or grate a 4-inch piece of ginger. Place the ginger in a jar and cover it with about 16 ounces of high-proof alcohol, such as vodka, ensuring the ginger is completely submerged. Seal the jar and store it in a cool, dark place for at least two weeks, shaking it every few days. After two weeks, strain the infusion through a fine mesh strainer or cheesecloth, discarding the ginger solids. Store the strained liquid in a clean, airtight container. Taking a small amount, typically 1 to 2 teaspoons, diluted in water or tea, can help stimulate circulation and provide warmth to the body.

Incorporating ginger into your diet or wellness practices offers a natural and effective way to combat inflammation, support digestive health, and improve circulation. Whether consumed as a tea, applied topically as a compress, or taken orally as an infusion, ginger's warming properties and ability to stimulate circulation make it a valuable herb for natural health and wellness.

Turmeric for Joint Health and Antioxidant Power

Turmeric, scientifically known as Curcuma longa, is a root herb that has garnered attention for its potent anti-inflammatory and antioxidant properties, primarily attributed to its active compound, curcumin. This vibrant yellow-orange spice has been a cornerstone in traditional medicine for thousands of years, offering a natural approach to treating various health conditions, including joint health and enhancing overall antioxidant power in the body. To fully leverage turmeric's benefits, it's crucial to understand how curcumin operates within the body and the most effective ways to incorporate turmeric into one's health regimen.

Curcumin's ability to combat inflammation is not only profound but operates on a molecular level, inhibiting several molecules known to play major roles in inflammation. This includes the blocking of NF-kB, a molecule that travels into the nuclei of cells and activates genes related to inflammation, which is believed to play a major role in many chronic diseases. For individuals experiencing joint pain or conditions such as arthritis, incorporating turmeric can help reduce symptoms by lowering inflammation and providing relief.

However, curcumin's bioavailability, or the body's ability to absorb and utilize the compound, is relatively low. To enhance absorption, it's recommended to consume turmeric alongside black pepper, which contains piperine, a natural substance that enhances the absorption of curcumin by 2,000%. A practical application involves adding a pinch of black pepper to turmeric-infused meals or health concoctions to ensure optimal absorption.

For joint health, creating a turmeric paste can serve as a powerful topical application. Combine 1 part turmeric powder with 2 parts water in a small saucepan, heating gently while stirring continuously until a thick paste forms. Once cooled, this paste can be applied directly to the affected area, providing direct anti-inflammatory benefits. For systemic effects, including the antioxidant benefits, integrating turmeric into the diet is key. This can be achieved by incorporating turmeric powder into smoothies, teas, or curries. A simple yet effective method is to prepare a turmeric tea by boiling 1 teaspoon of turmeric powder in 4 cups of water, simmering for 10 minutes. Strain and add honey or lemon to taste before consuming.

The antioxidant power of turmeric also plays a crucial role in overall health by neutralizing free radicals, chemicals that can cause damage to the body's cells. This oxidative stress is linked to a wide array of chronic conditions, including heart disease, cancer, and neurodegenerative diseases. Regular consumption of turmeric can help bolster the body's antioxidant capacity, protecting against cellular damage and supporting healthy aging.

For those looking to supplement with turmeric for its health benefits, standardized curcumin extract is available, offering a concentrated dose of the active compound. When selecting a supplement, opt for one that includes piperine or is formulated for enhanced absorption to ensure the body can effectively utilize curcumin. It's advisable to start with a lower dose to assess tolerance and gradually increase as needed, keeping in mind that consulting with a healthcare provider before starting any new supplement regimen is crucial, especially for individuals with existing health conditions or those taking medication.

Dandelion Root for Detoxification

Dandelion root, scientifically known as Taraxacum officinale, has been revered for centuries for its potent liver-cleansing effects and its ability to improve digestion. This humble weed, often overlooked and uprooted from gardens, harbors powerful medicinal properties in its roots. Rich in vitamins A, C, and K, as well as minerals like iron, potassium, and zinc, dandelion root offers a natural, effective solution for supporting liver function and promoting gastrointestinal health.

To harness these benefits, the dandelion root can be prepared in several ways, with the most common being a decoction, a tincture, or dried powder. Each preparation method extracts the root's beneficial compounds differently, providing various options for incorporation into daily wellness routines.

For a decoction, which is a concentrated liquid resulting from boiling the dandelion root, begin by thoroughly washing the roots to remove any dirt. Chop the clean roots into small pieces to increase the surface area for extraction. Place about one tablespoon of the chopped root into a pot with one cup of water. Bring the mixture to a boil, then simmer for 15 to 20 minutes. The resulting liquid should be dark and rich. Strain the decoction and consume it warm. This method is particularly effective for immediate digestive relief and can be taken two to three times a day before meals to stimulate digestion and support liver detoxification.

Creating a tincture involves soaking the dandelion root in alcohol to extract its active compounds. Fill a jar one-third full with dried, chopped dandelion root, then cover it completely with a high-proof alcohol, such as vodka or brandy, ensuring there are a couple of inches of alcohol above the root material. Seal the jar and store it in a cool, dark place for 4 to 6 weeks, shaking it every few days. After the steeping period, strain the liquid through a fine mesh strainer or cheesecloth into a clean bottle. Tinctures are concentrated and taken in small doses, typically 20-30 drops in water, up to three times daily. This method is beneficial for long-term liver support and detoxification.

For those preferring a non-alcoholic method, dandelion root powder offers a versatile alternative. The dried roots are ground into a fine powder using a coffee grinder or food processor. This powder can be encapsulated or added to smoothies, teas, or even sprinkled on foods. Taking 1-2 teaspoons of dandelion root powder daily can support digestive health, liver function, and detoxification processes.

Regardless of the preparation method chosen, it's important to source dandelion roots from areas free of pesticides and other chemicals to ensure the purity and efficacy of the remedy. Additionally, while dandelion root is generally considered safe for most people, it's advisable to consult with a healthcare provider before starting any new herbal regimen, especially for those with gallbladder disease, gallstones, or other serious health conditions, as well as those taking medications, to avoid potential interactions.

Ashwagandha Root Stress Relief Tonic

Beneficial effects

Ashwagandha Root Stress Relief Tonic utilizes the adaptogenic properties of Ashwagandha root, known for its ability to reduce stress and anxiety, improve concentration, and boost energy levels without causing drowsiness. This tonic can help in balancing the body's response to daily stressors, improving overall well-being and mental clarity.

Portions

Makes about 2 cups

Preparation time

15 minutes (plus overnight soaking)

Cooking time

15 minutes

Ingredients

- 1/4 cup dried Ashwagandha root
- 4 cups water
- 1 tablespoon honey (or to taste)

- 1/2 teaspoon ground cinnamon
- 1/4 teaspoon ground ginger
- A pinch of ground cardamom
- Lemon slices (for serving)

Instructions

1. Begin by placing the dried Ashwagandha root in a bowl. Cover it with water and let it soak overnight. This process helps to soften the root, making the active compounds more accessible.

2. The next day, drain the Ashwagandha root and place it in a medium-sized saucepan. Add 4 cups of fresh water to the saucepan.

3. Bring the mixture to a gentle boil over medium heat. Once boiling, reduce the heat to low and allow it to simmer for 15 minutes. This slow simmering process helps to extract the beneficial compounds from the Ashwagandha root.

4. After simmering, remove the saucepan from the heat. Strain the mixture through a fine mesh strainer into a heatproof container, discarding the solid pieces of root.

5. While the liquid is still warm, stir in the honey, ground cinnamon, ground ginger, and a pinch of ground cardamom. Mix well until the honey is fully dissolved and the spices are evenly distributed.

6. Allow the tonic to cool to room temperature. Once cooled, it can be served immediately with a slice of lemon in each cup, adding a refreshing twist and vitamin C to the tonic.

7. Any leftover tonic can be stored in a glass jar or bottle in the refrigerator for up to one week.

Variations

- For a vegan version, replace honey with maple syrup or agave nectar.
- Add a slice of fresh ginger while simmering the Ashwagandha root for an extra spicy kick and additional digestive benefits.
- Incorporate a teaspoon of vanilla extract for a subtly sweet and comforting flavor profile.

Storage tips

Keep the tonic refrigerated in a sealed glass jar or bottle to maintain freshness. Consume within one week for optimal benefits. Shake well before each use as natural sediment may occur.

Tips for allergens

For those with allergies to honey, maple syrup or agave nectar are suitable substitutes that maintain the tonic's natural sweetness without compromising its health benefits. Always ensure that the spices used are fresh and free from cross-contamination if you have specific spice allergies.

Scientific references

- "An Overview on Ashwagandha: A Rasayana (Rejuvenator) of Ayurveda" published in the African Journal of Traditional, Complementary and Alternative Medicines discusses the adaptogenic effects of Ashwagandha, including stress relief and improved cognitive function.
- "Efficacy and Safety of Ashwagandha (Withania somnifera) Root Extract in Insomnia and Anxiety: A Double-blind, Randomized, Placebo-controlled Study" in the journal Cureus highlights the benefits of Ashwagandha in reducing stress and anxiety levels.

CHAPTER 3: LEAVES AS HEALING TOOLS

Nettle for Energy and Detoxification

Nettle, scientifically known as **Urtica dioica**, is a powerhouse of nutrition and has been utilized for centuries due to its medicinal properties. This herb is particularly esteemed for its ability to **boost energy levels** and **aid in detoxification**, making it an invaluable addition to a natural health regimen. Rich in iron, vitamins A, C, and K, as well as various minerals like calcium and magnesium, nettle supports the body's natural detox processes and energy metabolism.

To harness the benefits of nettle for energy and detoxification, one can incorporate this herb into their diet through teas, tinctures, or supplements. Here's a detailed breakdown of how to prepare and use nettle for these specific purposes:

Preparing Nettle Tea for Energy Boost

1. **Harvesting**: Choose young nettle leaves, ideally in the spring when the plant's energy is concentrated in its foliage. Wear gloves to avoid the sting.
2. **Drying**: If not using fresh, dry the leaves in a well-ventilated, shaded area to preserve the nutrients. Once dry, store in an airtight container away from direct sunlight.
3. **Brewing**: Steep 1-2 teaspoons of dried nettle leaves in 8 ounces of boiling water for 10-15 minutes. This long infusion time allows the water to extract the iron and other vital nutrients effectively.
4. **Consumption**: Drink 1-2 cups daily, preferably in the morning or early afternoon to harness the herb's energizing properties without affecting nighttime sleep.

Using Nettle Tincture for Detoxification

1. **Preparation**: Fill a jar one-third full with dried nettle leaves and cover with vodka, ensuring that the leaves are completely submerged.
2. **Steeping**: Seal the jar and store it in a cool, dark place for 4-6 weeks, shaking it every few days to mix the contents.
3. **Straining**: After steeping, strain the liquid through a fine mesh strainer or cheesecloth into a clean, dark glass bottle.
4. **Dosage**: For detoxification, use 20-30 drops of nettle tincture in water, up to three times a day. This method supports the liver and kidneys in filtering and eliminating toxins from the body.

Nutritional Supplementation

- **Capsules**: Nettle is available in capsule form, providing a convenient option for those seeking to boost their iron intake and support energy levels. Follow the manufacturer's recommended dosage, typically 1-2 capsules daily.
- **Powder**: Nettle leaf powder can be added to smoothies, soups, or other dishes. Start with a small amount, about one teaspoon, and gradually increase to avoid digestive discomfort.

Addressing Seasonal Allergies

Nettle's anti-inflammatory properties make it beneficial for reducing the symptoms of seasonal allergies. Consuming nettle tea or taking supplements before and during allergy season can help mitigate the body's histamine response, providing natural allergy relief.

Safety and Considerations

While nettle is generally safe for most individuals, it's important to:
- Start with small doses to assess tolerance.

- Consult with a healthcare provider before using nettle if you are pregnant, nursing, or have existing health conditions, especially those related to blood sugar or blood pressure.
- Be aware of potential interactions with medications, particularly blood thinners, as nettle can affect blood clotting.

Incorporating nettle into your daily routine can significantly enhance energy levels and support the body's detoxification pathways, while also offering relief from seasonal allergies. Its nutritional profile and medicinal properties make it a versatile herb suitable for various health goals.

Sage: Cognitive Support & Antimicrobial Uses

Sage, scientifically known as Salvia officinalis, has been revered throughout history for its medicinal properties, particularly for its cognitive support and antimicrobial benefits. This herb, with its distinctive leaves and aromatic scent, offers a natural remedy for enhancing mental clarity and treating throat ailments. To fully harness the benefits of sage for cognitive support and antimicrobial purposes, it is essential to understand the specific methods of preparation and application that make sage an effective remedy.

For cognitive support, sage can be prepared as a simple tea. Begin by boiling one cup of water. Once boiling, add one to two teaspoons of dried sage leaves. Cover and steep for approximately 5-10 minutes. This allows the water to become infused with the essential oils and active compounds of the sage, which are thought to enhance cognitive function and memory. It is recommended to consume sage tea in the morning to kickstart the day with mental clarity. For a stronger cognitive boost, fresh sage leaves can also be used; however, the flavor will be more potent. When using fresh sage, lightly bruise the leaves with a mortar and pestle to release the essential oils before steeping.

In addition to its cognitive benefits, sage's antimicrobial properties make it an excellent remedy for throat health. A sage gargle can be prepared by following a similar method to the tea. Boil water and add dried or fresh sage leaves, steeping as directed above. Once the infusion has cooled to a warm temperature, strain the leaves and use the liquid as a gargle. Gargling with sage tea for 1-2 minutes helps to reduce throat inflammation, soothe soreness, and combat bacterial infections due to its antimicrobial properties. For enhanced antimicrobial effects, a teaspoon of sea salt can be dissolved in the sage infusion before gargling. This method is particularly beneficial during cold and flu season or at the first sign of throat discomfort.

When selecting sage for these remedies, ensure that the herb is sourced from a reputable supplier to guarantee purity and potency. Both dried and fresh sage can be used effectively, although fresh sage may offer a more robust flavor and potentially stronger therapeutic effects due to the higher content of essential oils. It is important to store sage properly, keeping dried leaves in an airtight container away from direct sunlight and moisture to preserve its medicinal qualities.

While sage is generally considered safe for most individuals, it is advisable to consult with a healthcare provider before incorporating it into a regular wellness routine, especially for those who are pregnant, nursing, or have existing health conditions. Sage contains thujone, a compound that can be toxic in high doses, so it is crucial to adhere to recommended amounts and not consume sage oil or excessive quantities of the herb.

Incorporating sage into one's diet and wellness practices offers a natural, time-honored approach to enhancing cognitive function and maintaining throat health. Through careful preparation and mindful consumption, the benefits of sage can be fully realized, providing a testament to the enduring wisdom of herbal remedies.

Bay Leaf: Digestion and Flavor Uses

Bay leaves, derived from the laurel tree, Laurus nobilis, have been a staple in culinary practices for their unique flavor and fragrance, enhancing dishes with a subtle depth. Beyond their culinary applications, bay leaves possess medicinal properties that support digestion and overall wellness. The leaves contain compounds such as cineole and eugenol, which have been shown to aid in digestive health and provide anti-inflammatory benefits. To leverage bay leaves for their digestive advantages while also infusing flavor into your meals, consider the following detailed methods for incorporating them into cooking and preparing medicinal teas.

When adding bay leaves to culinary dishes, it's essential to use them sparingly due to their potent flavor. Incorporate a single bay leaf into soups, stews, or broths at the beginning of the cooking process. This allows the heat to gently extract the oils and compounds from the leaf, infusing the dish with its distinctive aroma and flavor. For optimal release of flavor, the leaf should be slightly crushed or bruised before being added to the pot. However, ensure the leaf remains intact for easy removal before serving, as the leaves are not meant to be consumed whole due to their tough texture.

For a medicinal tea aimed at aiding digestion, a simple yet effective preparation can be employed. Begin by boiling water in a small pot or kettle. Once boiling, add one to two dried bay leaves to the water, reducing the heat to a simmer. Allow the leaves to steep in the simmering water for about five minutes. This duration is sufficient to extract the beneficial compounds without overly concentrating the tea, which might lead to a too strong or bitter taste. After steeping, remove the bay leaves with a spoon or strain the tea into a cup. The tea can be consumed as is or lightly sweetened with honey, which further complements the flavor and adds its own digestive benefits.

To ensure the quality and efficacy of the bay leaves used, whether for cooking or tea, sourcing from a reputable supplier is crucial. Look for organic bay leaves, which are less likely to have been treated with pesticides or other chemicals that could detract from their health benefits and flavor. Store the leaves in a cool, dry place, away from direct sunlight, in an airtight container to preserve their essential oils and potency.

While bay leaves are generally considered safe for most individuals, moderation is key, as with any herb. Incorporating bay leaf tea into your routine as a digestive aid should be done thoughtfully, paying attention to your body's responses. For those with specific health conditions or concerns, consulting with a healthcare provider before integrating bay leaves or any new herbal remedy into your health regimen is advisable to ensure compatibility with your health status and any medications you may be taking.

By understanding the dual role of bay leaves in both culinary and medicinal contexts, you can enrich your diet with flavors that not only tantalize the taste buds but also contribute to digestive wellness. The simplicity of adding a bay leaf to a simmering pot or steeping it in hot water for tea makes it an accessible and beneficial practice for enhancing both the enjoyment of meals and the health of the digestive system.

Mint and Basil Breath Freshener

Beneficial effects

This Mint and Basil Breath Freshener offers a natural and refreshing way to maintain oral hygiene and fresh breath throughout the day. Mint leaves contain menthol, which has a cooling effect and naturally neutralizes bad breath. Basil's antimicrobial properties help to reduce bacteria in the mouth that can cause odor. Together, these herbs create a potent, freshening spray that's convenient and effective for daily use.

Portions

Makes about 1 ounce (30 ml)

Preparation time
10 minutes
Cooking time
N/A
Ingredients
- 1/4 cup fresh mint leaves, tightly packed
- 1/4 cup fresh basil leaves, tightly packed
- 1 cup distilled water
- 1 teaspoon vodka (as a preservative)
- 3-5 drops peppermint essential oil (optional for extra freshness)
- A small spray bottle for storage

Instructions
1. Begin by thoroughly washing the mint and basil leaves to remove any dirt or pesticides. Pat them dry with a clean towel.
2. In a small saucepan, bring the distilled water to a boil. Once boiling, remove from heat.
3. Add the fresh mint and basil leaves to the hot water. Cover the saucepan with a lid and allow the leaves to steep for about 20 minutes. This process infuses the water with the flavors and beneficial properties of the herbs.
4. After steeping, strain the herb-infused water through a fine mesh sieve or cheesecloth into a clean bowl, pressing on the leaves to extract as much liquid as possible. Discard the leaves.
5. To the strained liquid, add 1 teaspoon of vodka. This acts as a preservative to extend the shelf life of your breath freshener. Stir well to combine.
6. If using, add 3-5 drops of peppermint essential oil to the mixture for additional freshness and antimicrobial benefits. Stir thoroughly to ensure the oil is well distributed.
7. Using a funnel, carefully pour the final mixture into a small spray bottle. Secure the lid tightly.
8. To use, simply spray 1-2 pumps directly into your mouth as needed for instant freshness.

Variations
- For a sweeter taste, add a few drops of stevia extract to the mixture.
- Replace peppermint essential oil with spearmint essential oil for a milder flavor.
- Add a teaspoon of glycerin for a slightly thicker consistency and smoother spray.

Storage tips
Store your Mint and Basil Breath Freshener in a cool, dark place, preferably in the refrigerator, to maintain its freshness. The vodka preservative allows for a shelf life of up to 2 weeks. Always shake well before use.

Tips for allergens
For those with sensitivities to essential oils, the peppermint essential oil can be omitted without significantly affecting the freshening properties of the spray.

Scientific references
- "Antimicrobial activity of essential oils and other plant extracts" published in the Journal of Applied Microbiology highlights the antimicrobial effects of peppermint oil, supporting its use in oral care products for reducing bacteria.

BOOK 6: RARE AND EXOTIC HERBS FOR HEALING

CHAPTER 1: ADAPTOGENS FOR STRESS AND ENERGY

Ashwagandha: Stress Relief and Sleep Aid

Ashwagandha, scientifically known as Withania somnifera, has been a cornerstone in traditional medicine for centuries, revered for its remarkable adaptogenic properties. This powerful herb plays a pivotal role in mitigating stress, enhancing restorative sleep, and bolstering adrenal health through its ability to modulate cortisol levels. Cortisol, often referred to as the stress hormone, is produced by the adrenal glands in response to stress and low blood-glucose concentration. In the fast-paced modern world, chronic stress can lead to persistently elevated cortisol levels, which in turn can wreak havoc on the nervous system and overall health. Ashwagandha steps in as a natural counterbalance to these challenges, offering a holistic approach to stress management and health restoration.

To harness the benefits of ashwagandha for stress reduction and improved sleep quality, it's crucial to understand the optimal dosage and method of consumption. The root extract of ashwagandha is commonly available in powdered form, capsules, or as a liquid extract, making it accessible for daily intake. For stress relief and adrenal support, a daily dosage of 300 to 500 mg of high-concentration ashwagandha extract is recommended, ideally taken with meals or a glass of water to enhance absorption. It's important to note that while ashwagandha is generally well-tolerated, starting with a lower dose and gradually increasing it allows the body to adapt and minimizes the risk of potential side effects.

Incorporating ashwagandha into the evening routine can significantly contribute to improved sleep quality. Its adaptogenic nature helps to stabilize the body's stress response, allowing for a more relaxed state that is conducive to sleep. A small, controlled study has shown that participants who consumed ashwagandha reported substantial improvements in sleep quality and mental alertness upon waking, underscoring its effectiveness as a sleep aid. For those looking to enhance sleep, taking ashwagandha with warm milk or a non-dairy alternative before bedtime can be particularly beneficial, as this combination has been traditionally used to promote relaxation and a restful night's sleep.

Beyond its stress-reducing and sleep-enhancing capabilities, ashwagandha also offers significant support for adrenal health. The adrenal glands, responsible for the production of cortisol, can become overtaxed due to prolonged stress, leading to adrenal fatigue. Ashwagandha aids in the modulation of cortisol production, thereby supporting adrenal function and helping to prevent the depletion of adrenal reserves. This adaptogenic herb not only helps in managing the body's stress response but also contributes to overall vitality and energy levels, making it a valuable ally in the pursuit of balance and wellness.

For individuals seeking to incorporate ashwagandha into their wellness regimen, it's advisable to consult with a healthcare provider, especially for those with thyroid conditions, autoimmune diseases, or those who are pregnant or breastfeeding. This ensures the safe and effective use of ashwagandha in harmony with one's health status and goals.

Rhodiola Rosea: Boosting Clarity and Stamina

Rhodiola Rosea, a remarkable adaptogen native to the cold, mountainous regions of Europe and Asia, has been utilized for centuries to enhance mental clarity, physical stamina, and resilience to stress. This herb, often found thriving in harsh climates, embodies a natural resilience that, when consumed, is imparted to the human body, offering a range of benefits particularly beneficial during periods of stress and fatigue.

The active compounds in Rhodiola Rosea, notably salidroside and rosavin, are credited with its potent adaptogenic properties. These compounds work synergistically to support the body's stress response system, helping to regulate the production of cortisol, a hormone released during stress. By modulating this response, Rhodiola Rosea aids in reducing the physical and mental fatigue associated with chronic stress, thereby enhancing endurance and stamina.

For individuals seeking to improve mental clarity and focus, Rhodiola Rosea offers significant benefits. The herb's ability to enhance cognitive functions is linked to its effect on neurotransmitter levels, including dopamine and serotonin, which play crucial roles in mood regulation, focus, and memory. Regular supplementation with Rhodiola Rosea can lead to improvements in concentration, mental performance, and a reduction in brain fog, particularly in individuals facing high levels of stress or cognitive demand.

Physical stamina, another key benefit of Rhodiola Rosea, is particularly evident in its capacity to increase the body's resistance to physical stress. This is achieved through its influence on physical performance and recovery, making it a popular supplement among athletes and those engaged in physically demanding activities. By enhancing oxygen transport and muscle energy status, Rhodiola Rosea helps improve endurance levels, reduce recovery times, and protect muscle tissue during exercise.

To incorporate Rhodiola Rosea into a wellness regimen, it is recommended to start with a dosage of 100 to 300 mg of a standardized extract, containing at least 1% salidroside and 3% rosavins, taken 30 minutes before breakfast and lunch. This timing helps maximize absorption and ensures that the adaptogenic effects are utilized throughout the day when they are most needed. It is important to note that Rhodiola Rosea's stimulating effects may interfere with sleep if taken late in the day.

Consistency is key when supplementing with Rhodiola Rosea, as the adaptogenic effects build over time. A cycle of several weeks of use followed by a break period is often recommended to maintain efficacy and prevent habituation. As with any supplement, individual responses can vary, and starting with a lower dose to assess tolerance is advisable.

Holy Basil: A Sacred Herb for Inner Harmony

Holy Basil, also known as Tulsi, is revered in many cultures for its profound healing properties, particularly its ability to foster inner harmony and balance. This sacred herb, native to the Indian subcontinent, is an adaptogen, meaning it helps the body adapt to stress and exerts a normalizing effect upon bodily processes. A key aspect of Holy Basil that makes it invaluable for health and wellness is its role in regulating blood sugar levels, reducing stress, and acting as a mild immune booster.

To understand the impact of Holy Basil on blood sugar regulation, it's essential to delve into its chemical composition. Holy Basil contains compounds such as eugenol, methyl eugenol, and caryophyllene. These compounds contribute to its ability to lower blood glucose levels, making it a significant herb for those managing diabetes or pre-diabetic conditions. Incorporating Holy Basil into one's diet can be done by preparing a simple tea: steep 1-2 teaspoons of dried Holy Basil leaves in boiling water for about 5 minutes. This tea can be consumed 2-3 times a day to help manage blood sugar levels. It's important to monitor blood sugar regularly when incorporating Holy Basil into your regimen, especially for those on blood sugar-lowering medication, to avoid hypoglycemia.

The stress-reducing properties of Holy Basil are attributed to its ability to modulate cortisol levels, the body's primary stress hormone. By keeping cortisol levels within a normal range, Holy Basil helps in mitigating the physical and psychological effects of stress. For stress relief, Holy Basil can be consumed as a tea or in capsule form, typically 300-600 mg of an extract, daily. The adaptogenic properties of Holy Basil not only help in reducing stress but also promote mental clarity and protect against the deleterious effects of stress on the body.

As a mild immune booster, Holy Basil supports the immune system through its antibacterial, antiviral, and antifungal properties. These properties make Holy Basil an excellent herb for supporting the body's natural defense mechanisms. To harness these benefits, incorporating Holy Basil leaves into cooking or consuming a daily tea made from the leaves can be effective. Additionally, Holy Basil essential oil can be used in a diffuser to purify the air and provide respiratory benefits, especially during cold and flu season.

For those looking to incorporate Holy Basil into their wellness routine, starting with a daily tea or supplement and observing the body's response over a few weeks is advisable. As with any herbal remedy, it's crucial to consult with a healthcare provider before beginning any new supplement, particularly for those with existing health conditions or those taking medication.

Holy Basil stands out as a versatile and powerful herb that offers a holistic approach to managing stress, regulating blood sugar, and boosting immunity. Its sacred status in various cultures is a testament to its profound benefits on physical, mental, and spiritual well-being. By incorporating Holy Basil into a daily wellness routine, individuals can tap into ancient wisdom to support modern health challenges, fostering a sense of balance and harmony in their lives.

Rhodiola Rosea Energy Elixir

Beneficial effects

Rhodiola Rosea Energy Elixir harnesses the adaptogenic powers of Rhodiola Rosea, a herb revered for its ability to enhance physical and mental energy, improve stress resilience, and support overall vitality. This elixir is designed to uplift and energize without the jitteriness associated with caffeine. Regular consumption can lead to improved endurance, mental clarity, and a balanced stress response, making it an ideal tonic for those facing high stress or demanding lifestyles.

Portions

Makes about 2 cups

Preparation time

10 minutes

Cooking time

5 minutes

Ingredients

- 2 tablespoons dried Rhodiola Rosea root
- 4 cups filtered water
- 1 tablespoon raw honey, or to taste
- Juice of 1 lemon
- A pinch of ground cinnamon (optional)

Instructions

1. Begin by bringing the filtered water to a boil in a medium saucepan.

2. Once boiling, reduce the heat to a simmer and add the dried Rhodiola Rosea root. Cover and let simmer for 5 minutes. This gentle simmering process helps to extract the adaptogenic compounds from the Rhodiola Rosea, making them bioavailable.

3. After simmering, remove the saucepan from heat and let it cool slightly for about 2-3 minutes, allowing the flavors and properties to meld together.

4. Strain the mixture using a fine mesh strainer or cheesecloth into a large pitcher or jar, pressing on the Rhodiola Rosea root to extract as much liquid as possible. Discard the used roots.

5. Stir in the raw honey while the elixir is still warm to ensure it dissolves completely. Adjust the sweetness according to your preference by adding more or less honey.

6. Add the fresh lemon juice and a pinch of ground cinnamon, if using. Stir well to combine. The lemon juice adds a refreshing zest and vitamin C, while cinnamon can enhance the warming, energizing effect of the elixir.

7. Serve the elixir warm, or allow it to cool and serve chilled for a refreshing tonic. It can be consumed immediately or stored in the refrigerator to enjoy cold.

Variations

- For a vegan version, substitute raw honey with maple syrup or agave nectar.
- Add a slice of fresh ginger during the simmering process for an extra kick and digestive benefits.
- Incorporate a few mint leaves for a cooling, refreshing twist.

Storage tips

Store any leftover Rhodiola Rosea Energy Elixir in a glass bottle or jar in the refrigerator for up to 5 days. Shake well before serving, as natural sediment may settle at the bottom.

Tips for allergens

For those with allergies or sensitivities to honey, maple syrup or agave nectar are excellent substitutes that won't compromise the elixir's beneficial properties. If you're sensitive to lemon or cinnamon, simply omit these ingredients; the elixir will still provide an energizing boost.

Scientific references

- "The effects of Rhodiola rosea L. extract on anxiety, stress, cognition and other mood symptoms" published in Phytotherapy Research highlights Rhodiola's efficacy in improving symptoms of stress and anxiety.

CHAPTER 2: HERBAL TONICS FOR LONGEVITY

Gotu Kola: The Brain Tonic

Gotu Kola, scientifically known as **Centella asiatica**, is a revered herb in the realm of natural health for its multifaceted benefits, particularly in enhancing cognitive clarity, memory improvement, boosting circulation, and aiding in skin regeneration. This herb, native to the wetlands of Asia, is not only a staple in traditional medicine but also a subject of interest in contemporary wellness practices for its potent therapeutic effects.

To harness the cognitive benefits of Gotu Kola, it's essential to understand the optimal methods of consumption and the recommended dosages. For improving memory and cognitive function, consuming **300 to 600 mg** of Gotu Kola extract daily is suggested. This can be taken in the form of capsules or a tincture. When selecting a Gotu Kola supplement, look for products that specify the concentration of **asiaticosides**, as these are the active compounds responsible for the herb's cognitive benefits. A product containing at least **20% asiaticosides** is ideal for achieving the desired effects on cognitive health.

Incorporating Gotu Kola into your diet can also be achieved through teas. To prepare Gotu Kola tea, steep **1 to 2 teaspoons** of dried Gotu Kola leaves in boiling water for about **10 minutes**. This herbal tea can be consumed twice daily to support mental clarity and memory enhancement. For those interested in topical applications, particularly for skin health, Gotu Kola can be applied externally in the form of creams or gels that contain Gotu Kola extract. These products often combine Gotu Kola with other skin-healing herbs to maximize the regenerative effects.

For enhancing circulation, Gotu Kola works by strengthening the capillaries and veins, which is beneficial for overall cardiovascular health and can aid in reducing the symptoms of varicose veins and chronic venous insufficiency. A daily intake of **300 to 600 mg** of Gotu Kola extract, divided into two or three doses, is recommended for circulatory support. It's crucial to maintain this regimen for at least **4 to 8 weeks** to observe significant improvements in circulation.

Gotu Kola's role in skin regeneration is attributed to its ability to stimulate collagen production, which is essential for healing wounds and reducing the appearance of scars and stretch marks. For topical use, applying a cream or gel containing Gotu Kola extract directly to the affected area twice daily can support the skin's healing process. Look for products that contain at least **1% Gotu Kola extract** for effective results.

When incorporating Gotu Kola into your wellness routine, whether for cognitive benefits, circulatory support, or skin health, it's important to start with the lower end of the recommended dosage and gradually increase it to assess your body's response.

Gotu Kola's versatility as a brain tonic, circulatory enhancer, and skin regenerator makes it a valuable addition to a holistic approach to health and wellness. By understanding the specific applications and recommended dosages, individuals can effectively utilize this ancient herb to support their cognitive and physical health.

Schisandra: Five-Flavor Herb for Vitality

Schisandra, scientifically known as Schisandra chinensis, is a powerful adaptogen that has been used for centuries in traditional Chinese medicine to promote whole-body vitality. This unique herb is characterized by its ability to present five distinct flavors: sweet, sour, salty, bitter, and pungent, a rarity in the plant world that symbolizes its comprehensive therapeutic impact on human health. Schisandra's adaptogenic properties make it an invaluable ally in enhancing the body's resistance to stress, fatigue, and various diseases by modulating the body's stress response systems. This includes supporting adrenal function, protecting against stress-induced damage, and enhancing mental and physical performance.

The liver detoxification process is crucial for maintaining overall health and vitality. Schisandra plays a significant role in this process by activating enzymes in liver cells that are responsible for detoxifying harmful substances. It achieves this through its bioactive compounds, including lignans such as schizandrin, which have been shown to increase the level of glutathione, a critical antioxidant in the body's detoxification system. This antioxidant not only neutralizes free radicals but also assists in the conversion of toxins into harmless substances that can be easily eliminated from the body. For optimal liver support, incorporating Schisandra into one's daily regimen involves consuming extracts or powdered forms of the berry. A common approach is to take 1-3 grams of Schisandra powder, mixed with water or tea, once or twice daily. It is also available in capsule form, with a recommended dose of 500-1000 mg daily, ideally taken with meals to enhance absorption.

Improving physical endurance is another remarkable benefit of Schisandra. Its adaptogenic effects contribute to enhanced physical performance by optimizing energy use and reducing fatigue. Schisandra achieves this by influencing the body's production and utilization of adenosine triphosphate (ATP), the primary energy currency of cells. This not only improves endurance and stamina but also supports recovery processes after physical exertion. Athletes and physically active individuals may find Schisandra particularly beneficial for increasing resistance to physical stress and accelerating recovery times. To harness Schisandra's endurance-enhancing properties, it is advisable to consume Schisandra extract or powder 30 minutes before engaging in physical activity. This timing allows the body to absorb and utilize the herb's active compounds effectively, providing an energy boost and enhanced performance during workouts or physical tasks.

For those incorporating Schisandra into their wellness routines, it's important to source high-quality products from reputable suppliers. The concentration of active compounds can vary significantly between products, so selecting standardized extracts that specify the percentage of key lignans ensures consistent and effective dosages. Additionally, while Schisandra is generally well-tolerated, it's wise to start with a lower dose to assess individual tolerance before gradually increasing to the recommended dosage. As with any supplement, consulting with a healthcare professional before adding Schisandra to your regimen, especially for individuals with pre-existing health conditions or those taking medications, is crucial to ensure safety and compatibility.

Astragalus: Immune Support & Cellular Repair

Astragalus, a perennial plant native to the northern and eastern parts of China as well as Mongolia and Korea, has been a cornerstone in traditional Chinese medicine for centuries. Its roots, harvested from plants that are at least four years old, are the primary medicinal component, known for their potent immune-boosting and disease-fighting capabilities. The active compounds within astragalus, including polysaccharides, saponins, flavonoids, amino acids, and trace minerals, work synergistically to enhance the body's resistance to diseases and promote longevity.

The immune-enhancing properties of astragalus are attributed primarily to its polysaccharides. These long-chain sugar molecules have been shown to stimulate the activity of white blood cells, which play a crucial role in the body's defense against pathogens. By activating these immune cells, astragalus helps to fortify the body's natural barriers against viruses and bacteria, potentially reducing the frequency and severity of common colds and respiratory infections.

Moreover, astragalus's saponins are recognized for their ability to support cardiovascular health. These compounds help to lower blood cholesterol levels and improve the overall function of the heart and blood vessels, thereby contributing to a reduced risk of heart disease. This cardiovascular support is essential not only for longevity but also for maintaining the body's ability to withstand the stresses of various diseases.

The flavonoids in astragalus, potent antioxidants, play a critical role in cellular repair and protection. They combat oxidative stress, a condition characterized by an imbalance between free radicals and antioxidants in the body. Oxidative stress is a common pathway for many chronic diseases, including cancer and heart disease, as well as aging. By neutralizing free radicals, the flavonoids in astragalus help to protect cells from damage, support the repair of damaged DNA, and slow down the aging process.

For those looking to incorporate astragalus into their wellness routine, it is available in various forms, including capsules, tinctures, and teas. When preparing astragalus tea, it is recommended to simmer the dried root in water for a period of time, usually between 30 to 60 minutes, to fully extract its beneficial compounds. This slow simmering process allows for the active ingredients to be released into the water, creating a potent immune-supporting beverage.

When selecting astragalus for use in homemade remedies or as a supplement, sourcing high-quality, organically grown astragalus root is crucial. The quality of the herb directly impacts its efficacy and safety. Organically grown astragalus ensures that the root is free from pesticides and other harmful chemicals that could detract from its health benefits.

Astragalus stands as a testament to the enduring wisdom of traditional herbal medicine, offering modern society a natural means to support the immune system, enhance cellular repair, and promote overall health and longevity. Its role in traditional Chinese medicine as a protector against illness and promoter of vitality continues to be validated by scientific research, making astragalus a valuable addition to a holistic approach to health and wellness.

Ginseng and Lemon Vitality Tonic

Beneficial effects

Ginseng and Lemon Vitality Tonic is a rejuvenating drink that combines the adaptogenic benefits of ginseng with the refreshing and detoxifying properties of lemon. Ginseng is renowned for its ability to increase energy levels, improve cognitive function, and support the immune system. Lemon, rich in vitamin C, aids in digestion and helps cleanse the body. This tonic is designed to boost vitality, enhance mental clarity, and promote overall well-being.

Portions

Makes about 4 cups

Preparation time

10 minutes

Cooking time

20 minutes

Ingredients

- 4 cups of water
- 2 tablespoons of dried ginseng root
- Juice of 2 large lemons
- 2 tablespoons of honey, or to taste
- A few slices of fresh ginger (optional for added flavor and digestive benefits)
- Lemon slices and mint leaves for garnish

Instructions

1. Pour 4 cups of water into a medium saucepan and bring to a simmer over medium heat.

2. Add the dried ginseng root to the simmering water. Cover the saucepan with a lid, reduce the heat to low, and let it simmer gently for 15 minutes to allow the ginseng to infuse.

3. After 15 minutes, remove the saucepan from the heat and let it cool slightly for about 5 minutes.

4. Strain the ginseng-infused water into a large pitcher or jar, discarding the ginseng roots.

5. Stir in the fresh lemon juice and honey into the ginseng water while it is still warm, ensuring the honey dissolves completely. Adjust the sweetness according to your taste by adding more or less honey.

6. If using, add a few slices of fresh ginger to the pitcher or jar for an extra layer of flavor and digestive benefits.

7. Refrigerate the tonic until it is thoroughly chilled, about 1-2 hours.

8. Serve the Ginseng and Lemon Vitality Tonic over ice, garnished with lemon slices and mint leaves for a refreshing and energizing drink.

Variations

- For a caffeine-free energy boost, add a teaspoon of matcha powder to the tonic once it has cooled.
- Incorporate a dash of cayenne pepper to the tonic for a metabolism-boosting effect.
- Substitute honey with maple syrup for a vegan-friendly sweetener option.

Storage tips

Store the Ginseng and Lemon Vitality Tonic in a sealed glass container in the refrigerator for up to 5 days. Shake well before serving as natural sediments from the ginseng and lemon may settle at the bottom.

Tips for allergens

For those with allergies to honey, maple syrup or agave nectar are excellent substitutes that won't compromise the tonic's beneficial properties. Ensure to use organic ginseng and lemons to minimize exposure to pesticides and other chemicals.

Scientific references

- "Ginseng, the 'Immunity Boost': The Effects of Panax ginseng on Immune System" in the Journal of Ginseng Research highlights the immune-boosting properties of ginseng.
- "Vitamin C and Immune Function" in Nutrients discusses the role of vitamin C, found in lemons, in supporting various cellular functions of both the innate and adaptive immune system.

CHAPTER 3: EXOTIC HERBS AND COMMON REMEDIES

Blending Rare Herbs with Adaptogens

Pairing rare herbs with everyday adaptogens creates a synergistic blend that can enhance energy levels, support stress resilience, and promote overall well-being. Ginseng, a revered adaptogen, is known for its ability to improve stamina, mental clarity, and immune function. When combined with nettle, an herb celebrated for its nutrient density and support of the body's natural defense mechanisms, the duo forms a potent remedy for balancing energy.

To create a balanced energy blend, start by sourcing high-quality, preferably organic, ginseng and nettle. Ginseng can be found in several varieties, including Panax ginseng (Asian ginseng) and Panax quinquefolius (American ginseng). Each type offers unique benefits, but all are known for their energizing properties. Nettle, on the other hand, is widely available and can be harvested in the wild or found at health food stores in dried form.

For the preparation of this blend, you will need:

- 1 part dried ginseng root, finely chopped or powdered
- 1 part dried nettle leaves
- A clean, dry jar for storage
- Boiling water if making a tea or an alcohol base (such as vodka) for a tincture

If opting to make a tea, measure equal parts of ginseng and nettle into a tea infuser or teapot. Pour boiling water over the herbs and allow them to steep for at least 15 minutes. This long steeping time ensures the maximum extraction of both the water-soluble and fat-soluble compounds from the ginseng and nettle, creating a potent brew. For those who prefer a tincture, fill a jar with equal parts of the dried herbs and cover them with a high-proof alcohol, ensuring the herbs are completely submerged. Seal the jar tightly and store it in a cool, dark place, shaking it daily for 4 to 6 weeks. This method extracts the active compounds into the alcohol, resulting in a concentrated liquid that can be taken in small doses.

When blending these herbs, it's important to consider the individual's constitution and any potential interactions with medications or health conditions. Ginseng, for instance, is a powerful herb that may not be suitable for everyone, especially those with high blood pressure, autoimmune diseases, or those who are pregnant. Nettle is generally considered safe but can interact with certain medications and conditions. Therefore, consulting with a healthcare provider or a knowledgeable herbalist before starting any herbal regimen is crucial.

The final product, whether a tea or tincture, offers a natural way to support the body's energy levels and adaptogenic response to stress. The combination of ginseng's invigorating properties with nettle's nutritional support provides a holistic approach to maintaining vitality and wellness. This blend can be consumed daily, preferably in the morning or early afternoon to harness its energizing effects without interfering with sleep patterns.

Incorporating this ginseng and nettle blend into a daily routine is a simple yet effective way to tap into the ancient wisdom of herbalism, leveraging the natural synergy between rare and common herbs for enhanced health and vitality.

Layering Herbs for Synergistic Benefits

Layering herbs for synergistic benefits involves a strategic combination of adaptogens, nervines, and tonics to create a holistic approach that addresses multiple body systems simultaneously. This method amplifies the individual effects of each herb, resulting in a compounded benefit that can enhance overall well-being, resilience to stress, and support for the body's natural healing processes. To effectively layer these herbs, it's essential to understand their unique properties and how they interact with each other.

Adaptogens, such as ashwagandha (Withania somnifera) and Rhodiola Rosea, are renowned for their ability to help the body resist and adapt to physical, chemical, and biological stressors. They work by modulating the release of stress hormones from the adrenal glands, helping to improve focus, energy, and stamina, while reducing anxiety and fatigue. When selecting adaptogens, opt for high-quality, organically grown herbs to ensure maximum potency and purity. For ashwagandha, a daily dosage of 300-500 mg of root extract is commonly recommended, while Rhodiola Rosea is often taken in 100-300 mg doses of extract, preferably in the morning to avoid potential interference with sleep.

Nervines, such as lemon balm (Melissa officinalis) and chamomile (Matricaria chamomilla), offer calming and soothing effects on the nervous system, making them ideal for reducing anxiety, promoting relaxation, and enhancing sleep quality. These herbs can be used in various forms, including teas, tinctures, and capsules. For a calming tea, steep 1-2 teaspoons of dried herb in boiling water for 10-15 minutes. For tinctures, a general guideline is to take 1-2 ml up to three times a day, but it's crucial to follow specific product recommendations or consult with a healthcare provider.

Tonics, such as dandelion (Taraxacum officinale) and nettle (Urtica dioica), support overall health by nourishing the body and promoting the optimal function of various organs and systems. They are particularly beneficial for the liver, kidneys, and blood, offering detoxifying effects and enhancing nutrient absorption. Dandelion root and nettle leaves can be consumed as teas, with 1-2 teaspoons of the dried herb steeped in hot water for about 10 minutes. These herbs are also available in tincture and capsule forms, with dosages varying based on the concentration of the product.

To create a layered herbal blend, start by identifying the primary health goal, such as stress reduction, immune support, or digestive health. Then, select one herb from each category (adaptogen, nervine, tonic) that aligns with this goal. For example, a blend aiming to reduce stress and support adrenal health might combine ashwagandha as an adaptogen, lemon balm as a nervine, and dandelion as a tonic. This combination works synergistically to modulate stress response, calm the nervous system, and support liver function, which can be particularly beneficial during times of increased stress.

When combining these herbs, it's important to consider the form in which they're being used (tea, tincture, capsule) and adjust the dosages accordingly to avoid potential overuse or interactions. Additionally, understanding the timing and method of administration can maximize the benefits of the blend. For instance, adaptogens are best taken in the morning or early afternoon to support daytime energy and focus, while nervines are more beneficial in the evening to promote relaxation and sleep.

Incorporating layered herbal blends into a daily wellness routine requires patience and experimentation, as the effects can be subtle and gradual. Monitoring one's response and adjusting the blend as needed can help achieve the desired health outcomes. Always consult with a healthcare provider before starting any new herbal regimen, especially for individuals with pre-existing health conditions or those taking medication, to ensure safety and compatibility.

Personalized Exotic Blends for Wellness

Crafting personalized exotic blends for specific needs such as **immunity, energy**, or **stress reduction** involves a thoughtful selection of herbs that target your unique health goals. Here's a detailed guide to creating these potent herbal formulas.

Immunity Boosting Blend

1. **Select Your Base Herb**: Start with **Astragalus Root**, known for its immune-boosting properties. Use about 1 part of dried, sliced astragalus root as the foundation of your blend. This adaptogen enhances the body's defense against stress and disease.

2. **Add Supporting Herbs**: Incorporate **Elderberry** (1/2 part), renowned for its antiviral effects, and **Echinacea** (1/2 part), which has been shown to increase white blood cell count, aiding in faster recovery from illnesses.

3. **Preparation Method**: Combine these dried herbs in a clean, dry jar. To make a tea, use 1 tablespoon of the blend per cup of boiling water, steeping for 15-20 minutes. For a tincture, fill a jar with the herb mixture and cover it with 40% alcohol, letting it sit for 4-6 weeks, shaking daily.

4. **Dosage**: Drink 1-2 cups of tea daily or take 1-2 ml of the tincture twice a day during flu season or when feeling under the weather.

Energy Enhancing Blend

1. **Select Your Base Herb**: **Rhodiola Rosea** serves as an excellent base for an energy blend due to its fatigue-fighting properties. Begin with 1 part of dried Rhodiola.

2. **Add Supporting Herbs**: Mix in **Ginseng** (1/2 part) to improve stamina and **Green Tea Leaves** (1/2 part) for a gentle caffeine boost and antioxidant support.

3. **Preparation Method**: For a tea, blend the dried herbs and steep 1 tablespoon in hot water for about 10 minutes. For an energy tincture, combine the herbs in alcohol as described above.

4. **Dosage**: Sip the tea in the morning or early afternoon to avoid disrupting sleep. Use the tincture in small doses (1 ml) in the morning or before physical activity.

Stress Reduction Blend

1. **Select Your Base Herb**: **Ashwagandha**, an adaptogen, is perfect for reducing stress and anxiety. Use 1 part of dried ashwagandha root.

2. **Add Supporting Herbs**: Incorporate **Lavender** (1/2 part) for its calming effect and **Holy Basil (Tulsi)** (1/2 part) to further reduce stress and balance the mind.

3. **Preparation Method**: To prepare a soothing tea, mix the herbs and steep 1 tablespoon in boiling water for about 10 minutes. For a stress-relief tincture, follow the general tincture preparation method.

4. **Dosage**: Enjoy a cup of tea in the evening to unwind before bed or take 1-2 ml of the tincture during stressful periods.

General Tips

- **Quality of Herbs**: Always source high-quality, organic herbs to ensure the purity and potency of your blend.

- **Storage**: Store your dried herb blends in airtight containers away from direct sunlight and moisture. Tinctures should be kept in amber or blue glass bottles to protect from light.

- **Consultation**: Before starting any new herbal regimen, especially if you have existing health conditions or are taking medications, consult with a healthcare professional.

By following these detailed steps and tailoring the herb selections to your specific needs, you can create powerful, personalized exotic blends that support your health and well-being.

Golden Milk with Ashwagandha

Beneficial effects

Golden Milk with Ashwagandha combines the soothing, anti-inflammatory properties of turmeric with the stress-reducing, vitality-boosting effects of Ashwagandha. This ancient remedy is revered for its ability to enhance mood, support joint and muscle health, and improve sleep quality. Turmeric, the main ingredient, contains curcumin, a compound with powerful antioxidant and anti-inflammatory benefits, while Ashwagandha is known for its adaptogenic properties that help the body resist stressors. Together, they create a potent drink that promotes overall well-being and relaxation.

Portions

2 servings

Preparation time

5 minutes

Cooking time

10 minutes

Ingredients

- 2 cups of almond milk (or any plant-based milk of your choice)
- 1 tablespoon of turmeric powder
- 1/2 teaspoon of ground Ashwagandha
- 1/4 teaspoon of black pepper (to enhance turmeric absorption)
- 1 tablespoon of coconut oil (for healthy fats and to aid absorption)
- 1-2 tablespoons of honey or maple syrup (to taste)
- A pinch of cinnamon (optional, for flavor)

Instructions

1. In a small saucepan, combine the almond milk, turmeric powder, ground Ashwagandha, and black pepper. Stir the mixture well to ensure the powders are fully dissolved in the milk.
2. Add the coconut oil to the saucepan. The fat from the coconut oil not only adds a creamy texture but also helps the body absorb the turmeric more efficiently.
3. Heat the mixture over medium heat, stirring occasionally, until it is hot but not boiling. This should take about 5-7 minutes. Avoid boiling to preserve the nutrients of the ingredients.
4. Once heated, remove the saucepan from the stove. Add honey or maple syrup to the golden milk, adjusting the amount to achieve your desired sweetness. Stir well to ensure it's fully mixed.
5. Pour the golden milk into two cups, using a fine mesh strainer if needed to catch any undissolved spices.
6. Sprinkle a pinch of cinnamon on top of each serving for added flavor and health benefits.
7. Serve warm and enjoy the calming, restorative effects of the drink.

Variations

- For a caffeine boost, add a shot of espresso or coffee to your golden milk, turning it into a turmeric latte.
- Include a piece of fresh ginger while heating the mixture to add a spicy kick and additional digestive benefits.
- Use vanilla almond milk for a subtly sweet, vanilla-flavored version without added sweeteners.

Storage tips

Golden Milk with Ashwagandha is best enjoyed fresh, but if you have leftovers, store them in an airtight container in the refrigerator for up to two days. Gently reheat on the stove or in the microwave before serving.

Tips for allergens

For those with nut allergies, coconut milk or oat milk are excellent alternatives to almond milk. Ensure to use pure ground Ashwagandha without any additives or fillers to avoid potential allergens. For a vegan version, opt for maple syrup instead of honey as the sweetener.

Scientific references

- "Curcumin: A Review of Its' Effects on Human Health," published in Foods, highlights the anti-inflammatory and antioxidant properties of curcumin found in turmeric.

- "An Overview on Ashwagandha: A Rasayana (Rejuvenator) of Ayurveda," published in the African Journal of Traditional, Complementary, and Alternative Medicines, discusses the adaptogenic effects of Ashwagandha, including stress relief and improved cognitive function.

BOOK 7: HERBAL REMEDIES FOR DIGESTIVE HEALTH

CHAPTER 1: CARMINATIVES FOR DIGESTIVE RELIEF

Peppermint and Fennel for Digestion

Peppermint (Mentha piperita) and fennel (Foeniculum vulgare) have been revered for their carminative properties, making them excellent natural remedies for gas, bloating, and digestive discomfort. To harness these benefits, one can prepare a simple yet effective herbal tea blend.

Peppermint, with its high menthol content, relaxes the smooth muscles of the digestive tract, which can alleviate spasms and discomfort associated with gas and bloating. **Fennel seeds**, on the other hand, contain compounds like anethole, fenchone, and estragole, which have antispasmodic and gas-relieving effects.

Preparation of Peppermint and Fennel Digestive Tea:

1. **Ingredients**:
   - 1 teaspoon of dried peppermint leaves
   - 1 teaspoon of fennel seeds
   - 8 ounces of boiling water

2. **Tools**:
   - A tea infuser or strainer
   - A mortar and pestle (optional, for crushing fennel seeds)
   - A kettle for boiling water
   - A teapot or a heat-resistant cup

3. **Instructions**:
   a. If using whole fennel seeds, lightly crush them with a mortar and pestle to release their volatile oils. This step is optional but recommended to maximize the therapeutic benefits.
   b. Place the crushed fennel seeds and dried peppermint leaves into a tea infuser or strainer.
   c. Boil 8 ounces of water using a kettle. Once boiling, pour the water over the peppermint and fennel in the teapot or cup.
   d. Cover and steep for 5 to 10 minutes. The longer it steeps, the stronger the flavor and therapeutic properties will be. However, do not exceed 10 minutes to avoid an overly bitter taste.
   e. Remove the infuser or strain the tea to remove the solid particles. The tea should have a pleasant, aromatic scent and a slightly sweet, minty flavor.

4. **Consumption**:
   - For best results, drink this tea 20 to 30 minutes before meals to prepare the digestive system or after meals to ease digestion.
   - It is advisable to start with one cup per day to assess tolerance and can be increased to 2-3 cups as needed, especially during times of increased digestive discomfort.

Additional Tips:

- Ensure the peppermint and fennel are of high quality and sourced from reputable suppliers to guarantee purity and potency.
- Individuals with GERD (gastroesophageal reflux disease) should proceed with caution when consuming peppermint, as it can relax the sphincter between the stomach and esophagus, potentially worsening symptoms.

- Pregnant women should consult with a healthcare provider before consuming fennel tea, as large quantities can be contraindicated during pregnancy.

This peppermint and fennel tea serves as a gentle, natural approach to mitigating digestive ailments such as gas and bloating. Its preparation and consumption are straightforward, making it an accessible remedy for those looking to incorporate herbal solutions into their digestive health regimen.

Ginger as a Digestive Stimulant

Ginger, scientifically known as **Zingiber officinale**, has been a cornerstone in traditional medicine for centuries, particularly for its effectiveness in promoting **healthy gastric motility** and reducing **nausea**. This root herb is rich in bioactive compounds, such as **gingerol**, which is primarily responsible for its potent digestive and anti-nausea properties.

To harness the benefits of ginger for digestive health, it's essential to understand how to select, prepare, and use this versatile herb. Fresh ginger root is preferable for most digestive remedies due to its higher concentration of active compounds compared to dried forms. Look for ginger root that is firm to the touch and free of mold or soft spots. Before use, the root should be washed thoroughly and peeled to remove the outer layer, which can be tough.

Preparation of Ginger Digestive Aid:

1. **Ingredients**:
   - 1 inch of fresh ginger root
   - 8 ounces of water
2. **Tools**:
   - A sharp knife or grater
   - A small pot for boiling
   - A strainer or cheesecloth
3. **Instructions**:

   a. Begin by slicing or grating the fresh ginger root to increase its surface area, enhancing the extraction of beneficial compounds.

   b. Add the prepared ginger to a pot containing 8 ounces of water. Bring the mixture to a boil, then reduce the heat, allowing it to simmer for about 10 minutes. This slow simmering process helps to extract the gingerol and other volatile oils into the water, creating a potent digestive tonic.

   c. After simmering, remove the pot from the heat and let it steep for an additional 5 minutes. This resting period allows the flavors to meld and the concoction to reach a palatable temperature.

   d. Strain the mixture through a strainer or cheesecloth into a cup, pressing or squeezing the ginger solids to extract as much liquid as possible.

Consumption:

- Drink the ginger tonic 20 to 30 minutes before meals to stimulate digestion or after meals to alleviate feelings of fullness or nausea. Starting with one cup per day is recommended, adjusting as needed based on personal tolerance and digestive response.

Additional Tips:

- For those sensitive to the strong taste of ginger, adding a teaspoon of honey or a slice of lemon can enhance the flavor, making it more enjoyable to consume.
- Ginger can also be incorporated into daily meals, such as soups, stews, or teas, to continuously support digestive health.

- While ginger is generally safe for most people, it's important to consider individual health conditions and consult with a healthcare provider if you're pregnant, nursing, or have a medical condition that could be affected by ginger's potent properties.

By incorporating ginger into your diet, you're not only adding a flavorful spice but also tapping into its powerful digestive and anti-nausea benefits. Its natural ability to promote gastric motility makes it an invaluable tool for maintaining optimal digestive health.

Cinnamon for Blood Sugar and Digestion

Cinnamon, derived from the inner bark of trees belonging to the genus Cinnamomum, stands out not only for its widespread culinary use but also for its potent medicinal properties, particularly in regulating blood sugar levels and supporting digestion. This spice's distinctive warming quality and sweet, woody aroma make it a favorite in various dishes, yet its health benefits, especially for digestive health, are equally remarkable.

To leverage cinnamon's benefits for blood sugar regulation, it's essential to understand its active components. Cinnamaldehyde, the compound responsible for cinnamon's unique flavor and smell, plays a pivotal role in influencing blood sugar control. It mimics insulin's action, improving glucose uptake by cells and thereby lowering blood sugar levels. For those managing conditions like type 2 diabetes or looking to maintain stable blood sugar levels, incorporating cinnamon into the diet can be particularly beneficial. A practical method is adding a quarter to a half teaspoon of ground cinnamon to morning oatmeal or smoothies. This not only enhances flavor but also contributes to a more regulated blood sugar level throughout the day.

In terms of digestion, cinnamon's warming properties stimulate saliva production and gastric juices, aiding in the breakdown of food more efficiently. This spice is particularly effective in relieving discomfort associated with indigestion, gas, and bloating. The essential oils in cinnamon have been found to reduce spasms in the gastrointestinal tract, soothing an upset stomach. A simple way to harness these digestive benefits is by preparing a cinnamon-infused tea. To do this, steep a cinnamon stick in boiling water for 10 minutes, allowing the volatile oils and compounds to infuse. Drinking this tea after meals can help ease digestive discomfort and promote a healthy digestive process.

Moreover, cinnamon's antimicrobial properties contribute to a healthy gut by reducing the growth of harmful bacteria while allowing beneficial gut flora to thrive. This balance is crucial for digestion and overall health, as an imbalance can lead to various digestive issues and decreased nutrient absorption.

For those incorporating cinnamon into their diet for health benefits, it's important to choose Ceylon cinnamon, also known as "true cinnamon," over Cassia cinnamon, commonly found in grocery stores. Ceylon cinnamon contains lower levels of coumarin, a compound that can be harmful in large doses, making it a safer choice for regular consumption.

Incorporating cinnamon into the diet for its blood sugar and digestive benefits can be as simple as sprinkling it on fruit, adding it to baking recipes, or even incorporating it into savory dishes for a touch of warmth and sweetness. The key is consistent and moderate use, as part of a balanced diet, to fully enjoy the health benefits cinnamon offers without overconsumption risks.

Remember, while cinnamon can be a valuable addition to a health-conscious diet, it should not replace medical treatment for chronic conditions. Always consult with a healthcare provider before making significant changes to your diet, especially if managing a health condition or taking medication.

Fennel and Ginger Digestive Tea

Beneficial effects

Fennel and Ginger Digestive Tea combines the soothing properties of fennel with the warming effects of ginger, creating a powerful digestive aid. Fennel seeds are known for their ability to relieve bloating and gas, thanks to their antispasmodic properties, while ginger has been widely recognized for its ability to alleviate nausea and promote gastric motility. This tea is perfect for soothing digestive discomfort and enhancing overall digestive health.

Portions

Makes about 4 cups

Preparation time

5 minutes

Cooking time

10 minutes

Ingredients

- 1 tablespoon fennel seeds
- 1 inch fresh ginger root, thinly sliced
- 4 cups water
- Honey or maple syrup to taste (optional)
- Fresh lemon slices for garnish (optional)

Instructions

1. Begin by crushing the fennel seeds lightly with a mortar and pestle to release their oils and flavor. If you don't have a mortar and pestle, the back of a spoon against a cutting board works as well.
2. Peel the ginger root and slice it thinly to maximize the surface area exposed to the water, enhancing the infusion of its flavors and beneficial compounds.
3. In a medium saucepan, bring the 4 cups of water to a boil. Once boiling, add the crushed fennel seeds and sliced ginger to the water.
4. Reduce the heat to low and let the mixture simmer gently for 10 minutes. This slow simmering process allows the water to become fully infused with the flavors and digestive benefits of the fennel and ginger.
5. After simmering, remove the saucepan from the heat. Strain the tea through a fine mesh sieve into a teapot or directly into cups, discarding the solids.
6. If desired, sweeten the tea with honey or maple syrup to taste. Stir well to ensure it dissolves completely in the warm tea.
7. Serve the tea warm, garnished with a slice of fresh lemon in each cup if using. The lemon not only adds a refreshing flavor but also contributes vitamin C and aids in digestion.

Variations

- For a cooler, refreshing version, allow the tea to cool to room temperature, then refrigerate until cold. Serve over ice.
- Add a cinnamon stick to the saucepan with the fennel and ginger for a subtly spiced flavor profile.
- Incorporate a few mint leaves into the tea after removing it from heat for a cooling, soothing effect.

Storage tips

Store any leftover tea in a glass container in the refrigerator for up to 2 days. Reheat gently on the stove or enjoy cold.

Tips for allergens

For those with allergies or sensitivities to honey, maple syrup is a suitable vegan alternative that provides natural sweetness without compromising the tea's digestive benefits.

Scientific references

- "The Effect of Fennel (Foeniculum Vulgare) Seed Oil Emulsion in Infantile Colic: A Randomized, Placebo-Controlled Study" published in Alternative Therapies in Health and Medicine highlights the antispasmodic and gas-relieving effects of fennel.

- "Ginger in Gastrointestinal Disorders: A Systematic Review of Clinical Trials" found in Food Science & Nutrition discusses ginger's effectiveness in enhancing gastrointestinal motility and alleviating nausea.

CHAPTER 2: HEALING THE GUT LINING

Slippery Elm Bark: Gut Soother

Slippery elm bark, derived from the inner bark of the Ulmus rubra tree, stands as a cornerstone in herbal medicine for its remarkable ability to soothe and protect the gastrointestinal tract. This efficacy is largely attributed to its rich mucilage content, a type of soluble fiber that becomes a slick gel when mixed with water. Upon ingestion, this mucilage coats the lining of the mouth, throat, stomach, and intestines, offering a protective layer that is particularly beneficial for those suffering from conditions like Irritable Bowel Syndrome (IBS) or acid reflux, also known as GERD (Gastroesophageal Reflux Disease).

To utilize slippery elm for its gut-soothing properties, it's essential to prepare it correctly. Begin by sourcing high-quality slippery elm powder, ensuring it comes from a reputable supplier to guarantee purity. For a basic slippery elm preparation, you will need:

- 1 to 2 tablespoons of slippery elm bark powder
- 1 cup (8 ounces) of hot water

The process is straightforward: Add the slippery elm powder to a cup of hot water and stir until it dissolves completely, transforming into a thick, gel-like substance. This can be consumed two to three times daily, preferably before meals to maximize the protective effect on the digestive tract.

For those dealing with acid reflux, incorporating slippery elm into your routine can help by forming a barrier against the upward flow of stomach acid, thereby reducing the irritation and burning sensation often experienced in the throat and chest. Meanwhile, individuals with IBS may find that slippery elm's mucilage helps regulate bowel movements and alleviate both diarrhea and constipation by adding bulk and softness to the stool, making it easier to pass.

In addition to its mucilage, slippery elm contains antioxidants and nutrients that further support digestive health. However, it's crucial to maintain hydration while taking slippery elm, as its high fiber content requires adequate water to ensure proper function and prevent potential blockages in the digestive system.

While slippery elm is generally considered safe for most people, it's advisable to start with a smaller dose to assess tolerance and gradually increase as needed. As with any herbal remedy, consulting with a healthcare provider before adding slippery elm to your regimen is wise, especially for those who are pregnant, nursing, or taking prescription medications, to avoid any potential interactions.

Remember, the effectiveness of slippery elm, like many herbal remedies, may vary from person to person. Consistent use over several weeks is often necessary to observe the full benefits. By incorporating slippery elm into a holistic approach to digestive wellness, including a balanced diet and stress management techniques, individuals can significantly enhance their gastrointestinal health and overall well-being.

Marshmallow Root for Digestive Health

Marshmallow root, scientifically known as Althaea officinalis, is a perennial herb that has been used for centuries to treat various digestive issues, including inflammatory bowel disorders and ulcers. Its healing properties stem from the high mucilage content, a sticky substance that when mixed with water forms a gel-like layer. This mucilage coats the lining of the digestive tract, providing a protective barrier that can soothe irritation, reduce inflammation, and promote healing. For individuals suffering from conditions such as irritable bowel syndrome (IBS), Crohn's disease, ulcerative colitis, and peptic ulcers, marshmallow root offers a natural and gentle approach to managing symptoms and supporting the body's healing processes.

To harness the benefits of marshmallow root for digestive health, it's essential to understand the proper preparation and dosage. The root can be used in several forms, including dried, powdered, or as a liquid extract. One of the most effective ways to prepare marshmallow root for digestive repair is by creating a cold infusion, which preserves the integrity of the mucilage and ensures maximum efficacy.

Preparation of Marshmallow Root Cold Infusion:

1. **Ingredients**:
   - 1-2 tablespoons of dried marshmallow root
   - 16 ounces (about 500 milliliters) of cold water

2. **Tools**:
   - A jar with a lid
   - A fine mesh strainer or cheesecloth

3. **Instructions**:

   a. Place the dried marshmallow root into the jar.

   b. Pour the cold water over the root, ensuring it is fully submerged.

   c. Seal the jar with the lid and let it sit at room temperature for at least 4 to 8 hours, or overnight. This slow infusion process allows the water to extract the mucilage from the root without degrading its soothing properties.

   d. After the infusion period, strain the liquid through a fine mesh strainer or cheesecloth into another container, pressing or squeezing the marshmallow root to extract as much liquid as possible.

The resulting infusion will have a slightly thick, slippery texture, indicative of the mucilage content. For digestive repair, it's recommended to drink this infusion 2-3 times daily, preferably before meals to allow the mucilage to coat the digestive tract effectively.

Additional Tips:

- For individuals with acute conditions or flare-ups, increasing the amount of marshmallow root to 3 tablespoons per 16 ounces of water can enhance the soothing effects.
- Marshmallow root infusion can be stored in the refrigerator for up to 2-3 days. Shake well before use as the mucilage may settle at the bottom.
- While marshmallow root is generally safe for most people, it's important to consult with a healthcare provider before starting any new herbal remedy, especially for those who are pregnant, nursing, or taking prescription medications, as it may interact with certain drugs by affecting their absorption.

Marshmallow root's ability to soothe and protect the digestive lining makes it a valuable ally in the natural treatment of digestive disorders. Its gentle action and minimal side effects make it suitable for long-term use as part of a comprehensive approach to digestive health. Incorporating marshmallow root into a daily regimen can help manage symptoms of digestive discomfort, promote healing of ulcers, and support overall digestive function.

Calendula for Gut Inflammation

Calendula, scientifically known as **Calendula officinalis**, is renowned for its potent anti-inflammatory and healing properties, making it an invaluable ally in combating gut inflammation.

This vibrant, golden-hued flower harbors a wealth of compounds including flavonoids, saponins, and mucilage, which collectively contribute to its therapeutic efficacy in soothing the digestive tract.

To harness the benefits of calendula for gut health, one can prepare a simple yet effective **calendula tea**. Begin by sourcing high-quality, dried calendula flowers, ensuring they are free from pesticides and contaminants to maximize the purity and potency of your remedy. For each cup of boiling water, add approximately 1 to 2 teaspoons of dried calendula flowers. Cover and steep for 10 to 15 minutes. This steeping time allows for the extraction of the beneficial compounds into the water, creating a therapeutic infusion. Strain the tea to remove the flowers, and consume the tea warm. For optimal results, it's recommended to drink calendula tea 2 to 3 times daily, especially before meals to prepare the digestive system for food intake and to maximize absorption of nutrients.

In addition to its consumption as tea, calendula can be incorporated into meals. **Calendula petals** are edible and can be sprinkled over salads or blended into smoothies, offering a nourishing and anti-inflammatory boost to your diet. When using calendula culinarily, ensure the petals are clean and free from any chemical treatments.

Maintaining a clean and organized space for the preparation of calendula remedies is crucial. Ensure all utensils, such as teapots and strainers, are thoroughly cleaned to prevent contamination. Storing dried calendula flowers in airtight containers away from direct sunlight and moisture will help preserve their quality and medicinal properties.

Slippery Elm and Marshmallow Root Gut Soothing Tea

Beneficial effects

Slippery Elm and Marshmallow Root Gut Soothing Tea is a gentle, effective remedy for various digestive issues, including irritation of the digestive tract, heartburn, and indigestion. Slippery elm contains mucilage, a gel-like substance that coats and soothes the mouth, throat, stomach, and intestines, making it ideal for easing gastrointestinal discomfort. Marshmallow root also contains mucilage, along with anti-inflammatory properties, providing relief from irritation and inflammation within the digestive system. Together, these herbs create a soothing tea that supports the healing of the gut lining and promotes overall digestive health.

Portions

Makes about 2 cups

Preparation time

5 minutes

Cooking time

15 minutes

Ingredients

- 1 tablespoon dried slippery elm bark
- 1 tablespoon dried marshmallow root
- 2 cups water
- Honey or maple syrup to taste (optional)

Instructions

1. Combine the dried slippery elm bark and dried marshmallow root in a small saucepan.
2. Add 2 cups of water to the saucepan, and gently bring the mixture to a simmer over low heat. Avoid boiling to preserve the herbs' beneficial properties.

3. Once simmering, cover the saucepan with a lid and allow the mixture to simmer gently for 15 minutes. This slow simmering process allows the mucilage from the herbs to release and infuse into the water.

4. After 15 minutes, remove the saucepan from heat and let it sit, covered, for an additional 5 minutes to further steep and enhance the infusion.

5. Strain the tea through a fine mesh sieve or cheesecloth into a mug or teapot, pressing on the herbs to extract as much liquid as possible. Discard the used herbs.

6. If desired, sweeten the tea with honey or maple syrup to taste. Stir well to ensure it dissolves completely in the warm tea.

7. Serve the tea warm for immediate soothing relief, or allow it to cool for a refreshing, gut-healing beverage.

Variations

- For added digestive support, include a slice of fresh ginger or a pinch of cinnamon to the simmering water with the herbs.
- Lemon zest or a squeeze of lemon juice can be added after straining the tea for a refreshing twist and additional digestive benefits.

Storage tips

This tea is best enjoyed fresh, but if you have leftovers, they can be stored in a sealed glass container in the refrigerator for up to 2 days. Reheat gently on the stove or enjoy cold.

Tips for allergens

For those with sensitivities or allergies to honey, maple syrup is a suitable vegan alternative that provides natural sweetness without compromising the tea's soothing properties.

Scientific references

- "Mucilage from Slippery Elm Bark and Marshmallow Root: Extraction, Characterization, and Anti-inflammatory Properties" published in the Journal of Ethnopharmacology discusses the mucilage's role in soothing the digestive tract and its potential anti-inflammatory benefits.

CHAPTER 3: LIVER AND GALLBLADDER SUPPORT

Milk Thistle: Liver Detox and Regeneration

Milk thistle, scientifically known as Silybum marianum, has been recognized for centuries as a powerful herb for liver health. Its active ingredient, silymarin, is a complex of flavonolignans that has been extensively studied for its hepatoprotective properties. Silymarin acts as an antioxidant, anti-inflammatory, and antifibrotic agent, making milk thistle an essential component of any regimen aimed at supporting liver function and detoxification processes.

To effectively harness the benefits of milk thistle for liver detoxification and cell regeneration, it's crucial to understand the optimal form and dosage. Silymarin is poorly soluble in water, so traditional tea preparations may not yield significant therapeutic benefits. Instead, standardized extracts in the form of capsules, tablets, or liquid tinctures are recommended to ensure adequate bioavailability of silymarin. Look for products that specify the percentage of silymarin or silybin, another active compound, and aim for a daily dosage of 140 to 210 milligrams of silymarin, divided into two or three doses.

For those interested in incorporating milk thistle into their daily routine, starting with a lower dose and gradually increasing it allows the body to adjust and minimizes the risk of any gastrointestinal discomfort, a common side effect. It's also advisable to consult with a healthcare provider before beginning any new supplement, especially for individuals with existing liver conditions, pregnant or nursing women, or those taking medications that could interact with milk thistle.

In addition to supplementation, incorporating milk thistle into your diet can be another avenue to explore. While the seeds are the most potent part of the plant, containing the highest concentration of silymarin, the leaves can be used fresh in salads or as a garnish. For those who prefer a hands-on approach, milk thistle seeds can be ground and added to smoothies, oatmeal, or homemade bread, providing a nutty flavor along with its liver-boosting benefits.

Maintaining liver health is a multifaceted endeavor that involves not only supplementation but also lifestyle choices that support liver function. This includes a diet rich in fruits, vegetables, lean proteins, and whole grains, regular physical activity, and avoiding excessive alcohol consumption and exposure to environmental toxins. Incorporating milk thistle as part of a holistic approach to liver health can amplify the liver's natural detoxification processes, aid in the regeneration of damaged liver cells, and provide a protective effect against liver diseases.

When storing milk thistle supplements, keep them in a cool, dry place away from direct sunlight to preserve their potency. As with any herb, the quality of milk thistle products can vary widely between brands. Opting for products that have been third-party tested and verified for purity and potency can provide additional assurance of their effectiveness.

Dandelion Root and Bile Production

Dandelion root, scientifically known as **Taraxacum officinale**, plays a crucial role in supporting liver health and enhancing bile production. Bile, a fluid produced by the liver and stored in the gallbladder, is essential for the digestion and absorption of fats in the diet. It acts as a natural emulsifier, breaking down fats into smaller droplets, which enzymes can more easily digest. An increase in bile flow can aid in this process, making dandelion root a valuable herb for those looking to improve their digestive health and fat metabolism.

To utilize dandelion root for its bile-enhancing properties, one can prepare a **dandelion root decoction**. Begin by sourcing high-quality, organic dandelion root, either fresh or dried. If using fresh root, clean it thoroughly and chop it into small pieces. For dried root, a coarse grind will suffice. Measure one teaspoon of dried root or one tablespoon of fresh root per cup of water. Place the root into a saucepan and add the water. Bring the mixture to a boil, then reduce the heat and simmer for about 15 to 20 minutes. This process extracts the bitter compounds responsible for stimulating bile production. Strain the decoction and consume it warm. Drinking one to two cups daily, preferably before meals, can optimize digestive processes and support liver function.

For those who prefer a more convenient approach, **dandelion root tinctures** are available. Look for tinctures that specify they are made from the root rather than the flower or leaf, as it's the root that contains the properties beneficial for liver support and bile production. The typical dosage for a tincture is 1-2 ml, taken three times a day. However, starting with a lower dose and adjusting based on individual tolerance can be wise.

Incorporating **dandelion root into your diet** is another way to reap its benefits. The root can be roasted and ground to make a caffeine-free coffee substitute. This preparation retains the root's beneficial properties and provides a pleasant, earthy beverage that can be enjoyed any time of day. Adding a pinch of cinnamon or cardamom can enhance the flavor and further support digestive health.

When selecting dandelion root, whether fresh, dried, or in tincture form, opting for organic sources ensures the product is free from pesticides and other contaminants that could undermine its health benefits. Store dried dandelion root in an airtight container in a cool, dark place to maintain its potency.

Regular consumption of dandelion root, alongside a balanced diet rich in fiber, healthy fats, and lean proteins, can support the body's natural detoxification processes, improve fat digestion, and enhance overall digestive health. Remember, while dandelion root is generally considered safe for most people, those with gallbladder disease, bile duct obstructions, or on medications should consult with a healthcare provider before adding it to their regimen to avoid potential interactions or adverse effects.

Artichoke for Cholesterol and Digestion

Artichoke, scientifically known as **Cynara scolymus**, is a nutrient-rich plant that has been used for centuries to support digestive health and manage cholesterol levels. The leaves of the artichoke plant contain a variety of bioactive compounds, including cynarin and luteolin, which are believed to be the primary contributors to its health benefits. These compounds have been shown to stimulate bile production, which is essential for digesting fats and the absorption of vitamins from the diet. Increased bile production can also help to reduce symptoms of indigestion and improve overall digestive function.

To utilize artichoke for its cholesterol-lowering and digestive benefits, consider incorporating artichoke leaves or extracts into your diet. **Artichoke leaf extract** is available in capsule or liquid form and is standardized to contain a certain percentage of cynarin. The recommended dosage for cholesterol management and digestive support is typically 300-600 mg of artichoke leaf extract, taken three times daily with meals. This dosage can vary depending on the concentration of the extract, so it's important to follow the manufacturer's instructions or consult with a healthcare provider.

For those who prefer whole food sources, fresh or frozen artichoke hearts can be incorporated into a variety of dishes. When preparing fresh artichokes, it's important to trim the thorns and remove the outer leaves to reveal the heart, which is the most nutrient-dense part of the plant. Artichoke hearts can be steamed, boiled, or grilled and are often used in salads, dips, and as a topping for pizzas and pastas.

Steaming artichokes is a simple method that preserves their nutritional content. To steam, place trimmed artichokes in a steaming basket over boiling water, cover, and steam for approximately 25-45 minutes, or until the leaves can be easily pulled off. You can enhance the flavor by adding garlic, lemon slices, or herbs to the steaming water.

Another way to incorporate artichokes into your diet is through **artichoke tea**, which can be made by boiling dried artichoke leaves for about 15 minutes and then straining the liquid. This tea can be consumed once or twice daily to support liver function and aid digestion.

When selecting artichokes, whether fresh or in supplement form, look for products that are free from pesticides and other contaminants to ensure the highest quality and health benefits. Fresh artichokes should feel heavy for their size and have tightly packed leaves. Store them in a plastic bag in the refrigerator to maintain freshness for up to a week.

Regular consumption of artichokes or artichoke extract can support liver health by promoting the production of bile, aiding in the digestion of fats, and facilitating the removal of toxins from the body. Additionally, the antioxidant properties of artichokes can help protect the liver from oxidative stress and inflammation. For individuals with high cholesterol, artichokes may offer a natural way to help manage levels and improve cardiovascular health.

As with any dietary supplement or significant change to your diet, it's advisable to consult with a healthcare provider, especially for those with pre-existing health conditions or those taking medications, to ensure that artichokes are an appropriate and safe option.

Dandelion and Milk Thistle Liver Detox Tea

Beneficial effects

Dandelion and Milk Thistle Liver Detox Tea is a powerful blend designed to support liver health and detoxification. Dandelion root is celebrated for its liver-cleansing properties and ability to promote bile production, which helps the liver detoxify more efficiently. Milk thistle is renowned for its silymarin content, a compound that has been shown to protect liver cells from damage and enhance liver function. Together, these herbs work synergistically to cleanse, protect, and support liver health, making this tea an excellent choice for those looking to naturally support their liver's detoxification processes.

Portions

Makes about 4 cups

Preparation time

5 minutes

Cooking time

15 minutes

Ingredients

- 2 tablespoons dried dandelion root
- 2 tablespoons dried milk thistle seeds
- 4 cups water
- Honey or lemon to taste (optional)

Instructions

1. Begin by coarsely grinding the milk thistle seeds with a mortar and pestle or a coffee grinder to increase their surface area and enhance the extraction of beneficial compounds. Be careful not to pulverize them into a fine powder; a coarse grind is sufficient.
2. Combine the ground milk thistle seeds and dried dandelion root in a medium saucepan.

3. Add 4 cups of water to the saucepan and bring the mixture to a gentle boil over medium heat.

4. Once boiling, reduce the heat to low, cover the saucepan, and simmer for 15 minutes. This slow simmer allows the water to become infused with the liver-supporting compounds from the dandelion and milk thistle.

5. After simmering, remove the saucepan from the heat and let it steep, covered, for an additional 5 minutes to further enhance the potency of the tea.

6. Strain the tea through a fine mesh strainer or cheesecloth into a large pitcher or directly into cups, pressing on the herbs to extract as much liquid as possible. Discard the used herbs.

7. If desired, add honey or a squeeze of lemon to the tea for flavor. Stir well to ensure any added sweeteners are fully dissolved.

8. Serve the tea warm, or allow it to cool and then refrigerate for a refreshing cold beverage.

Variations

- For a more complex flavor profile, add a cinnamon stick or a few slices of fresh ginger to the saucepan along with the dandelion root and milk thistle seeds.
- Incorporate a teaspoon of turmeric powder to the blend for additional anti-inflammatory benefits.

Storage tips

Store any leftover tea in a glass container in the refrigerator for up to 3 days. Reheat gently on the stove or enjoy cold for a revitalizing liver detox support.

Tips for allergens

For those with allergies or sensitivities to honey, maple syrup is a great vegan alternative that can add a touch of sweetness without compromising the detoxifying benefits of the tea.

Scientific references

- "The diuretic effect in human subjects of an extract of Taraxacum officinale folium over a single day" published in the Journal of Alternative and Complementary Medicine highlights the diuretic properties of dandelion, which can support liver detoxification.
- "Silymarin, the Antioxidant Component and Silybum marianum Extracts Prevent Liver Damage" in the journal Fitoterapia discusses the hepatoprotective effects of milk thistle, underscoring its role in supporting liver health and function.

BOOK 8: RESPIRATORY HEALTH WITH HERBS

CHAPTER 1: NATURAL DECONGESTANTS AND MUCOLYTICS

Eucalyptus for Respiratory Relief

Eucalyptus, known for its potent essential oil, plays a crucial role in respiratory health, particularly in opening airways and alleviating sinus and lung congestion. The active component, **eucalyptol**, possesses anti-inflammatory, antispasmodic, and decongestant properties, making it an ideal remedy for those suffering from colds, flu, or bronchitis. Here, we will detail how to utilize eucalyptus in steam baths and chest rubs for effective respiratory relief.

Creating a Eucalyptus Steam Bath:

1. **Materials Needed:**
   - Fresh or dried eucalyptus leaves (1 cup) or Eucalyptus essential oil (5-10 drops)
   - Large pot or kettle
   - Heat-resistant bowl
   - Towel

2. **Procedure:**
   - Begin by boiling water in a large pot or kettle. Once boiling, carefully pour the water into a heat-resistant bowl.
   - If using fresh or dried eucalyptus leaves, add them directly to the boiling water. For those opting for eucalyptus essential oil, wait for the water to slightly cool before adding 5-10 drops to prevent the oil from evaporating too quickly.
   - Lean over the bowl, ensuring you are at a comfortable distance to prevent steam burns. Drape a towel over your head and the bowl to create a tent that traps the steam.
   - Inhale deeply for 5-10 minutes, allowing the eucalyptus-infused steam to penetrate your respiratory system. This method helps to loosen mucus, clear congestion, and open up the airways.

Formulating a Eucalyptus Chest Rub:

1. **Ingredients:**
   - Eucalyptus essential oil (10-15 drops)
   - Carrier oil (e.g., coconut oil, jojoba oil) (1/4 cup)
   - Beeswax (optional for thicker consistency) (2 tablespoons)

2. **Equipment:**
   - Double boiler
   - Small container or jar for storage

3. **Method:**
   - If using beeswax, melt it with the carrier oil in a double boiler over low heat until fully dissolved. This creates a thicker base for the chest rub, which aids in longer-lasting application.
   - Remove from heat and allow the mixture to cool slightly before adding the eucalyptus essential oil. Stir well to ensure even distribution of the oil.
   - Pour the mixture into a small container or jar and allow it to solidify. If you did not use beeswax, simply mix the eucalyptus oil with the carrier oil and store it in a container.

- To use, apply a small amount of the chest rub on the chest, throat, and back, massaging gently. The eucalyptus scent will help to clear congestion and ease breathing.

Safety Precautions:

- Always perform a patch test before applying the chest rub to ensure no allergic reactions occur.
- Eucalyptus essential oil is potent; always dilute it with a carrier oil before topical application.
- The steam bath is not recommended for children under the age of 10 or individuals with asthma without prior consultation from a healthcare provider.

By incorporating eucalyptus into your respiratory health regimen through steam baths and chest rubs, you can harness its natural decongestant properties to support clear breathing and relief from congestion.

Thyme for Clearing Mucus

Thyme, a powerful herb with a long history of use in traditional medicine, is renowned for its ability to break up mucus and soothe inflammation, making it an invaluable ally in the fight against respiratory ailments. This herb contains thymol, one of its primary active compounds, which possesses strong expectorant and antibacterial properties. Thymol helps in thinning and loosening phlegm in the respiratory tract, facilitating its expulsion and thereby clearing congestion. Additionally, thyme exhibits anti-inflammatory effects that can alleviate the swelling and irritation in the throat and bronchial tubes, providing relief from coughing and soreness.

To harness the benefits of thyme for respiratory health, one can prepare a simple yet effective thyme tea. Begin by boiling water, about one cup (approximately 240 milliliters), and then add one to two teaspoons (approximately 5 to 10 grams) of dried thyme leaves. Allow the leaves to steep in the boiling water for about 10 to 15 minutes, ensuring that the volatile oils and active compounds are adequately extracted. Strain the leaves from the infusion and, if desired, sweeten the tea with honey, which adds its own antimicrobial and soothing properties to the concoction.

For those dealing with acute respiratory conditions, inhaling the steam from thyme-infused water can be particularly beneficial. Add a handful of dried thyme or several drops of thyme essential oil to a bowl of hot water. Lean over the bowl, covering the head and bowl with a towel to trap the steam, and inhale deeply for 5 to 10 minutes. This method helps in directly delivering thymol and other beneficial compounds to the respiratory system, enhancing the herb's decongestant and anti-inflammatory effects.

It's important to source high-quality, organic thyme, whether using dried leaves or essential oil, to ensure the potency and safety of the remedy. When using thyme essential oil, always dilute it with a carrier oil, such as coconut or olive oil, to prevent irritation when applied topically or used in steam inhalation. Typically, a safe dilution ratio is about three to five drops of essential oil per ounce (approximately 30 milliliters) of carrier oil.

While thyme is generally safe for most people, those who are pregnant, nursing, or have specific health conditions should consult with a healthcare provider before incorporating it into their health regimen. Additionally, it's crucial to pay attention to the body's reactions when using herbal remedies and discontinue use if any adverse effects occur.

Licorice Root for Respiratory Healing

Licorice root, scientifically known as Glycyrrhiza glabra, has been a cornerstone in herbal medicine for thousands of years, revered for its extensive healing properties, particularly in the realm of respiratory health. This powerful herb acts as a demulcent, meaning it forms a soothing film over mucous membranes, alleviating irritation and dryness in the throat and lungs. Additionally, its anti-inflammatory properties make it an effective remedy for reducing swelling and irritation in the respiratory tract, offering relief for conditions such as bronchitis, sore throats, and coughs.

To harness the respiratory healing benefits of licorice root, one can prepare a simple licorice root tea. Begin by obtaining high-quality, dried licorice root from a reputable source to ensure potency and safety. Measure approximately one teaspoon (roughly 5 grams) of the dried root and add it to a cup (about 240 milliliters) of boiling water. Cover and steep for 10 to 15 minutes, allowing the water to extract the root's medicinal properties. Strain the tea to remove the solid pieces of root, and consider adding a natural sweetener like honey, which can further soothe the throat and enhance the tea's flavor.

For those experiencing acute respiratory discomfort, creating a licorice root gargle can provide direct relief to the throat. Dissolve a small amount of licorice root powder in warm water and gargle with the solution for a few minutes, being careful not to swallow. This method delivers the herb's soothing and anti-inflammatory effects directly to the irritated throat area.

It's important to note that while licorice root is generally safe for most people, it should be used with caution. Licorice root can cause adverse effects, such as elevated blood pressure and lowered potassium levels, when consumed in large quantities or over extended periods. Individuals with hypertension, kidney disease, or those who are pregnant or breastfeeding should avoid licorice root or consult with a healthcare provider before use.

For topical application, particularly for chest congestion, a licorice root poultice can be made by mixing licorice root powder with enough warm water to form a paste. Spread this paste on a clean cloth and apply it to the chest area, covering it with plastic wrap and a warm towel to keep it in place. This method allows the anti-inflammatory properties of licorice root to penetrate the skin and help reduce chest congestion.

Incorporating licorice root into a holistic approach to respiratory health can significantly alleviate symptoms and improve overall well-being. Whether consumed as a tea, used as a gargle, or applied topically, licorice root offers a natural, effective remedy for a wide range of respiratory issues. Always ensure to source licorice root from reputable suppliers and adhere to recommended dosages to maximize its healing benefits while minimizing potential risks.

Eucalyptus and Peppermint Chest Rub

Beneficial effects

Eucalyptus and Peppermint Chest Rub offers a natural way to ease respiratory discomfort, clear nasal passages, and promote easier breathing. Eucalyptus oil is known for its ability to reduce symptoms of coughs, colds, and congestion due to its anti-inflammatory, antispasmodic, and decongestant properties. Peppermint oil complements eucalyptus by providing a cooling sensation that can relieve sore throats and act as a mild analgesic to reduce discomfort. Together, these essential oils create a synergistic blend that helps to open up the airways and facilitate better respiratory health.

Ingredients

- ¼ cup coconut oil
- ¼ cup shea butter
- 20 drops eucalyptus essential oil
- 15 drops peppermint essential oil
- Small jar or container for storage

Instructions

1. Begin by gently melting the coconut oil and shea butter together. Use a double boiler method for controlled, even heating. Fill a pot with a couple of inches of water and place a heat-safe bowl on top, ensuring the bottom of the bowl does not touch the water. Add the coconut oil and shea butter to the bowl, stirring occasionally until fully melted.

2. Once melted, remove the mixture from heat and allow it to cool slightly, for about 5 minutes, to prevent the essential oils from evaporating when added.

3. Add the eucalyptus and peppermint essential oils to the melted oil and butter mixture. Stir thoroughly to ensure the essential oils are well distributed throughout the mixture.

4. Carefully pour the mixture into your chosen container. Allow it to set and solidify. This can be expedited by placing the container in the refrigerator for about an hour.

5. To use, rub a small amount of the chest rub on your chest, throat, and back as needed to relieve congestion and ease breathing. Avoid applying too close to the face, especially near the eyes.

Variations

- For extra respiratory support, add 5 drops of thyme essential oil to the mixture. Thyme is known for its antibacterial properties and can help fight respiratory infections.
- For a softer rub, increase the amount of shea butter to ⅓ cup. This will make the rub more spreadable, especially in cooler temperatures.

Storage tips

Store the eucalyptus and peppermint chest rub in a cool, dry place. If stored in the refrigerator, it will have a firmer consistency but will melt upon contact with skin. The rub should last for up to 6 months when stored properly.

Tips for allergens

If you are allergic to coconut oil, you can substitute it with another carrier oil such as almond oil or olive oil. Always perform a patch test on a small area of skin before applying the rub more broadly, especially if you have sensitive skin or are prone to allergies.

Scientific references

- "Eucalyptus Essential Oil: A Review of the Literature on Current Research, Safety, and Use in Clinical Practice" in the Journal of Essential Oil Research highlights the antimicrobial and anti-inflammatory properties of eucalyptus oil.
- "Peppermint Oil: Clinical Uses in the Treatment of Gastrointestinal Diseases" published in the Journal of Gastrointestinal and Liver Diseases discusses the antispasmodic and analgesic effects of peppermint oil, supporting its use in relieving discomfort and aiding respiratory conditions.

CHAPTER 2: HERBS FOR RESPIRATORY HEALTH

Mullein for Chronic Bronchitis and Asthma

Mullein (**Verbascum thapsus**) is a valuable herb in the treatment of respiratory conditions such as chronic bronchitis and asthma due to its ability to strengthen lung tissue and reduce inflammation. This plant, characterized by its tall, dense spike of yellow flowers and soft, velvety leaves, has been used for centuries in herbal medicine for its therapeutic properties.

To utilize mullein for respiratory support, the leaves and flowers are the primary parts used, both of which contain mucilage, saponins, and flavonoids. These compounds contribute to mullein's expectorant, anti-inflammatory, and demulcent actions, making it an effective remedy for easing coughs, reducing inflammation in the airways, and promoting the expulsion of mucus.

Preparation of Mullein Tea:

1. **Materials Needed:**
   - Dried mullein leaves and/or flowers (1-2 teaspoons)
   - Boiling water (1 cup, approximately 240 milliliters)
   - Strainer or tea infuser

2. **Procedure:**
   - Place the dried mullein leaves and/or flowers into a tea infuser or directly into a cup.
   - Pour boiling water over the mullein and cover the cup to prevent the steam, which contains beneficial volatile compounds, from escaping.
   - Allow the tea to steep for 10 to 15 minutes. This duration ensures that the water becomes well-infused with the herb's active compounds.
   - Strain the tea to remove the plant material. Mullein leaves can be fine and hairy, and it's crucial to strain the tea properly to avoid ingesting these fine hairs, which can be irritating to the throat.

Mullein Tincture:

For those who prefer a more concentrated form or require a more portable option, a mullein tincture can be beneficial, especially during flare-ups of chronic bronchitis or asthma.

1. **Materials Needed:**
   - Dried mullein leaves and flowers
   - High-proof alcohol (e.g., vodka or brandy, at least 40% alcohol by volume)
   - Glass jar with a tight-fitting lid

2. **Procedure:**
   - Fill a glass jar about halfway with dried mullein leaves and flowers.
   - Pour the alcohol over the herbs until they are completely submerged. Leave about an inch of space at the top of the jar.
   - Seal the jar tightly and place it in a cool, dark place for 4 to 6 weeks, shaking it every few days to ensure the alcohol extracts the active constituents from the mullein.
   - After the maceration period, strain the tincture through a fine mesh strainer or cheesecloth into a clean, dark glass bottle. Label the bottle with the date and contents.

Dosage and Usage:

- For mullein tea, it is recommended to drink 1 to 2 cups daily, especially during periods of respiratory discomfort.

- The mullein tincture can be taken in doses of 1/4 to 1/2 teaspoon (1-2 milliliters) up to three times a day. Due to its potency, the tincture should be diluted in water or tea before consumption.

Safety Considerations:

While mullein is generally considered safe for most individuals, it is always prudent to start with small doses to monitor for any potential allergic reactions. Pregnant or breastfeeding women should consult with a healthcare provider before using mullein due to limited research on its use during these periods.

Incorporating mullein into a respiratory health regimen can offer supportive care for those dealing with chronic bronchitis and asthma, aiding in the reduction of inflammation and facilitating easier breathing.

Nettle for Seasonal Allergy Relief

Nettle, scientifically known as Urtica dioica, has been utilized for centuries in herbal medicine for its wide array of health benefits, including its ability to mitigate the symptoms of seasonal allergies. This plant's efficacy in combating hay fever stems from its natural antihistamine properties, which help to reduce the body's allergic response. Bioactive compounds found in nettle, such as flavonoids, carotenoids, and vitamin C, contribute to its anti-inflammatory and immune-boosting effects, making it an excellent remedy for those seeking natural relief from the sneezing, itching, and congestion associated with seasonal allergies.

To harness the benefits of nettle for allergy relief, it is commonly prepared as a tea or taken in capsule form. For tea preparation, one would typically use dried nettle leaves. To make nettle tea, add one to two tablespoons of dried nettle leaves to a cup of boiling water. It's important to cover the cup while the tea steeps to ensure that the volatile oils and other therapeutic compounds do not escape with the steam. After allowing the tea to steep for 10 to 15 minutes, strain the leaves and consume the beverage. Drinking nettle tea two to three times a day during allergy season can significantly alleviate symptoms.

For those preferring a more concentrated form, nettle capsules are available and provide a convenient alternative to tea. The recommended dosage for nettle capsules varies, but typically one to two capsules taken two to three times a day with water during meals is effective for reducing allergy symptoms. It's crucial to consult the product's label for specific dosage recommendations and to ensure that it does not exceed the manufacturer's suggested daily intake.

Another method to utilize nettle for seasonal allergies is through a nettle leaf tincture, which involves extracting the plant's medicinal properties using alcohol. To create a tincture, fill a jar with dried nettle leaves and cover them with a high-proof alcohol, such as vodka, ensuring that the leaves are completely submerged. Seal the jar and store it in a cool, dark place, shaking it daily for about four to six weeks. After this period, strain the liquid through a fine mesh strainer or cheesecloth into a clean, dark glass bottle. The resulting tincture can be taken in small doses, typically 1-2 milliliters, up to three times a day diluted in water.

When sourcing nettle, whether for tea, capsules, or tincture preparation, it's essential to choose high-quality, organically grown nettle to avoid potential contaminants and to ensure the highest potency of its active compounds. Fresh nettle can also be used when in season; however, one must handle it with gloves to avoid the plant's characteristic sting.

Despite its natural efficacy, individuals considering nettle for allergy relief should first consult with a healthcare provider, especially those who are pregnant, nursing, or taking prescription medications, to avoid potential interactions or contraindications. Starting with smaller doses and gradually increasing to gauge tolerance can also help minimize any adverse effects.

Plantain for Coughs and Lung Healing

Plantain (Plantago major) is a versatile herb known for its remarkable healing properties, especially beneficial for respiratory health. It acts as both an expectorant, helping to clear mucus from the lungs, and a demulcent, soothing irritated mucous membranes. This dual action makes plantain an invaluable remedy for coughs and lung tissue healing.

To harness plantain's benefits for coughs and lung health, you can prepare a simple tea or infusion. Begin by sourcing **high-quality dried plantain leaves** from reputable suppliers to ensure potency. For making plantain tea, you will need:

- 1-2 teaspoons of dried plantain leaves
- 1 cup (about 240 ml) of boiling water
- A strainer or tea infuser
- Honey or lemon to taste (optional)

Steps for Preparing Plantain Tea:

1. Place the dried plantain leaves in a tea infuser or directly in a cup.
2. Pour boiling water over the leaves, ensuring they are fully submerged.
3. Cover the cup with a lid or a small plate to retain heat and allow the leaves to steep for 10-15 minutes. This steeping time allows the therapeutic compounds in the plantain leaves to infuse into the water.
4. After steeping, remove the tea infuser or strain the tea to remove the leaves.
5. Optionally, add honey or lemon to taste. Honey provides additional soothing properties, while lemon can enhance the tea's flavor and offer vitamin C.

Consuming Plantain Tea:

For coughs and respiratory discomfort, drink the plantain tea 2-3 times daily. The tea works by moistening the respiratory tract and facilitating the removal of mucus, while its soothing properties reduce irritation caused by coughing.

Additional Uses and Applications:

Beyond tea, plantain can be used in various forms, including tinctures and poultices, for external applications. A poultice of fresh plantain leaves can be applied to the chest to help ease congestion and soothe the skin.

Precautions:

While plantain is generally safe for most people, it's essential to start with small doses to gauge individual sensitivity. Those with known allergies to plantain or related plants should avoid its use. Additionally, consult with a healthcare provider before using plantain, especially for individuals on medication, pregnant or breastfeeding women, and children.

CHAPTER 3: IMMUNE-BOOSTING RESPIRATORY SUPPORT

Elderberry for Colds and Flu

Elderberry, scientifically known as Sambucus nigra, is a plant that has been used for centuries to combat colds and flu due to its potent antiviral properties. The active components in elderberry include flavonoids and anthocyanins, which are powerful antioxidants that help to strengthen the immune system and reduce inflammation. These components have been shown to inhibit the replication of viruses, making elderberry an effective remedy for respiratory illnesses. To harness the benefits of elderberry for fighting colds and flu, one can prepare elderberry syrup or tea at home with detailed precision.

For elderberry syrup, you will need dried elderberries, water, raw honey, and optional ingredients such as ginger root, cinnamon sticks, and cloves for additional flavor and health benefits. Begin by measuring out one cup of dried elderberries and placing them in a medium saucepan. Add four cups of water to the saucepan, along with one inch of ginger root sliced, two cinnamon sticks, and five cloves if using. Bring the mixture to a boil, then reduce the heat and allow it to simmer for about 45 minutes to an hour, or until the liquid has reduced by half. This slow simmering process allows for the extraction of the elderberries' medicinal properties.

After the mixture has reduced, remove it from the heat and let it cool until it is safe to handle. Mash the elderberries gently using a spoon or a potato masher to release any remaining juice. Strain the mixture through a fine mesh strainer or cheesecloth into a large bowl, pressing on the solids to extract as much liquid as possible. Discard the solids and allow the liquid to cool to lukewarm. Once cooled, add raw honey to the elderberry liquid, using one cup of honey for every cup of liquid. Stir the honey into the liquid until it is fully dissolved. The honey not only adds sweetness but also contributes additional antimicrobial and soothing properties to the syrup.

For elderberry tea, the process is simpler. You will need dried elderberries, boiling water, and optional additions such as lemon juice or a cinnamon stick for flavor. Measure out one tablespoon of dried elderberries per cup of boiling water. If desired, add a slice of lemon or a cinnamon stick to the cup. Pour the boiling water over the elderberries and optional ingredients, then cover and allow the mixture to steep for at least 15 to 20 minutes. This steeping time ensures the extraction of the elderberries' antiviral components. Strain the tea to remove the elderberries and any added ingredients. The tea can be sweetened with honey if desired, but it is recommended to add the honey after the tea has cooled slightly to preserve its beneficial enzymes.

Both elderberry syrup and tea can be consumed daily during the cold and flu season to support the immune system and prevent respiratory illnesses. It is recommended to start taking elderberry at the first sign of illness to maximize its antiviral effects. However, it's important to note that while elderberry is generally safe for most people, it should not be consumed by pregnant or breastfeeding women without consulting a healthcare provider.

Additionally, those with autoimmune diseases should exercise caution, as the immune-stimulating properties of elderberry may exacerbate their condition. Always source high-quality, organic dried elderberries from reputable suppliers to ensure the safety and efficacy of your homemade remedies.

Garlic as a Natural Antimicrobial

Garlic, scientifically known as **Allium sativum**, has been revered for centuries not only as a staple in global cuisines but also for its potent antimicrobial properties. Its ability to fight a wide range of infections and bolster the immune system makes it an invaluable component of any immune-boosting regimen, particularly for respiratory health.

The active compound in garlic responsible for its antimicrobial effects is **allicin**. When garlic cloves are crushed, chopped, or chewed, this compound is formed, releasing garlic's characteristic pungent aroma and offering powerful antimicrobial activity against bacteria, viruses, fungi, and parasites. Allicin is thought to disrupt the metabolic functions of pathogens, effectively inhibiting their growth and proliferation.

To harness garlic's benefits for respiratory support and immune defense, consider the following detailed methods of preparation and use:

1. **Raw Garlic Consumption**:
   - Begin by selecting fresh, organic garlic bulbs with firm cloves. Avoid bulbs that are soft, shriveled, or sprouting.
   - Peel one clove of garlic and finely mince, chop, or crush it to activate the allicin. Let it sit for 5-10 minutes to maximize the allicin formation.
   - Consume the raw garlic by itself or mix it with a teaspoon of honey to ease the strong taste. Honey also adds its own antimicrobial and soothing properties, making this combination particularly beneficial for coughs and sore throats.

2. **Garlic Infusion for Tea**:
   - Peel and crush 2-3 garlic cloves and add them to a pot containing 1 quart (about 950 ml) of boiling water.
   - Lower the heat and let the garlic simmer for 5 minutes to infuse the water.
   - Strain the garlic from the water and pour the warm garlic-infused tea into a mug. If desired, enhance the flavor and therapeutic benefits with a teaspoon of honey and a squeeze of lemon juice, which provides vitamin C.

3. **Garlic Oil**:
   - Peel and gently crush 5-6 garlic cloves.
   - Combine the crushed garlic with 1 cup (about 240 ml) of olive oil in a small saucepan and heat gently over low heat for 2-3 minutes. Do not allow the oil to simmer or the garlic to brown, as this can reduce the effectiveness of the allicin.
   - Remove from heat and let the mixture cool. Strain the garlic pieces from the oil.
   - Store the garlic-infused oil in a sealed glass container in the refrigerator. Use it to massage the chest and back to help relieve congestion. This method combines the antimicrobial properties of garlic with the soothing warmth of the oil.

Precautions:

While garlic is generally safe for most individuals, consuming it in large quantities may lead to digestive discomfort or irritation. Those on blood-thinning medications should consult with a healthcare provider due to garlic's natural blood-thinning properties. Additionally, the application of garlic oil should be patch tested on a small skin area first to ensure there is no sensitivity or allergic reaction.

Incorporating garlic into your daily diet or as part of a targeted approach to boost respiratory health can be a simple yet effective strategy. Whether consumed raw, as part of a soothing tea, or used externally in oil form, garlic's natural antimicrobial and immune-enhancing properties make it a powerful ally in maintaining respiratory health and overall wellness.

Oregano Oil for Stubborn Infections

Oregano oil, derived from the leaves and flowers of the oregano plant, Origanum vulgare, contains powerful compounds like carvacrol and thymol that are known for their antibacterial and antifungal properties. These compounds work synergistically to combat stubborn infections, particularly those affecting the respiratory system. The effectiveness of oregano oil in fighting off pathogens makes it a valuable addition to any immune-boosting regimen, especially for those seeking natural remedies for respiratory health.

To utilize oregano oil for respiratory support, it's essential to source a high-quality, therapeutic-grade oil that guarantees the presence of active constituents in significant amounts. When selecting oregano oil, look for products that specify the percentage of carvacrol, as this is a key indicator of the oil's potency and effectiveness. A concentration of 70% or higher is ideal for medicinal purposes.

For respiratory infections, oregano oil can be used in several ways. One method is to add a few drops of the oil to a diffuser or vaporizer. This method allows the therapeutic compounds to be inhaled directly into the respiratory system, providing relief from congestion, inflammation, and infection. When setting up your diffuser, ensure it's placed in a well-ventilated area and limit the diffusion time to 30 minutes to prevent irritation of mucous membranes.

Another effective application is creating a steam inhalation blend. Add 2-3 drops of oregano oil to a bowl of boiling water, cover your head with a towel, and inhale the steam for 5-10 minutes. This method helps to open up the airways, loosen mucus, and deliver the antimicrobial properties of oregano oil directly to the lungs and sinuses. It's crucial to close your eyes during steam inhalation to avoid irritation from the potent vapors.

For those who prefer a more direct approach, oregano oil can also be taken internally. However, due to its potent nature, it must be diluted before ingestion. Mix 1-2 drops of oregano oil with a teaspoon of a carrier oil, such as olive or coconut oil, and place it under the tongue for a few minutes before swallowing. This method allows the oil to enter the bloodstream quickly, providing systemic support against infections. Alternatively, the diluted oregano oil can be added to a capsule to avoid the strong taste. It's important to start with a low dose to assess tolerance and gradually increase as needed, not exceeding 4 drops per day.

When using oregano oil, especially for the first time, it's essential to monitor for any signs of an allergic reaction or irritation, such as rash, itching, or digestive discomfort. Pregnant or breastfeeding women and individuals with certain health conditions should consult a healthcare provider before using oregano oil due to its potent effects.

Incorporating oregano oil into your respiratory health regimen offers a natural and effective way to enhance immune function and combat stubborn infections. Its broad-spectrum antimicrobial properties make it a versatile remedy for various respiratory conditions, from common colds to more persistent bacterial and fungal infections. By following proper dilution guidelines and usage methods, you can safely harness the benefits of oregano oil for respiratory support and overall wellness.

Elderberry and Echinacea Immune Support Syrup

Beneficial effects

Elderberry and Echinacea Immune Support Syrup combines the immune-boosting power of elderberries with the infection-fighting properties of echinacea. Elderberries are rich in antioxidants and vitamins that can help combat colds and flu, while echinacea is known for its ability to enhance the immune system and reduce inflammation. This syrup is an effective, natural remedy for supporting respiratory health and bolstering the body's defenses against common pathogens.

Portions

Approximately 16 ounces

Preparation time

10 minutes

Cooking time

1 hour

Ingredients

- 3/4 cup dried elderberries
- 1/2 cup dried echinacea purpurea (flowers and leaves)
- 4 cups water
- 1 cup raw honey
- 2 tablespoons fresh ginger, grated
- 1 cinnamon stick
- 1 teaspoon whole cloves

Instructions

1. Combine the dried elderberries, dried echinacea, grated ginger, cinnamon stick, and whole cloves in a medium saucepan. Pour the 4 cups of water over the herbs and spices.

2. Bring the mixture to a boil over high heat. Once boiling, reduce the heat to low, allowing the mixture to simmer. Cover the saucepan with a lid, leaving it slightly ajar to let steam escape.

3. Let the mixture simmer for about 45 minutes to 1 hour, or until the liquid has reduced by almost half. This slow simmering process helps to extract the medicinal properties from the elderberries and echinacea.

4. After the mixture has reduced, remove the saucepan from the heat. Carefully strain the liquid through a fine mesh strainer or cheesecloth into a large bowl, pressing on the solids to extract as much liquid as possible. Discard the solids.

5. Allow the liquid to cool to lukewarm. Once it's cool enough, add the raw honey to the elderberry and echinacea liquid. Stir well until the honey is completely dissolved. The honey not only sweetens the syrup but also adds its own antibacterial properties.

6. Pour the finished syrup into a clean, airtight glass bottle or jar. Seal the container and label it with the date.

Variations

- For added immune support, include a tablespoon of dried rosehips in the simmering process for a boost of vitamin C.
- If you prefer a thicker syrup, reduce the liquid further to your desired consistency before adding the honey.

Storage tips

Store the Elderberry and Echinacea Immune Support Syrup in the refrigerator. It will keep for up to 2-3 months when stored properly. For longer storage, consider freezing the syrup in an ice cube tray and then transferring the frozen cubes to a freezer bag for easy single servings.

Tips for allergens

For those with honey allergies or vegan preferences, substitute the honey with maple syrup or agave nectar. Adjust the sweetness to taste, as these alternatives may be sweeter or less sweet than honey.

Scientific references

- "The effect of Sambucus nigra L. (black elderberry) on the immune system: a systematic review" published in the journal Phytotherapy Research discusses the immune-modulating effects of elderberry.
- "Echinacea purpurea: Pharmacology, phytochemistry and analysis methods" found in Pharmacognosy Reviews highlights echinacea's role in immune system support and its anti-inflammatory properties.

BOOK 9: EMOTIONAL HEALING WITH HERBS

CHAPTER 1: ADAPTOGENS FOR STRESS RELIEF

Ashwagandha for Cortisol Balance

Ashwagandha, scientifically known as **Withania somnifera**, is a powerful adaptogen that has been used for centuries in Ayurvedic medicine to help the body manage stress. It's renowned for its ability to **balance cortisol levels**, which are often referred to as the body's stress hormone. Elevated cortisol levels over prolonged periods can lead to a myriad of health issues, including chronic fatigue, impaired cognitive function, and weakened immune response.

To harness the benefits of Ashwagandha for cortisol balance, it's crucial to understand the optimal dosage and method of consumption. The recommended dosage typically ranges from **300 to 500 mg** of a root extract, standardized to contain **1.5 to 5% withanolides**, which are the active compounds believed to contribute to Ashwagandha's stress-reducing effects. It is advisable to start with a lower dose to assess tolerance and gradually increase as needed.

For daily consumption, Ashwagandha root extract can be taken in capsule or powder form. The powder can be mixed into a beverage, such as a smoothie or warm milk, before bedtime to promote relaxation and sleep quality. When selecting Ashwagandha supplements, look for products that have been **third-party tested** for purity and potency to ensure you are receiving a high-quality product.

Incorporating Ashwagandha into your daily routine requires consistency for the best results. It may take several weeks to notice a significant reduction in stress levels and improvement in overall well-being. It's also important to consider lifestyle factors that contribute to elevated cortisol levels, such as sleep quality, diet, and exercise, and to use Ashwagandha as part of a comprehensive approach to stress management.

For individuals with certain health conditions, such as autoimmune diseases, thyroid disorders, or those who are pregnant or breastfeeding, consulting a healthcare professional before starting Ashwagandha is recommended to avoid potential adverse effects.

In summary, Ashwagandha offers a natural and effective way to help balance cortisol levels and manage stress. By understanding the proper dosage, method of consumption, and ensuring the selection of a high-quality supplement, individuals can safely incorporate this ancient herb into their wellness routine to support their body's ability to cope with stress.

Holy Basil for Emotional Balance

Holy Basil, scientifically known as Ocimum sanctum or Tulsi, has been revered for centuries in traditional Ayurvedic medicine for its profound healing properties, particularly in the realm of emotional balance and stress relief. This herb is not only a cornerstone in holistic wellness practices but also a subject of interest in contemporary research for its adaptogenic qualities, which are substances that help the body adapt to stress and exert a normalizing effect upon bodily processes.

To fully harness the benefits of Holy Basil for emotional balance, it's essential to understand its active compounds, optimal consumption methods, and practical applications. The plant contains a rich profile of bioactive compounds including eugenol, ursolic acid, and rosmarinic acid, which contribute to its anti-stress, anxiolytic (anxiety-reducing), and antidepressant properties. These compounds work synergistically to enhance the body's natural response to physical and emotional stress, promoting mental clarity and calmness.

For daily consumption, Holy Basil can be prepared in several forms, the most popular being herbal tea. To prepare Holy Basil tea, use fresh or dried leaves — approximately one teaspoon of dried leaves or three to five fresh leaves per cup of boiling water. Steep the leaves for about 5 to 6 minutes to allow the water to extract the herb's essential oils and active compounds. This tea can be consumed two to three times a day to support mood regulation and stress relief. For those who prefer not to drink tea, Holy Basil is also available in capsule and tincture forms, providing a convenient alternative for daily intake. When selecting supplements, look for products that specify the concentration of active compounds to ensure potency.

Incorporating Holy Basil into your daily routine involves more than just consuming the herb; it's about creating a holistic approach to stress management. This includes integrating other stress-reduction techniques such as mindfulness meditation, regular physical activity, and a balanced diet, alongside Holy Basil consumption. By doing so, individuals can enhance the herb's efficacy in promoting emotional balance and overall well-being.

When cultivating Holy Basil at home, choose a location that receives full sunlight for at least six hours per day. The plant thrives in well-drained soil with a neutral to slightly acidic pH. Regular watering, especially during dry periods, will ensure the plant's health and potency. Harvesting the leaves just before the plant flowers will yield the highest concentration of essential oils.

For those new to Holy Basil, it's advisable to start with a lower dosage and gradually increase it to assess individual tolerance. While Holy Basil is generally considered safe for most people, pregnant or nursing women and individuals on medication should consult a healthcare professional before adding it to their regimen. This precaution ensures that Holy Basil does not interact adversely with existing conditions or medications.

By understanding the nuances of Holy Basil's adaptogenic properties and incorporating it mindfully into daily life, individuals can effectively leverage this ancient herb's potential to foster emotional equilibrium, reduce stress, and enhance mood regulation.

Rhodiola Rosea for Stress and Focus

Rhodiola Rosea, often hailed as the golden root, is a remarkable adaptogen known for its potent ability to enhance stress resilience and mental clarity. This herb thrives in the cold, mountainous regions of Europe and Asia, where it has been traditionally used for centuries to combat fatigue and improve cognitive function during challenging times. The efficacy of Rhodiola Rosea in bolstering mental performance and endurance under stress is attributed to its active compounds, namely salidroside and rosavin. These compounds play a pivotal role in regulating the body's stress response system, thereby reducing the impact of stress hormones like cortisol on the body.

To leverage Rhodiola Rosea for stress resilience and mental clarity, it's crucial to understand the optimal dosage and method of consumption. Studies suggest that a daily intake of 200 to 600 mg of Rhodiola Rosea extract, standardized to contain 1% salidroside and 3% rosavin, is effective for enhancing cognitive function and reducing mental fatigue. It is recommended to start with a lower dose to assess individual tolerance and gradually increase as needed. For maximum absorption and efficacy, Rhodiola Rosea should be taken on an empty stomach approximately 30 minutes before breakfast and lunch. Avoiding intake in the evening is advisable to prevent potential interference with sleep patterns.

Incorporating Rhodiola Rosea into one's daily regimen involves consistent use over a period of at least four to six weeks to observe significant improvements in stress management, mental clarity, and energy levels. It is also important to select high-quality Rhodiola Rosea supplements that have been third-party tested for purity and potency. Look for products that explicitly list the percentage of active compounds, ensuring you receive a product capable of delivering therapeutic benefits.

Beyond supplementation, embracing a holistic approach to stress management can amplify the benefits of Rhodiola Rosea. This includes maintaining a balanced diet rich in antioxidants and omega-3 fatty acids, engaging in regular physical activity, and practicing mindfulness or meditation to enhance emotional resilience. Together, these practices, coupled with Rhodiola Rosea supplementation, form a comprehensive strategy for combating stress and fostering a state of mental clarity and well-being.

For individuals seeking natural remedies to support mental performance and adaptability in the face of stress, Rhodiola Rosea stands out as a scientifically backed option. Its adaptogenic properties not only aid in reducing fatigue but also in enhancing cognitive functions, making it a valuable ally for anyone looking to thrive in today's fast-paced and often stressful environment.

Ashwagandha and Holy Basil Stress Relief Tea

Beneficial effects

Ashwagandha and Holy Basil Stress Relief Tea harnesses the adaptogenic powers of Ashwagandha and the stress-relieving properties of Holy Basil (Tulsi) to create a soothing, calming beverage ideal for reducing stress and anxiety. Ashwagandha is known for its ability to balance cortisol levels, thus reducing the physical and psychological effects of stress, while Holy Basil has been used for centuries in Ayurvedic medicine to promote emotional well-being and resilience against stress. Together, they form a potent herbal remedy that can help enhance mood, improve sleep quality, and support overall mental health.

Portions

Makes about 4 cups

Preparation time

5 minutes

Cooking time

15 minutes

Ingredients

- 1 tablespoon dried Ashwagandha root
- 1 tablespoon dried Holy Basil (Tulsi) leaves
- 4 cups water
- Honey or maple syrup to taste (optional)
- Lemon slices for garnish (optional)

Instructions

1. Begin by bringing 4 cups of water to a boil in a medium-sized saucepan.

2. Once the water is boiling, reduce the heat to low and add 1 tablespoon of dried Ashwagandha root to the saucepan.

3. Simmer the Ashwagandha root on low heat for 10 minutes to allow for a thorough infusion. This slow simmer helps to extract the root's adaptogenic properties effectively.

4. After 10 minutes, add 1 tablespoon of dried Holy Basil leaves to the saucepan. Cover and simmer for an additional 5 minutes. The Holy Basil leaves require less time to infuse, preserving their essential oils and flavor.

5. Remove the saucepan from the heat and let it sit for 2 minutes, allowing the flavors to meld together.

6. Strain the tea through a fine mesh strainer into a teapot or directly into cups, ensuring to press on the herbs to extract their full benefits. Discard the used Ashwagandha root and Holy Basil leaves.

7. If desired, sweeten the tea with honey or maple syrup according to taste. Stir well to ensure the sweetener is fully dissolved.

8. Serve the tea warm, garnished with a slice of lemon in each cup if using. The lemon not only adds a refreshing flavor but also provides a vitamin C boost.

Variations

- For a spicier kick, add a small piece of fresh ginger to the saucepan along with the Ashwagandha root.
- Incorporate a cinnamon stick during the simmering process for a warming, aromatic flavor.
- For a caffeine boost, add a bag of green tea to the saucepan during the last 3 minutes of simmering.

Storage tips

Store any leftover tea in a glass container in the refrigerator for up to 2 days. Gently reheat on the stove or enjoy cold for a refreshing, stress-relieving beverage.

Tips for allergens

For those with honey allergies or following a vegan diet, maple syrup serves as a delicious plant-based sweetener alternative that complements the earthy flavors of the tea.

Scientific references

- "An Overview on Ashwagandha: A Rasayana (Rejuvenator) of Ayurveda" published in the African Journal of Traditional, Complementary, and Alternative Medicines discusses Ashwagandha's adaptogenic and stress-reduction properties.
- "Tulsi - Ocimum sanctum: A herb for all reasons" in the Journal of Ayurveda and Integrative Medicine highlights Holy Basil's efficacy in mitigating stress and promoting mental clarity.

CHAPTER 2: NERVINES FOR CALMNESS

Chamomile for Restful Sleep and Anxiety

Chamomile, scientifically known as Matricaria chamomilla or Chamomilla recutita, is a herb renowned for its gentle sedative properties, making it an excellent choice for those seeking natural remedies to enhance sleep quality and alleviate mild anxiety. The active compounds in chamomile, including bisabolol, apigenin, and matricin, contribute to its calming effects by interacting with the body's central nervous system in a way that promotes relaxation and drowsiness. To effectively utilize chamomile for restful sleep and mild anxiety relief, it's essential to understand the preparation methods, optimal consumption times, and additional supportive practices that can amplify its benefits.

Preparing chamomile tea involves steeping dried chamomile flowers in hot water to extract the plant's essential oils and active compounds. For a potent brew, use about 2 to 3 teaspoons of dried chamomile flowers per cup of boiling water. Place the chamomile in a tea infuser or directly in the cup, then pour boiling water over the flowers and cover the cup with a saucer to trap the steam, enhancing the infusion process. Allow the tea to steep for 5 to 10 minutes, depending on your taste preference and the desired strength. The longer the steeping time, the more potent the calming effects may be. After steeping, remove the chamomile flowers or infuser and, if desired, add a natural sweetener like honey to taste. Honey not only improves the flavor but also offers additional soothing properties that can enhance the tea's overall calming effect.

For those dealing with mild anxiety or seeking to improve sleep quality, consuming chamomile tea approximately 30 minutes to an hour before bedtime can help ease the transition into a restful state, making it easier to fall asleep. This timing allows the body to begin metabolizing the active compounds in chamomile, setting the stage for relaxation and drowsiness by the time you're ready to sleep.

Incorporating chamomile tea into a nightly routine can signal to your body that it's time to wind down, creating a psychological association between the tea and sleep. To further enhance the calming effects of chamomile tea, consider adopting additional relaxation practices in the evening, such as dimming the lights, reading a book, or practicing gentle yoga or meditation. These activities can help reduce stress and prepare the mind and body for sleep, working synergistically with chamomile tea to promote a deeper and more restorative night's rest.

While chamomile tea is generally safe for most people, it's important to be aware of potential allergies, especially for those who are allergic to plants in the daisy family, as chamomile is a member of this family. Additionally, pregnant or nursing women and individuals taking sedative medications should consult with a healthcare professional before incorporating chamomile tea into their routine to ensure safety and avoid any potential interactions.

Valerian Root for Deep Relaxation

Valerian root, scientifically known as Valeriana officinalis, has been revered for centuries for its sedative qualities and ability to promote relaxation and improve sleep. This powerful herb works by increasing the levels of gamma-aminobutyric acid (GABA) in the brain, a neurotransmitter responsible for regulating nerve impulses, which in turn helps to calm the nervous system. The root of the valerian plant contains a number of compounds that contribute to its effectiveness, including valerenic acid, isovaleric acid, and a variety of antioxidants.

For individuals seeking to incorporate valerian root into their nightly routine to combat insomnia or an overactive mind, it is crucial to understand the optimal form and dosage for consumption.

Valerian root can be consumed in several forms, including capsules, tinctures, and teas. Each form has its own advantages, and the choice largely depends on personal preference and the desired speed of onset.

Capsules are a convenient and straightforward method of consumption, offering a precise dosage and minimal taste. The recommended dosage for adults is between 400 to 900 milligrams, taken approximately one hour before bedtime. It is important to start with the lower end of the dosage range and gradually increase if necessary, to assess individual tolerance.

Tinctures, another popular form, allow for more immediate absorption and can be particularly effective for those who have difficulty swallowing capsules. When using a valerian root tincture, it is advisable to start with 1 to 2 teaspoons, diluted in water or juice, taken 30 minutes to an hour before bedtime.

Valerian tea offers a soothing and ritualistic approach to relaxation, ideal for those who appreciate the process of brewing and sipping tea as a way to unwind. To prepare valerian root tea, steep 2 to 3 grams of dried valerian root in hot water for 10 to 15 minutes. The longer steeping time allows for a stronger extraction of the root's active ingredients. Adding honey or lemon can enhance the flavor, making the herbal remedy more palatable.

While valerian root is generally considered safe for most adults, it is essential to be mindful of potential side effects, such as dizziness, drowsiness, or stomach upset. These effects are typically mild and decrease with continued use. However, valerian root should not be used in conjunction with alcohol, other sleep-inducing medications, or by individuals with liver disease without consulting a healthcare provider.

To ensure the effectiveness of valerian root for promoting deep relaxation and improving sleep, it is also recommended to maintain good sleep hygiene practices. This includes establishing a consistent bedtime routine, limiting exposure to screens and blue light before sleep, and creating a comfortable, dark, and quiet sleeping environment.

Passionflower for Anxiety Relief

Passionflower, scientifically known as **Passiflora incarnata**, is a perennial climbing vine renowned for its beautiful flowers and medicinal properties, particularly in alleviating anxiety and nervous tension. The key components of passionflower that contribute to its calming effects include flavonoids, alkaloids, and gamma-aminobutyric acid (GABA), which work synergistically to enhance GABA levels in the brain, thus promoting relaxation without inducing sedation. This makes passionflower an excellent choice for individuals seeking a natural remedy to soothe their anxious minds while maintaining alertness and cognitive function.

To harness the benefits of passionflower for anxiety and nervous tension, it can be prepared in several forms, such as teas, tinctures, capsules, or extracts. For making a **passionflower tea**, which is a gentle way to experience its calming effects, follow these steps:

1. **Tea Preparation**: Use one teaspoon of dried passionflower herb per cup of boiling water. Steep the herb in hot water for 10 to 15 minutes. This long steeping time allows the water to extract a broad range of phytochemicals from the dried plant material.

2. **Dosage**: For managing anxiety, drink one cup of passionflower tea 2 to 3 times daily. It's especially beneficial when consumed in the evening to ease nervous tension and facilitate a restful night's sleep.

3. **Tincture Use**: If opting for a passionflower tincture, a typical dosage is 1 to 2 ml, three times a day. Tinctures offer a more concentrated form of passionflower and can be a convenient option for those with a busy lifestyle.

4. **Capsules and Extracts**: When using capsules or standardized extracts, follow the manufacturer's recommended dosage, usually around 400 to 800 mg per day, divided into two or three doses.

It's crucial to source **high-quality passionflower** products from reputable suppliers to ensure the efficacy of the remedy. Look for organic certification to avoid contaminants that could detract from the herb's therapeutic value.

While passionflower is generally considered safe for most adults, it's important to consult with a healthcare provider before incorporating it into your routine, especially for pregnant or nursing women, children, and those on medication. Interactions with sedatives, blood thinners, and other medications affecting the central nervous system could occur.

Incorporating passionflower into a holistic approach to anxiety management can also include lifestyle modifications such as regular exercise, a balanced diet, adequate sleep, and stress reduction techniques like meditation and deep breathing exercises. Together, these strategies can help create a comprehensive plan for reducing anxiety and enhancing overall well-being.

Lavender and Valerian Root Relaxation Tea

Beneficial effects

Lavender and Valerian Root Relaxation Tea is a natural remedy designed to alleviate stress, promote relaxation, and enhance sleep quality. Lavender is renowned for its calming and soothing properties, helping to reduce anxiety and induce a peaceful state of mind. Valerian root complements lavender by acting as a powerful sedative that enhances GABA (gamma-aminobutyric acid) in the brain, which helps to regulate nerve impulses and quiet the nervous system. This combination makes the tea an ideal beverage for those seeking to unwind after a stressful day or prepare for a restful night's sleep.

Portions

Makes about 2 cups

Preparation time

5 minutes

Cooking time

10 minutes

Ingredients

- 1 tablespoon dried lavender flowers
- 1 tablespoon dried valerian root
- 2 cups boiling water
- Honey or stevia to taste (optional)

Instructions

1. Boil 2 cups of water in a kettle or saucepan. While waiting for the water to boil, gather the dried lavender flowers and dried valerian root.

2. Place the dried lavender and valerian root into a tea infuser or directly into a teapot. If you're using a teapot, ensure it's one that can accommodate the infusion and easy straining of the herbs.

3. Once the water has reached a rolling boil, carefully pour it over the lavender and valerian root in the teapot or into the cup containing the tea infuser.

4. Cover the teapot or cup with a lid or a small plate to trap the steam and allow the herbs to steep. Let them infuse for 10 minutes. This steeping time allows the hot water to extract the active compounds from the herbs, creating a potent herbal tea.

5. After 10 minutes, remove the tea infuser from the cup, or if using a teapot, strain the tea into a cup. Press on the herbs lightly to extract as much liquid and beneficial properties as possible.

6. Taste the tea and, if desired, add honey or stevia to sweeten it. Stir well to ensure the sweetener dissolves completely.

7. Enjoy the tea warm, taking slow sips to experience its calming effects fully.

Variations

- For a citrus note, add a slice of lemon or a few strips of lemon zest to the tea while it steeps.
- Combine with chamomile flowers for an even more relaxing blend. Use ½ tablespoon of chamomile flowers along with the lavender and valerian root.

Storage tips

If you have leftover tea, it can be stored in a sealed glass container in the refrigerator for up to 2 days. Reheat gently on the stove or enjoy chilled.

Tips for allergens

For those with allergies to honey, stevia serves as a great alternative sweetener that does not trigger common allergies.

Scientific references

- "Lavender and the Nervous System," published in Evidence-Based Complementary and Alternative Medicine, highlights lavender's anxiolytic (anxiety-reducing) effects and its potential for treating sleep disorders.
- "Valerian Root in Treating Sleep Problems and Associated Disorders—A Systematic Review and Meta-Analysis," in the Journal of Evidence-Based Integrative Medicine, discusses valerian root's role in improving sleep quality and its use as a sedative.

CHAPTER 3: UPLIFTING HERBS FOR EMOTIONAL WELLBEING

St. John's Wort for Depression

St. John's Wort (**Hypericum perforatum**) has been utilized for centuries as a natural remedy for various ailments, with its use as an antidepressant being one of the most valued. This herb contains active compounds such as hyperforin and hypericin that are thought to contribute to its therapeutic effects, particularly in the treatment of mild to moderate depression. The mechanism is believed to involve the inhibition of serotonin reuptake, similar to how conventional SSRIs (Selective Serotonin Reuptake Inhibitors) work, thereby increasing the availability of serotonin in the brain—a neurotransmitter associated with mood regulation.

For those considering St. John's Wort as a natural antidepressant, it is typically available in several forms, including capsules, tablets, tinctures, and teas. The standard dosage for treating mild to moderate depression is generally 300 mg of standardized extract (0.3% hypericin content), taken three times daily. It is crucial to use standardized extracts to ensure consistent dosing of the active ingredients.

Preparation of St. John's Wort Tea:

1. **Ingredients**: Use 1-2 teaspoons of dried St. John's Wort per cup of boiling water.

2. **Steeping**: Pour boiling water over the herb and steep for 10-15 minutes. This long steeping time allows for the maximal extraction of the beneficial compounds.

3. **Consumption**: It is recommended to drink one cup of tea three times a day for therapeutic effects.

St. John's Wort Tincture:

- **Preparation**: A tincture can be made by soaking the dried herb in alcohol (usually vodka or brandy) for several weeks, shaking the container periodically.

- **Dosage**: The typical dose of St. John's Wort tincture is 1-2 ml, taken three times daily.

When sourcing St. John's Wort, look for products that are certified organic to avoid exposure to pesticides and ensure the highest quality. Given the herb's potential to interact with a wide range of medications, including but not limited to antidepressants, birth control pills, and blood thinners, it is imperative to consult with a healthcare provider before starting treatment, especially if you are currently taking any medications.

It is also important to note that while St. John's Wort can be effective for mild to moderate depression, it may not be suitable for severe depression or bipolar disorder. Monitoring by a healthcare professional is advisable to assess its effectiveness and adjust treatment as necessary.

Despite its potential benefits, users should be aware of possible side effects, such as photosensitivity, which can lead to skin irritation when exposed to sunlight. Therefore, wearing protective clothing and applying sunscreen when outdoors is recommended while using St. John's Wort.

Lemon Balm for Mood and Clarity

Lemon balm, scientifically known as Melissa officinalis, is a perennial herb from the mint family and has been widely recognized for its mood-enhancing and cognitive benefits. This herb possesses a lemony scent and flavor, making it not only a delightful addition to various culinary dishes but also a powerful remedy in herbal medicine, particularly for improving emotional well-being and mental focus. The primary compounds in lemon balm, including rosmarinic acid, citronellal, and geraniol, contribute to its therapeutic properties by positively affecting the nervous system, thereby offering a dual action of calming anxiety and boosting cognitive functions.

To utilize lemon balm for its emotional lift and focus-enhancing properties, one can prepare it in several forms, such as teas, tinctures, capsules, or even as a fresh herb in culinary recipes. However, the preparation and use of lemon balm tea and tincture will be detailed here, as these are common methods to harness its benefits for mood and mental clarity.

Lemon Balm Tea Preparation:

1. **Ingredients**: For making lemon balm tea, use fresh or dried lemon balm leaves. If using fresh leaves, a handful (approximately ¼ cup) is sufficient for one cup of tea. For dried leaves, use about 2 teaspoons per cup of water.

2. **Steeping**: Boil water and pour it over the lemon balm leaves in a cup or teapot. Cover and steep for at least 5 to 10 minutes. The longer you steep, the more potent the tea will be. Covering the cup or teapot prevents the essential oils, which contain the therapeutic properties, from evaporating.

3. **Strain and Serve**: After steeping, strain the leaves from the tea and serve. If desired, honey or lemon can be added for flavor, but it's best enjoyed plain to fully appreciate its natural lemony essence.

Lemon Balm Tincture Preparation:

1. **Ingredients and Equipment**: To prepare a lemon balm tincture, you will need fresh lemon balm leaves, high-proof alcohol (such as vodka or brandy, at least 40% alcohol by volume), a clean glass jar, and a strainer or cheesecloth.

2. **Preparation**: Fill the glass jar about ¾ full with fresh lemon balm leaves, then pour the alcohol over the leaves until the jar is nearly full, ensuring all leaves are submerged to prevent mold growth. Seal the jar tightly.

3. **Storage**: Store the jar in a cool, dark place for about 4 to 6 weeks, shaking it every few days to help the extraction process.

4. **Straining**: After the steeping period, strain the liquid through a strainer or cheesecloth into another clean glass jar or bottle, squeezing the leaves to extract as much liquid as possible.

5. **Usage**: The standard dose for a lemon balm tincture is 1-2 milliliters (approximately 30-60 drops), taken 3 times daily or as needed. It can be added to water, tea, or taken directly under the tongue.

Lemon balm's efficacy in enhancing mood and mental clarity can be attributed to its ability to act as a mild sedative, reducing anxiety and promoting a sense of calm, while simultaneously improving attention and cognitive function. This makes it particularly useful for those experiencing stress, anxiety, or needing a mental focus boost without the side effects often associated with pharmaceuticals.

For individuals looking to incorporate lemon balm into their wellness routine, it's important to source high-quality, organic lemon balm leaves or products to ensure the best results. While lemon balm is generally considered safe for most people, it's advisable to consult with a healthcare provider before starting any new herbal remedy, especially for those who are pregnant, nursing, or on medication, as lemon balm may interact with certain medications.

Incorporating lemon balm into one's daily routine can be a simple yet effective way to enhance emotional well-being and cognitive performance. Whether enjoyed as a soothing tea in the evening or taken as a tincture for a midday mental clarity boost, lemon balm offers a natural, accessible solution for those seeking to improve their mood and focus through the gentle power of herbs.

Saffron for Mood Regulation

Saffron, scientifically known as **Crocus sativus**, is a highly valued spice derived from the dried stigmas of the saffron crocus flower. Beyond its culinary uses, saffron has been recognized for its potential in mood regulation and the alleviation of depressive symptoms. This section delves into the mechanisms through which saffron contributes to emotional stability and outlines practical guidelines for incorporating this potent herb into a natural wellness regimen.

The mood-enhancing effects of saffron can be attributed to its rich content of bioactive compounds, including **crocin**, **crocetin**, **safranal**, and **picrocrocin**. These compounds interact with the brain's neurotransmitter systems, particularly serotonin, which plays a key role in mood regulation. By modulating the levels of serotonin in the brain, saffron acts similarly to conventional antidepressants but with fewer side effects.

Dosage and Preparation: For mood regulation, the recommended dosage of saffron extract ranges from **30 to 50 mg daily**, divided into two doses. It's crucial to use a standardized extract to ensure consistent potency. Saffron can be consumed in capsule form or as a tea. To prepare saffron tea:

1. **Steep**: Use about 15-30 mg (a pinch) of saffron threads in one cup of boiling water.
2. **Time**: Allow the saffron to steep for up to 10 minutes. The water will turn a golden-yellow hue as the saffron infuses.
3. **Strain**: If desired, strain the tea to remove the threads, although leaving them in can enhance the tea's therapeutic benefits.
4. **Frequency**: Drink saffron tea once or twice daily, preferably in the morning and evening.

Quality Considerations: When purchasing saffron, opt for threads rather than powdered form to ensure purity and avoid adulteration. The threads should have a deep red color, which indicates a high concentration of active compounds. Store saffron in a cool, dark place to preserve its potency.

Safety and Interactions: While saffron is generally safe for most individuals, high doses may cause side effects such as dry mouth, dizziness, or nausea. Pregnant women should avoid high doses of saffron due to its potential uterine-stimulating effects. Always consult with a healthcare provider before adding saffron to your regimen, especially if you are taking medication for depression or other conditions, as interactions may occur.

Integrating Saffron into Daily Life: Beyond its use as a supplement, saffron can be incorporated into daily meals and snacks. Add saffron to rice dishes, soups, and teas for an emotional boost. Combining saffron with other mood-supportive herbs like **lavender** or **chamomile** can enhance its calming effects.

In summary, saffron offers a natural, effective option for mood regulation and the alleviation of depressive symptoms. By understanding the proper dosage, preparation methods, and quality considerations, individuals can safely incorporate saffron into their wellness routine to promote emotional stability and overall well-being.

Lemon Balm and St. John's Wort Mood Lifting Tea

Beneficial effects

Lemon Balm and St. John's Wort Mood Lifting Tea combines the soothing properties of Lemon Balm with the mood-stabilizing effects of St. John's Wort. Lemon Balm is known for its ability to ease stress, anxiety, and promote a sense of calm, while St. John's Wort is recognized for its potential to alleviate symptoms of depression and boost mood. This herbal blend creates a synergistic tea that can help lift spirits, improve emotional well-being, and enhance overall mental health.

Portions

Makes about 4 cups

Preparation time

10 minutes

Cooking time

15 minutes

Ingredients

- 2 tablespoons dried Lemon Balm leaves
- 2 tablespoons dried St. John's Wort flowers
- 4 cups water
- Honey or stevia to taste (optional)

Instructions

1. Bring 4 cups of water to a boil in a medium-sized saucepan.
2. Once the water is boiling, reduce the heat to low and add the dried Lemon Balm leaves and St. John's Wort flowers to the saucepan.
3. Cover the saucepan with a lid and simmer the mixture on low heat for 15 minutes. This gentle simmering process allows the water to extract the active compounds from the herbs effectively.
4. After 15 minutes, remove the saucepan from the heat and let it sit, still covered, for an additional 5 minutes to further infuse.
5. Strain the tea through a fine mesh strainer into a large pitcher or directly into cups, pressing on the herbs with a spoon to extract as much liquid as possible. Discard the used herbs.
6. If desired, sweeten the tea with honey or stevia according to taste. Stir well to ensure the sweetener is fully dissolved.
7. Serve the tea warm to enjoy its full therapeutic benefits.

Variations

- For a citrus twist, add a few slices of fresh lemon to the tea while it steeps.
- Incorporate a cinnamon stick during the simmering process for added warmth and complexity to the flavor profile.
- To enhance relaxation effects, add a tablespoon of dried chamomile flowers to the blend.

Storage tips

Store any leftover tea in a glass container in the refrigerator for up to 2 days. Reheat gently on the stove or enjoy chilled for a refreshing and uplifting beverage.

Tips for allergens

For those with allergies or sensitivities to honey, stevia provides a sweetening alternative that does not trigger common allergies. Ensure to use pure stevia extract to avoid any fillers that might contain allergens.

Scientific references

- "Melissa officinalis L. – A Review of its Traditional Uses, Phytochemistry and Pharmacology" in the Journal of Ethnopharmacology discusses the anxiolytic effects of Lemon Balm.
- "St. John's Wort and its Active Principles in Depression and Anxiety" in the journal Molecular Psychiatry highlights the mood-enhancing properties of St. John's Wort.

BOOK 10: HERBAL REMEDIES FOR ATHLETES

CHAPTER 1: PRE-WORKOUT HERBS FOR ENERGY

Ginseng for Sustained Energy

Ginseng, recognized for its remarkable ability to enhance physical stamina and mitigate fatigue, stands as a cornerstone herb in the realm of natural remedies aimed at athletes and individuals leading active lifestyles. This potent root, primarily sourced from the Panax genus, embodies a synergy of bioactive compounds, notably ginsenosides, which are credited with its energy-boosting properties. To harness ginseng's full potential for sustained energy, it's imperative to delve into the specifics of its selection, preparation, and optimal dosage.

Selecting high-quality ginseng is the first critical step toward ensuring the efficacy of this herb in energy enhancement. Look for roots that are at least four to six years old, as maturity significantly influences the concentration of ginsenosides. The root should appear firm, unblemished, and have a natural ivory to yellowish tint. Preference should be given to organically grown ginseng to avoid the intake of pesticides and herbicides, which can negate the root's health benefits.

Preparation of ginseng can be approached in several ways, with the method of decoction being the most traditional and widely recommended. To prepare a ginseng decoction, slice approximately 3 to 5 grams of the root thinly. These slices are then simmered in about 350 to 500 milliliters of water for 45 to 60 minutes, until the liquid is reduced by half. This process extracts the vital ginsenosides into the water, creating a potent tonic. For those leading a fast-paced lifestyle, ginseng can also be consumed in the form of powder, capsules, or tinctures, though it's essential to adhere to the manufacturer's recommended dosages to avoid possible side effects.

The optimal dosage of ginseng varies depending on the individual's body weight, health condition, and tolerance. However, a general guideline suggests starting with a lower dose of 200 to 400 milligrams of extract per day, gradually increasing as needed, without exceeding 2 grams per day to prevent overstimulation and potential insomnia. It's crucial to cycle the use of ginseng, typically following a regimen of taking it for 2 to 3 weeks followed by a 1 to 2-week break. This cycling helps maintain the herb's effectiveness and reduces the risk of developing tolerance.

While ginseng is generally considered safe for most individuals, it's advisable to consult with a healthcare professional before incorporating it into your regimen, especially for those with underlying health conditions or those taking prescription medications, as ginseng can interact with certain drugs. By adhering to these guidelines on selection, preparation, dosage, and timing, individuals can effectively leverage ginseng's natural prowess to sustain energy, improve stamina, and enhance overall athletic performance, all while steering clear of synthetic stimulants and their associated side effects.

Beetroot for Athletic Performance

Beetroot, scientifically known as Beta vulgaris, has garnered attention in the realm of sports nutrition for its potential to enhance athletic performance and endurance through increased oxygen efficiency. This root vegetable is rich in dietary nitrates, compounds that the body converts into nitric oxide, a molecule that plays a crucial role in regulating blood flow and oxygen delivery to muscles during physical exertion. The process begins when dietary nitrates from beetroot are ingested and subsequently absorbed into the bloodstream. Once absorbed, these nitrates are converted into nitrites by the action of bacteria found in the oral cavity. As the nitrites are further broken down during digestion, they form nitric oxide, which exerts vasodilatory effects—meaning it relaxes and widens blood vessels, improving blood flow.

This enhanced blood flow allows for a more efficient delivery of oxygen and nutrients to working muscles, which is vital for athletes and individuals engaged in high-intensity physical activities. By optimizing the oxygen-carrying capacity of the blood, beetroot consumption can help reduce the oxygen cost of exercise, meaning less oxygen is required to maintain a certain level of exercise intensity. This can translate into improved endurance, as athletes may find they can sustain higher levels of performance for longer periods.

For those looking to incorporate beetroot into their pre-workout regimen, it's essential to understand the most effective forms and timing of consumption to maximize its potential benefits. Fresh beetroot juice is often considered the most efficient way to consume dietary nitrates, as juicing increases the bioavailability of nitrates. Approximately 250 to 500 milliliters (about 8 to 16 ounces) of beetroot juice consumed 2 to 3 hours before exercise is suggested to allow sufficient time for nitrate conversion and nitric oxide formation. This timing window is critical as it aligns with the peak plasma nitrate levels, ensuring optimal nitric oxide availability during physical activity.

For those who prefer solid food or are looking for a more convenient option, beetroot powder is an alternative. When selecting beetroot powder, aim for a product that specifies a high nitrate content to ensure its efficacy. The recommended dose can vary based on the concentration of the powder, but generally, mixing 1 to 2 teaspoons of beetroot powder with water or a smoothie approximately 2 to 3 hours before exercise can provide similar benefits to fresh juice.

It's also worth noting that regular consumption of beetroot or beetroot supplements can have a cumulative effect on nitric oxide levels, potentially leading to long-term improvements in cardiovascular health, exercise performance, and endurance. However, individual responses to dietary nitrates can vary, and it's advisable to experiment with beetroot supplementation during training sessions before incorporating it into pre-competition routines.

While beetroot is generally safe for consumption, individuals with conditions that affect nitrate levels, such as those taking nitrate-based medications, should consult with a healthcare provider before adding high-nitrate foods like beetroot to their diet. Additionally, due to its potent color, consuming large amounts of beetroot can lead to temporary changes in urine or stool color, a harmless condition known as beeturia.

Cordyceps for Enhanced Physical Stamina

Cordyceps, a unique fungus known for its extraordinary health benefits, particularly shines in the realm of enhancing physical stamina and energy levels. This fungus, which naturally grows on the larvae of insects in the high mountain regions of China, has been harnessed in traditional Chinese medicine for centuries. Today, it is available in various forms, including powders, capsules, and tinctures, making it accessible for athletes and those seeking a natural boost in physical performance.

The primary mechanism through which cordyceps enhances physical stamina lies in its ability to improve oxygen utilization. Studies have shown that the active components in cordyceps, including adenosine and cordycepin, contribute to increased production of ATP (adenosine triphosphate), which is crucial for energy transfer within cells. This increase in ATP production helps to improve the way the body uses oxygen, especially during exercise. Essentially, cordyceps can help the body to utilize oxygen more efficiently, thereby delaying the onset of fatigue and allowing for improved endurance and performance.

For those looking to incorporate cordyceps into their pre-workout regimen, it is recommended to start with a **dose of 3 to 6 grams** of the dried mushroom or 300 to 500 milligrams of an extract. This should be taken approximately 30 to 60 minutes before physical activity to allow the body to metabolize the active compounds effectively. It's important to source high-quality cordyceps supplements, as the concentration of active ingredients can vary significantly between products.

Look for products that specify the level of active compounds, such as adenosine and cordycepin, to ensure potency.

When preparing cordyceps, if using the dried form, it can be steeped in hot water to make a tea. This method allows for the extraction of the water-soluble active compounds. Alternatively, cordyceps powder can be added to smoothies or shakes, providing a convenient and effective way to consume the fungus. For those opting for a tincture, following the manufacturer's dosing recommendations is crucial to achieve the desired effects.

It's also worth noting that consistency is key when using cordyceps for enhancing physical stamina. Regular consumption can lead to cumulative benefits, making it a valuable addition to the dietary regimen of athletes and active individuals. However, as with any supplement, it's advisable to consult with a healthcare professional before starting, especially for those with underlying health conditions or those taking medication, as cordyceps can interact with certain drugs.

Ginseng and Maca Pre-Workout Elixir

Beneficial effects
Ginseng and Maca Pre-Workout Elixir is designed to enhance energy, endurance, and focus during workouts. Ginseng is known for its ability to fight fatigue and improve physical performance, while Maca root offers benefits such as increased energy and mental clarity. Together, they create a powerful elixir that can help maximize your workout potential.

Portions
Makes about 2 servings

Preparation time
5 minutes

Cooking time
No cooking required

Ingredients
- 1 teaspoon of powdered Ginseng
- 1 teaspoon of powdered Maca root
- 2 cups of cold water or coconut water
- 1 tablespoon of honey or agave syrup (optional for sweetness)
- Juice of ½ lemon
- A pinch of sea salt (to replenish electrolytes)
- Ice cubes (optional)

Instructions
1. In a blender, combine the powdered Ginseng and Maca root with the cold water or coconut water. The choice between water and coconut water depends on your preference for added electrolytes and a slight sweetness from the coconut water.

2. Add the honey or agave syrup to the blender if you prefer a sweeter taste. This step is optional and can be adjusted based on personal preference.

3. Squeeze the juice of ½ lemon into the blender. The lemon juice adds a refreshing taste and vitamin C, which can help with the absorption of the herbs.

4. Add a pinch of sea salt to the mixture. This is especially beneficial for longer or more intense workouts where electrolyte replenishment is crucial.

5. Blend all the ingredients on high speed until fully mixed and the powder is completely dissolved. This should take about 30 seconds to ensure a smooth texture.

6. If desired, add ice cubes to the blender and pulse a few times to chill the elixir. Alternatively, you can serve the elixir over ice in a glass.

7. Pour the elixir into a glass or a reusable water bottle if you're heading to the gym or outdoors for your workout.

Variations

- For an extra energy boost, add a shot of espresso or ½ cup of strong brewed coffee to the elixir. This is particularly useful for early morning workouts.
- Incorporate a scoop of your favorite protein powder to support muscle repair and growth.
- Add a teaspoon of chia seeds for added fiber, omega-3s, and protein. Let the elixir sit for a few minutes after blending to allow the chia seeds to swell.

Storage tips

It's best to consume the Ginseng and Maca Pre-Workout Elixir immediately after preparation to benefit from the energy-boosting properties. However, if you need to store it, keep the elixir in a sealed bottle in the refrigerator for up to 24 hours. Shake well before consuming if the ingredients have settled.

Tips for allergens

For those with sensitivities to honey or agave, the sweetener can be omitted or substituted with a few drops of stevia for a low-glycemic alternative. Ensure the Ginseng and Maca powders are pure and free from fillers or additives that could trigger allergies.

Scientific references

- "Effects of Panax Ginseng C.A. Meyer saponins on exercise performance in mice" in the journal Phytotherapy Research discusses the fatigue-fighting and performance-enhancing effects of Ginseng.
- "Subjective well-being in healthy men after the administration of gelatinized Maca root" in the journal Andrologia highlights the benefits of Maca root on mood and energy.

CHAPTER 2: HERBAL POST-WORKOUT RECOVERY

Turmeric for Reducing Inflammation

Turmeric, a vibrant yellow-orange spice, has been used for centuries in traditional medicine for its anti-inflammatory properties, primarily attributed to its active compound, **curcumin**. For athletes and individuals engaged in regular physical activity, incorporating turmeric into their post-workout recovery routine can significantly aid in reducing inflammation, enhancing muscle recovery, and supporting joint health.

To leverage turmeric's benefits for inflammation and recovery, it's essential to understand the optimal forms, dosages, and methods of consumption. Curcumin, while powerful, has low bioavailability, which means it's not easily absorbed by the body. However, combining turmeric with certain substances can enhance its absorption and effectiveness.

Forms of Turmeric for Consumption:

- **Powdered Turmeric:** Easily added to smoothies, teas, or post-workout meals. When using powdered turmeric, aim for a dosage of 1 to 3 grams per day.
- **Turmeric Supplements:** Available in capsules, these can provide a more concentrated dose of curcumin. Look for supplements containing piperine (black pepper extract), which can increase curcumin absorption by up to 2000%.
- **Turmeric Tinctures:** Liquid extracts offer another method for consuming turmeric, with the advantage of being easily adjustable for dosage. Typically, 20-40 drops can be taken in water or juice, up to three times daily.

Enhancing Absorption:

- **Pair with Black Pepper:** The piperine in black pepper enhances curcumin absorption. When adding turmeric to food or drinks, sprinkle in a little black pepper.
- **Combine with Fats:** Curcumin is fat-soluble, so consuming it with healthy fats like coconut oil, olive oil, or avocados can improve its uptake.
- **Heat Increases Bioavailability:** Cooking with turmeric or gently heating it in milk or a fat-based carrier can help unlock its benefits.

Application in Post-Workout Recovery:

- **Turmeric Golden Milk:** A traditional drink made with warm milk (dairy or plant-based), turmeric, a pinch of black pepper, and healthy fats like coconut oil. This beverage can be consumed post-exercise to support recovery and reduce inflammation.
- **Turmeric Infused Smoothie:** Add 1 teaspoon of turmeric powder along with a pinch of black pepper to your post-workout smoothie. Combine with ingredients rich in protein and healthy fats to aid muscle repair and enhance curcumin absorption.
- **Topical Application:** For localized joint or muscle soreness, a paste made from turmeric powder, water, and a little coconut oil can be applied directly to the skin. Wrap with a cloth to keep the area warm and enhance absorption.

Safety and Considerations:

While turmeric is generally safe for most individuals, high doses or long-term use of supplements should be approached with caution, especially for those with gallbladder disease, bleeding disorders, or those on blood-thinning medications. Always consult with a healthcare professional before introducing a new supplement, particularly at higher doses.

By incorporating turmeric into your post-workout routine through dietary consumption or topical application, you can harness its anti-inflammatory and recovery-enhancing benefits. Whether you're an athlete looking to optimize recovery or someone engaging in regular physical activity, turmeric can be a valuable addition to your wellness regimen.

Arnica for Sore Muscles

Arnica, a potent herb known for its anti-inflammatory and pain-relieving properties, is a cornerstone in natural remedies for athletes and individuals experiencing muscle soreness and bruising from physical activities. The active compounds in arnica, such as helenalin and flavonoids, contribute to its effectiveness in reducing inflammation and accelerating healing processes. Creating arnica-based salves and gels offers a practical approach to harnessing these benefits for post-workout recovery.

To craft an arnica salve, begin by sourcing high-quality dried arnica flowers. These are the primary ingredient for infusing oil, which serves as the base for the salve. For the infusion, combine approximately one cup of dried arnica flowers with two cups of a carrier oil such as coconut oil, olive oil, or almond oil in a double boiler. Heat the mixture gently for two to three hours, ensuring the temperature does not exceed 140°F to preserve the therapeutic properties of the oil. After heating, strain the oil using a fine mesh sieve or cheesecloth to remove all plant material, ensuring a pure infusion.

The next step involves the preparation of the salve. For every cup of infused arnica oil, add a quarter cup of beeswax pellets to the mixture. Return the mixture to the double boiler and heat gently, stirring continuously until the beeswax is completely dissolved. This combination, when cooled, forms the base of the salve. For enhanced pain relief and aromatic qualities, consider adding essential oils such as lavender or peppermint oil to the mixture. Approximately 10-20 drops per cup of infused oil should suffice, depending on personal preference and sensitivity to essential oils.

Pour the final mixture into clean, dry containers such as small jars or metal tins and allow it to cool and solidify. Label each container with the date and ingredients to keep track of the preparation and ensure proper usage.

For those preferring a gel format, which can be more cooling and easier to apply, the process begins similarly with the creation of an arnica-infused oil. Instead of beeswax, incorporate a natural gel base such as aloe vera gel into the infused oil. A common ratio is three parts aloe vera gel to one part arnica-infused oil, adjusted as needed to achieve the desired consistency. Essential oils can also be added to the gel for additional therapeutic benefits. Mix thoroughly to ensure an even distribution of the arnica oil throughout the gel. Store the gel in airtight containers, preferably in a cool, dark place to maintain its potency.

When applying arnica salve or gel to sore muscles or bruises, use a small amount and gently massage it into the affected area. It is crucial to avoid applying arnica to broken skin or open wounds as it can cause irritation. Always perform a patch test on a small area of skin before widespread use to ensure there is no adverse reaction.

By incorporating arnica salves or gels into post-workout routines, athletes and active individuals can benefit from a natural, effective method for managing muscle soreness and accelerating recovery. This approach not only leverages the healing power of arnica but also provides a soothing, therapeutic experience that supports overall well-being after physical exertion.

Ashwagandha for Post-Exercise Energy

Ashwagandha, scientifically known as Withania somnifera, stands out as a powerful adaptogen with profound benefits for athletes and individuals engaging in rigorous physical activities. This ancient herb, deeply rooted in Ayurvedic medicine, is renowned for its ability to enhance the body's resilience to stress and physical exertion, making it an invaluable asset for post-workout recovery. The adaptogenic properties of Ashwagandha work by modulating the body's stress response systems, thereby aiding in the restoration of energy and promoting overall well-being after intense exercise sessions.

To harness the benefits of Ashwagandha for energy restoration post-exercise, it is crucial to understand the optimal dosage and method of consumption. A daily intake of 300 to 500 mg of a high-concentration Ashwagandha extract, standardized to contain at least 5% withanolides (the active compounds), is recommended for significant results. This dosage can be taken in capsule or powder form, ideally with meals to enhance absorption. For athletes or individuals with higher physical demands, consulting a healthcare provider for personalized dosage advice is advisable to ensure safety and efficacy.

Incorporating Ashwagandha into the post-workout routine involves more than just consuming the herb; it's about understanding the timing for optimal benefits. Taking Ashwagandha immediately after exercise may help in reducing cortisol levels, which spike during physical stress, and support the body's recovery process. Additionally, consuming Ashwagandha before bedtime can contribute to improved sleep quality, further facilitating muscle recovery and energy restoration.

Beyond its adaptogenic effects, Ashwagandha also offers anti-inflammatory and antioxidant benefits, which are crucial for athletes dealing with muscle soreness and oxidative stress from intense workouts. These properties not only aid in reducing inflammation and pain but also accelerate the repair of muscle tissues, thus enhancing recovery speed.

For those looking to integrate Ashwagandha into their post-exercise regimen, incorporating the powder form into smoothies or shakes can be an effective way to consume the herb. This method allows for easy digestion and absorption, ensuring that the body can utilize the herb's benefits efficiently. Alternatively, Ashwagandha capsules provide a convenient option for those with a busy lifestyle or those who prefer not to taste the herb.

It's important to source Ashwagandha from reputable suppliers to ensure the product's purity and potency. Look for organic certifications and third-party testing to guarantee that the Ashwagandha supplement is free from contaminants and accurately labeled in terms of withanolide content.

In conclusion, Ashwagandha's adaptogenic properties make it a powerful tool for restoring energy and supporting recovery post-exercise. By incorporating this ancient herb into a well-rounded recovery plan, athletes and active individuals can enhance their resilience to physical stress, improve recovery times, and optimize their overall performance. Remember, while Ashwagandha offers remarkable benefits for post-workout recovery, it should be used as part of a holistic approach to health and wellness, including proper nutrition, hydration, and rest.

Arnica and Ginger Muscle Recovery Balm

Beneficial effects

Arnica and Ginger Muscle Recovery Balm is designed to soothe sore muscles, reduce inflammation, and accelerate recovery after workouts or physical strain. Arnica is widely recognized for its anti-inflammatory and pain-relieving properties, making it a staple in natural remedies for bruises, aches, and sprains. Ginger complements arnica by promoting circulation and warmth to the affected area, further aiding in the healing process. This balm is an excellent addition to any athlete's post-workout routine or for anyone looking to alleviate muscular discomfort naturally.

Portions

Approximately 100 grams (3.5 oz)

Preparation time

15 minutes

Cooking time
10 minutes

Ingredients
- ¼ cup arnica oil
- 2 tablespoons grated beeswax
- 1 tablespoon coconut oil
- 1 teaspoon ginger powder
- 10 drops of peppermint essential oil
- 5 drops of lavender essential oil

Instructions
1. Begin by setting up a double boiler: Fill a pot with a couple of inches of water and place it on the stove over medium heat. Rest a heat-safe glass bowl on top of the pot, ensuring the bottom of the bowl does not touch the water.
2. Add the arnica oil, grated beeswax, and coconut oil to the glass bowl. Stir the mixture gently as the beeswax and coconut oil melt, combining with the arnica oil into a smooth, unified liquid.
3. Once fully melted and mixed, carefully remove the bowl from the heat. Be sure to use oven mitts or a towel to protect your hands from the heat.
4. Stir in the ginger powder to the melted oil mixture. Ensure it is thoroughly dispersed throughout the liquid.
5. Allow the mixture to cool for a minute or two but not solidify. Then, add the peppermint and lavender essential oils, stirring well to ensure they are evenly distributed throughout the balm.
6. Before the mixture begins to solidify, carefully pour it into a clean, dry container with a lid. A small metal tin or glass jar works well for storage.
7. Let the balm cool and solidify completely at room temperature. This may take a few hours. Avoid moving the container too much during this time to ensure a smooth surface on the balm.
8. Once solidified, close the container with its lid. Label the container with the product name and date made for future reference.

Variations
- For extra pain relief, add 5 drops of eucalyptus essential oil to the mixture for its analgesic properties.
- If beeswax is too hard or not preferred, substitute it with the same amount of candelilla wax as a vegan alternative.

Storage tips
Store the Arnica and Ginger Muscle Recovery Balm in a cool, dry place away from direct sunlight. The balm should remain effective for up to 12 months if stored properly. If the balm becomes too soft in warm temperatures, refrigerate it for a short time to harden.

Tips for allergens
For those with coconut oil sensitivities, substitute it with an equal amount of shea butter or jojoba oil, both of which are gentle on the skin and have similar moisturizing properties.

Scientific references
- "Arnica montana L. – a plant of healing: review" in the Journal of Pharmacy and Pharmacology discusses arnica's effectiveness in reducing bruising and pain.
- "Ginger (Zingiber officinale) reduces muscle pain caused by eccentric exercise" in The Journal of Pain highlights ginger's role in alleviating muscle pain.

Chapter 3: Long-Term Athletic Health Support

Nettle for Mineral Replenishment

Nettle, scientifically known as Urtica dioica, is a powerhouse of nutrients essential for athletes and individuals leading active lifestyles. This herb, often overlooked due to its stinging nature when raw, transforms into a nutritional treasure when processed correctly. Nettle is rich in minerals such as iron, magnesium, potassium, and calcium, which are crucial for replenishing the body's stores depleted during intense physical activity. These minerals play vital roles in various bodily functions, including muscle contraction, hydration, and energy production, making nettle an excellent supplement for long-term athletic health support.

To effectively incorporate nettle into an athlete's diet for mineral replenishment, it's important to understand the optimal preparation methods that will maximize the bioavailability of these nutrients. One of the most effective ways to consume nettle is by preparing a nettle infusion or tea. To do this, one should use dried nettle leaves, which can be sourced from reputable suppliers ensuring they are free from contaminants and have been harvested sustainably. Approximately one tablespoon of dried nettle leaves should be steeped in one cup of boiling water for 10 to 15 minutes. This long steeping time allows for the extraction of the maximum amount of minerals and other beneficial compounds.

Another method to harness the benefits of nettle is through incorporating it into smoothies. Fresh nettle leaves, once blanched to remove the sting, can be blended into a nutrient-dense smoothie alongside fruits and vegetables high in vitamin C, such as oranges or kiwis. Vitamin C enhances the absorption of iron from plant sources, making this combination ideal for maximizing the nutritional benefits of nettle.

For athletes interested in a more direct approach to supplementing with nettle, nettle leaf capsules are available. These should be taken according to the manufacturer's instructions, typically with meals to improve absorption. It's crucial to choose capsules that are standardized to contain a specific amount of plant material, ensuring a consistent dose of the herb's beneficial compounds with each intake.

Incorporating nettle into the diet can also be achieved through culinary uses. Nettle leaves, when young and tender, can be cooked similarly to spinach and added to soups, stews, and sautés. This not only enriches the dishes with minerals but also adds a unique flavor profile. When cooking with nettle, it's important to remember that the leaves should be harvested wearing gloves to avoid the sting and should be washed thoroughly before use.

Athletes looking to benefit from nettle's mineral-replenishing properties should aim to include this herb in their diet regularly. Consistency is key in experiencing the full range of benefits, including reduced fatigue and improved recovery times. However, as with any supplement, it's advisable to consult with a healthcare provider before adding nettle to the diet, especially for those with existing health conditions or those taking medications, as nettle can interact with certain drugs.

Horsetail for Joint and Bone Health

Horsetail, scientifically known as Equisetum arvense, is a perennial fern that has been utilized for centuries due to its high silica content, making it an exceptional herb for supporting joint and bone health. Silica, a trace mineral found abundantly in horsetail, plays a crucial role in the formation and maintenance of connective tissues, as well as in the strengthening of bones and joints. This mineral contributes to the optimal assimilation of calcium in the body, which is vital for bone density and overall skeletal strength.

For athletes and individuals engaged in regular physical activity, incorporating horsetail into their wellness regimen can be particularly beneficial for enhancing the body's resilience against the wear and tear associated with rigorous exercises and sports. The silica in horsetail not only aids in the repair of cartilage and connective tissues but also helps in reducing inflammation and improving the flexibility and mobility of joints. This makes horsetail an invaluable herb for long-term athletic health support, especially for those looking to maintain peak physical condition and prevent injuries.

To effectively leverage the benefits of horsetail for joint and bone strength, it is essential to understand the most efficient methods of preparation and consumption. One common method is to prepare a horsetail tea or infusion. To do this, add one to two teaspoons of dried horsetail herb to a cup of boiling water and allow it to steep for 10 to 15 minutes. This process extracts the silica and other beneficial compounds from the herb, resulting in a tea that can be consumed two to three times daily for optimal benefits. It's important to note that the taste of horsetail tea can be somewhat bland or slightly bitter, so individuals may choose to enhance the flavor with honey or lemon.

Another effective way to incorporate horsetail into the diet is through the use of tinctures or extracts, which provide a concentrated dose of the herb's beneficial compounds. When selecting a horsetail tincture, look for products that are alcohol-free and have been standardized to ensure a consistent level of silica content. The recommended dosage for horsetail extract is typically a few drops, taken with water, up to three times a day. However, dosages can vary depending on the concentration of the product, so it's advisable to follow the manufacturer's instructions or consult with a healthcare professional.

For those interested in a more holistic approach, incorporating horsetail into homemade salves or ointments can provide targeted support for joint and bone health. By infusing a carrier oil with dried horsetail and then blending it with beeswax, one can create a soothing topical application. This salve can be applied directly to the skin over joints and bones, providing localized benefits and aiding in the absorption of silica through the skin.

When sourcing horsetail, it's crucial to opt for high-quality, organically grown herbs to ensure the absence of contaminants and pesticides, which can detract from the herb's health benefits. Additionally, while horsetail is generally considered safe for most individuals, it's important to be aware of potential contraindications. Due to its diuretic properties, horsetail should be used with caution by those with kidney issues or those taking diuretic medications. As with any supplement, consulting with a healthcare provider before adding horsetail to your regimen is recommended, especially for those with existing health conditions or those who are pregnant or breastfeeding.

Incorporating horsetail into one's wellness routine offers a natural and effective way to support joint and bone health, particularly for athletes and active individuals seeking to maintain their physical performance and prevent injuries. Through consistent and mindful use, the benefits of horsetail can contribute significantly to long-term skeletal strength and resilience.

Ginger for Circulation and Flexibility

Ginger, scientifically known as Zingiber officinale, is a potent herb renowned for its ability to enhance circulation and reduce stiffness, making it an invaluable resource for athletes and individuals engaged in regular physical activity. The active compounds in ginger, particularly gingerols and shogaols, have been shown to have significant anti-inflammatory and blood-thinning effects, which contribute to its efficacy in promoting blood flow and improving flexibility. These properties not only aid in the prevention of muscle stiffness and soreness post-exercise but also support the body's natural healing processes, facilitating quicker recovery from workouts and injuries.

To leverage ginger's benefits for enhancing circulation and reducing stiffness, it's essential to incorporate it effectively into one's diet or wellness routine. One of the most straightforward methods is the consumption of fresh ginger tea. To prepare this, thinly slice or grate approximately one inch of fresh ginger root, then steep it in boiling water for about 10 to 15 minutes. This method allows for the extraction of ginger's active compounds. Drinking ginger tea two to three times daily can help in alleviating muscle stiffness and improving blood circulation throughout the body.

Another practical application of ginger for athletes is through topical application. Creating a ginger-infused oil for massage can provide targeted relief to stiff and sore muscles. To prepare, finely grate ginger and simmer it in a carrier oil such as coconut or jojoba oil over low heat for 30 to 60 minutes. After cooling and straining, this infused oil can be gently massaged into the skin, focusing on areas prone to stiffness and soreness. The topical application of ginger oil not only soothes the muscles but also stimulates blood flow to the affected area, enhancing flexibility and mobility.

For those seeking a more concentrated form of ginger's benefits, ginger supplements are available in capsules or tablets. These supplements are particularly beneficial for individuals with a busy lifestyle or those who may not enjoy the taste of ginger. When selecting a ginger supplement, opting for a product standardized to contain a specific percentage of gingerols and shogaols is crucial, as these are the primary active compounds. The recommended dosage can vary, but generally, 500 to 1000 mg of ginger extract taken daily, divided into two or three doses, is effective for enhancing circulation and reducing stiffness. However, it's advisable to consult with a healthcare provider before starting any new supplement regimen, especially for individuals on blood-thinning medications, as ginger can enhance these effects.

Incorporating ginger into post-workout smoothies is another excellent way to benefit from its properties. Combining ginger with other anti-inflammatory foods like turmeric and omega-3 rich flaxseeds can amplify its effects, aiding in muscle recovery and flexibility. A simple smoothie recipe might include a small piece of fresh ginger, turmeric, banana, flaxseed oil, and almond milk. Blend these ingredients until smooth and consume immediately after workouts to support muscle recovery and circulation.

It's important to source ginger from reputable suppliers to ensure it's free from contaminants and pesticides, which can negate its health benefits. Whether using fresh ginger, ginger oil, or supplements, quality is key to achieving the desired therapeutic effects.

By understanding the specific mechanisms through which ginger enhances circulation and reduces stiffness, individuals can tailor their use of this powerful herb to fit their unique health and wellness goals. Regular consumption or application of ginger, combined with a balanced diet and proper exercise regimen, can significantly contribute to improved athletic performance, reduced recovery times, and enhanced overall well-being.

Beetroot and Tart Cherry Recovery Smoothie

Beneficial effects

The Beetroot and Tart Cherry Recovery Smoothie is a powerhouse of nutrients designed to support muscle recovery, reduce inflammation, and boost endurance. Beetroot is rich in nitrates, which the body converts into nitric oxide, improving blood flow and oxygen delivery to muscles, enhancing exercise performance, and reducing recovery time. Tart cherries are packed with antioxidants and anti-inflammatory compounds, helping to minimize post-exercise muscle pain and soreness. Together, these ingredients create a delicious, natural remedy for athletes and active individuals looking to optimize their recovery process and overall athletic health.

Portions
Makes about 2 servings

Preparation time
10 minutes

Ingredients
- 1 medium-sized beetroot, peeled and chopped
- 1 cup frozen tart cherries
- 1 banana, sliced
- 1/2 cup unsweetened almond milk (or any plant-based milk of your choice)
- 1/2 cup orange juice, freshly squeezed
- 1 tablespoon chia seeds
- 1 teaspoon fresh ginger, grated
- Ice cubes (optional, for a colder smoothie)

Instructions

1. Start by preparing the beetroot. Peel it with a vegetable peeler, then chop it into small pieces. This will help it blend more easily and create a smoother texture in your smoothie.

2. Place the chopped beetroot, frozen tart cherries, and sliced banana into a high-speed blender. These ingredients form the base of your smoothie, offering a mix of vitamins, minerals, and antioxidants essential for recovery.

3. Add the unsweetened almond milk to the blender. This will give your smoothie a creamy texture without the need for dairy. If you prefer a thinner consistency, you can add more almond milk as needed.

4. Pour in the freshly squeezed orange juice. This not only adds a natural sweetness to your smoothie but also provides a good dose of vitamin C, which is crucial for repairing tissue and reducing inflammation.

5. Sprinkle the chia seeds into the blender. Chia seeds are a great source of omega-3 fatty acids, fiber, and protein, all of which are beneficial for muscle recovery and overall health.

6. Add the grated fresh ginger. Ginger is known for its anti-inflammatory properties, which can help reduce muscle soreness and pain after intense workouts.

7. If desired, add a handful of ice cubes to the blender for a colder, more refreshing smoothie.

8. Blend all the ingredients on high speed until the mixture is smooth and creamy. Depending on the power of your blender, this may take between 30 seconds to 1 minute.

9. Once blended to your liking, pour the smoothie into two glasses and enjoy immediately for the best flavor and nutritional benefits.

Variations

- For an extra protein boost, add a scoop of your favorite plant-based protein powder. This is especially beneficial if you're consuming this smoothie post-workout.
- Swap out almond milk for coconut water for added electrolytes, which are essential for hydration and recovery.
- Add a handful of spinach or kale for an extra serving of greens without significantly altering the taste of the smoothie.

Storage tips

It's best to consume the Beetroot and Tart Cherry Recovery Smoothie immediately after blending to maximize its nutritional benefits. However, if you need to store it, keep the smoothie in a sealed container in the refrigerator for up to 24 hours. Give it a good shake or stir before drinking, as separation may occur.

Tips for allergens

For those with nut allergies, substituting almond milk with oat milk or hemp milk can provide a similar creamy texture without the allergens. Always ensure that the plant-based milk you choose is fortified with calcium and vitamin D for added health benefits.

Scientific references

- "Dietary nitrate supplementation reduces the O2 cost of low-intensity exercise and enhances tolerance to high-intensity exercise in humans," published in the Journal of Applied Physiology, discusses the benefits of beetroot on exercise performance and recovery.

- "Efficacy of tart cherry juice in reducing muscle pain during running: a randomized controlled trial," published in the Journal of the International Society of Sports Nutrition, highlights the effectiveness of tart cherries in reducing post-exercise pain.

BOOK 11: WOMEN'S HEALTH AND HERBAL SUPPORT

CHAPTER 1: HORMONAL BALANCE & REPRODUCTIVE HEALTH

Vitex for PMS and Menstrual Regulation

Vitex, commonly known as chasteberry, has been a cornerstone in herbal medicine for centuries, particularly in the realm of women's health. Its efficacy in mitigating premenstrual syndrome (PMS) symptoms and aiding menstrual regulation is rooted in its ability to modulate hormonal imbalances, a common cause of discomfort for many. The active compounds in vitex act directly on the pituitary gland, the body's master endocrine gland, which controls the release of luteinizing hormone (LH). By increasing LH levels, vitex indirectly promotes progesterone production, a hormone often found in lower levels during PMS. This hormonal adjustment is crucial for alleviating symptoms like mood swings, cramps, breast tenderness, and irritability.

To harness the benefits of vitex for PMS and menstrual regulation, it's essential to understand the proper preparation and dosage. The most effective form of vitex is the dried berry, which can be used to make a decoction or an infusion. To prepare a vitex tea, take one teaspoon of dried berries and steep them in boiling water for 10 to 15 minutes. This allows the water to extract the active compounds effectively. For those seeking convenience, vitex is also available in capsule and tincture forms. The standard dosage for managing PMS symptoms ranges from 160 to 240 milligrams of extract daily, ideally taken in the morning to align with the body's natural hormonal rhythm.

Consistency is key when using vitex, as its benefits are cumulative and may take several cycles to become fully apparent. It's not uncommon for improvements in PMS symptoms and menstrual regularity to be observed after three months of consistent use. However, it's important to note that while vitex is generally well-tolerated, it may not be suitable for everyone. Women who are pregnant, breastfeeding, or those who are on hormonal medications should consult with a healthcare provider before incorporating vitex into their regimen.

In addition to its hormonal benefits, vitex also exhibits dopaminergic effects, which may contribute to its mood-stabilizing properties. By acting on dopamine receptors, vitex helps alleviate the emotional symptoms associated with PMS, offering a holistic approach to menstrual health.

When sourcing vitex, look for products that specify the concentration of active compounds, ensuring you receive a standardized dose. Quality matters, as the potency of herbal supplements can vary widely between brands. Opt for reputable manufacturers that provide third-party testing to guarantee the purity and strength of their products.

Incorporating vitex into a broader lifestyle approach that includes a balanced diet, regular exercise, and stress management techniques can further enhance its effectiveness in managing PMS and promoting menstrual health. Remember, while vitex is a powerful tool for hormonal balance, it works best when part of a comprehensive approach to wellness.

Black Cohosh for Menopause Relief

Black Cohosh, scientifically known as **Actaea racemosa**, is a perennial plant that has been traditionally used for centuries to support women's health, particularly during the menopausal transition. This herb is renowned for its ability to alleviate some of the most common and uncomfortable symptoms associated with menopause, such as **hot flashes, mood swings, and sleep disturbances**.

The active compounds in Black Cohosh, including **triterpene glycosides**, have been studied for their estrogen-like effects, which can help balance hormone levels without the use of hormone replacement therapy. For women seeking natural alternatives, Black Cohosh presents a viable option.

To effectively use Black Cohosh for menopause support, it's essential to understand the recommended forms and dosages. The root and rhizome of the plant are the parts used for medicinal purposes, available in several forms including **capsules, tinctures, and teas**.

For those opting for capsules, a common dosage is **20 to 40 milligrams twice daily**. It's important to look for products that are standardized to contain 2.5% triterpene glycosides, ensuring a consistent dose of the active compounds. When using a tincture, **1 to 2 milliliters** can be taken up to three times a day, diluted in water or juice. For tea, steeping 1 gram of dried Black Cohosh root in 240 milliliters (about a cup) of boiling water for 20 to 30 minutes offers a gentler approach, though the exact dosage may be more difficult to measure compared to standardized extracts.

While Black Cohosh is generally well-tolerated, it's crucial to be aware of potential side effects, such as gastrointestinal upset or headaches. Long-term safety beyond six months of use has not been extensively studied, so it's advisable to consult with a healthcare provider before incorporating Black Cohosh into your regimen, especially for those with liver issues, or who are taking medications for blood pressure or blood thinners.

Quality and sourcing are paramount when selecting a Black Cohosh supplement. Opt for products from reputable manufacturers that adhere to Good Manufacturing Practices (GMP) and provide transparency about sourcing and standardization. This ensures that the product is free from contaminants and accurately labeled.

Incorporating Black Cohosh into a holistic approach to menopause management, including a balanced diet rich in phytoestrogens, regular physical activity, and stress-reduction techniques, can enhance overall wellbeing during this transition. While Black Cohosh can offer relief for many, it's important to remember that individual responses may vary, and adjustments to the approach may be necessary to find the most effective relief.

Shatavari for Fertility and Hormonal Balance

Shatavari, scientifically known as **Asparagus racemosus**, is a revered herb in traditional Ayurvedic medicine, often hailed as a potent adaptogen with a special affinity for enhancing women's reproductive health. Its roots contain a rich blend of phytochemicals, including saponins, flavonoids, and steroidal glycosides, which contribute to its efficacy in balancing hormones and supporting fertility.

To leverage **Shatavari** for fertility and hormonal harmony, it's crucial to understand its adaptogenic properties. Adaptogens are substances that help the body resist physical, chemical, and biological stressors. Shatavari's adaptogenic effects stem from its ability to modulate the body's production of stress hormones, which can impact menstrual cycles and fertility.

For those looking to incorporate Shatavari into their wellness routine, it is available in various forms, including **powders, capsules, and liquid extracts**. The powdered root can be mixed with water or milk and taken once or twice daily. The recommended dosage for powdered Shatavari is typically **1/4 to 1/2 teaspoon**, while capsules often come in doses ranging from **500 to 1000 milligrams** per capsule, taken with water.

When preparing Shatavari as a tea, steep 1 teaspoon of the powdered root in 10 ounces of hot water for about 10 minutes. This method allows for a gentle extraction of the herb's beneficial compounds. For those preferring convenience, Shatavari capsules can be taken with water, usually one to two capsules twice daily, or as directed by a healthcare provider.

Quality is paramount when selecting a Shatavari supplement. Look for products that are certified organic and tested for purity and strength. Reputable brands will provide third-party testing results to confirm the absence of heavy metals and contaminants.

It's important to note that while Shatavari is generally considered safe, it may not be suitable for everyone. Women who are pregnant or nursing, or those with a history of estrogen-sensitive conditions, should consult with a healthcare professional before adding Shatavari to their regimen. Additionally, because of its potential to interact with certain medications, including diuretics and insulin, a healthcare provider should be consulted to ensure compatibility.

Incorporating Shatavari into a daily routine for fertility and hormonal balance is a practice supported by centuries of traditional use. However, it's most effective when part of a holistic approach to wellness that includes a balanced diet, regular exercise, and stress management techniques. Consistency and patience are key, as the full benefits of Shatavari may take several weeks to manifest.

Chasteberry and Red Clover Hormone Balancing Tea

Beneficial effects

Chasteberry and Red Clover Hormone Balancing Tea is crafted to naturally support hormonal balance and reproductive health. Chasteberry, also known as Vitex, has been shown to help regulate menstrual cycles, relieve PMS symptoms, and support fertility by balancing estrogen and progesterone levels in the body. Red Clover is rich in isoflavones, plant-based compounds that mimic estrogen, making it beneficial for easing menopause symptoms like hot flashes and bone density loss. Together, these herbs create a synergistic blend that promotes overall hormonal health and well-being.

Portions

Makes about 4 cups

Preparation time

5 minutes

Cooking time

15 minutes

Ingredients

- 2 tablespoons dried Chasteberry (Vitex agnus-castus)
- 2 tablespoons dried Red Clover flowers (Trifolium pratense)
- 4 cups of water
- Honey or stevia to taste (optional)

Instructions

1. Begin by bringing 4 cups of water to a boil in a medium-sized saucepan. While waiting for the water to boil, measure out the dried Chasteberry and Red Clover flowers.

2. Once the water reaches a rolling boil, add the Chasteberry and Red Clover directly to the water. Reduce the heat to low, allowing the herbs to simmer gently. This slow simmer helps extract the active compounds from the herbs without destroying their delicate balance.

3. Cover the saucepan with a lid and let the herbs steep in the hot water for 15 minutes. Keeping the saucepan covered helps to trap the steam and essential oils from the herbs, enhancing the tea's therapeutic properties.

4. After 15 minutes, remove the saucepan from the heat. Strain the tea through a fine mesh sieve into a large pitcher or directly into tea cups, pressing on the herbs with the back of a spoon to extract as much liquid and beneficial properties as possible.

5. If desired, sweeten the tea with honey or stevia according to your taste preferences. Stir well to ensure the sweetener is fully dissolved.

6. Serve the tea warm, or allow it to cool and enjoy it chilled. This tea can be consumed daily to support hormonal balance and reproductive health.

Variations

- For added flavor and benefits, include a cinnamon stick or a few slices of fresh ginger in the saucepan while simmering the herbs.
- Combine with a tablespoon of dried peppermint or lemon balm leaves for a refreshing twist and additional digestive support.

Storage tips

Store any leftover tea in a glass container in the refrigerator for up to 48 hours. Reheat gently on the stove or enjoy chilled. For best results, consume within 24 hours to ensure the potency of the active compounds.

Tips for allergens

For those with allergies or sensitivities to honey, stevia serves as a natural, low-glycemic alternative sweetener that does not trigger common allergies. Ensure the dried herbs are sourced from reputable suppliers to avoid contamination with allergens.

Scientific references

- "Chasteberry: A Systematic Review of its Efficacy in Women's Health." This study, published in the journal Herbal Medicine, provides a comprehensive review of Chasteberry's benefits for menstrual disorders, fertility, and menopause symptoms.
- "The Role of Isoflavones in Menopausal Health: Consensus Opinion of The North American Menopause Society." Published in Menopause, this article discusses the benefits of isoflavones found in Red Clover for managing menopause symptoms and supporting hormonal health.

Chapter 2: Herbs for Pregnancy & Postpartum

Red Raspberry Leaf for Uterine Health

Red Raspberry Leaf, scientifically known as Rubus idaeus, holds a venerable place in the realm of herbal remedies, particularly for its uterine health benefits. This herb, rich in vitamins and minerals such as magnesium, potassium, iron, and vitamins B, C, and E, has been traditionally used to strengthen and tone the uterine muscles, preparing the uterus for labor and aiding in the recovery process postpartum. Its use is grounded in both historical practice and contemporary herbalism, offering a natural approach to supporting women through the challenges of pregnancy and beyond.

The mechanism by which Red Raspberry Leaf exerts its effects on the uterus can be attributed to its fragarine and tannin compounds. Fragarine, an alkaloid, works by toning the muscles of the pelvic region, including the uterus, which can contribute to a more efficient labor by enhancing contractions and potentially reducing labor time. Tannins, on the other hand, possess astringent properties that can help reduce bleeding and inflammation, supporting the body's recovery after childbirth.

To harness the benefits of Red Raspberry Leaf for uterine health, it is commonly consumed in the form of a tea. Preparing this tea involves steeping one to two teaspoons of dried Red Raspberry leaves in boiling water for about 10 to 15 minutes. This method allows for the extraction of the beneficial compounds into the water, creating a therapeutic infusion. For those approaching labor, it is often recommended to start with one cup of tea a day, gradually increasing to three cups as the due date approaches. This gradual increase allows the body to adjust to the herb's effects and can maximize the toning benefits on the uterus.

In addition to tea, Red Raspberry Leaf is also available in capsule and tincture forms, providing alternative methods for consumption. Capsules may offer a convenient option for those who prefer not to drink tea or are seeking a more concentrated form of the herb. The typical dosage for capsules is around 400 to 500 milligrams taken twice daily, but it is crucial to follow the specific recommendations provided by the product manufacturer or a healthcare provider.

While Red Raspberry Leaf is widely regarded as safe for most pregnant women, it is essential to consult with a healthcare provider before incorporating it into a prenatal regimen, especially for those with a history of miscarriage, preterm labor, or other pregnancy complications. This precaution ensures that the herb's use is appropriate for an individual's specific health circumstances.

Quality and sourcing are critical considerations when selecting Red Raspberry Leaf products. Opting for organic leaves or products certified free from pesticides and contaminants can provide peace of mind regarding the purity of the herb. Additionally, purchasing from reputable suppliers that specialize in medicinal herbs can ensure that the Red Raspberry Leaf is harvested at the optimal time for medicinal use, preserving its potency and efficacy.

Nettle for Postpartum Recovery

Nettle (Urtica dioica), a nutrient-rich plant, plays a crucial role in postpartum recovery, particularly in replenishing iron and boosting energy levels. After childbirth, many new mothers experience fatigue and iron deficiency, making nettle an invaluable herb during this recovery phase. Its high iron content aids in the replenishment of lost blood during childbirth, while its array of vitamins and minerals supports overall vitality and wellness.

To incorporate nettle into a postpartum recovery regimen, start with **nettle tea**, which is gentle on the stomach and easy to prepare. Use 1-2 tablespoons of dried nettle leaves per cup of boiling water. Steep the leaves in the water, covered, for 10-15 minutes to ensure that the water becomes rich in the plant's soluble vitamins and minerals. This method allows for a maximum extraction of nutrients, making the tea not only a rich source of iron but also of magnesium, calcium, and vitamins A, C, and K, which are essential for recovery and energy.

For those who prefer a more concentrated form, **nettle tincture** can be an alternative. A typical dosage for postpartum recovery might start at 1-2 milliliters, taken three times a day. However, it's crucial to consult with a healthcare provider for personalized advice, especially when breastfeeding, to ensure the dosage is appropriate.

Nettle can also be incorporated into meals; **nettle soup** is a traditional and nourishing option. To prepare, sauté a diced onion and garlic in olive oil until soft. Add a large handful of fresh nettle leaves (wearing gloves to handle), and sauté until they wilt. Add vegetable broth and simmer for 15-20 minutes. Blend until smooth for a rich, iron-packed soup.

For direct supplementation, **nettle leaf capsules** are available and provide a straightforward way to include this herb in your daily routine. The typical dosage is around 300-500 milligrams per day, but as with tinctures, it's important to verify the dosage with a healthcare provider, particularly for breastfeeding mothers.

When selecting nettle products, look for **organic certification** to ensure the herbs are free from pesticides and other contaminants. This is especially important during the postpartum period, as toxins can affect both the mother's and baby's health.

Incorporating nettle into the diet postpartum should be done gradually, starting with small doses and increasing as tolerated. This approach allows the body to adjust and minimizes the risk of any adverse reactions. Always ensure adequate hydration, particularly when increasing dietary fiber through nettle consumption, to support digestive health and nutrient absorption.

Remember, while nettle offers significant benefits for postpartum recovery, it is one component of a holistic approach to postnatal care. A balanced diet, adequate rest, and medical consultation are paramount to a healthy recovery period.

Calendula for Postpartum Healing

Calendula, scientifically known as Calendula officinalis, is a remarkable herb recognized for its potent healing properties, particularly beneficial during the postpartum period. This vibrant, orange-yellow flower harbors anti-inflammatory, antimicrobial, and soothing qualities, making it an invaluable ally for new mothers experiencing skin irritations, tears, or other discomforts following childbirth.

For the effective use of calendula in postpartum healing, it's essential to understand the preparation of topical applications such as infused oils, salves, and compresses. To begin with, creating a calendula-infused oil is a foundational step. Select high-quality, dried calendula petals and submerge them in a carrier oil - for instance, organic olive oil or sweet almond oil are excellent choices due to their gentle nature and skin-nourishing benefits. The mixture should be placed in a glass jar and left to infuse in a warm, sunny spot for 4 to 6 weeks, allowing the oil to draw out the healing compounds of the calendula petals. It's crucial to shake the jar gently every few days to ensure the even distribution of the petals' properties.

Once the infusion process is complete, the oil should be strained using a fine mesh sieve or cheesecloth to remove the calendula petals, resulting in a richly colored, potent oil. This calendula-infused oil can be applied directly to sensitive areas, or it can serve as a base for further preparations.

To enhance the healing effects, particularly for tears or deeper skin irritations, transforming the infused oil into a calendula salve adds a protective layer that promotes skin regeneration. This involves gently heating the infused oil and combining it with beeswax, which solidifies the mixture upon cooling. The ratio typically recommended is one part beeswax to four parts calendula-infused oil by volume. Once the beeswax is fully melted and mixed with the oil, the liquid salve can be poured into sterilized jars or tins and allowed to cool and solidify. This salve can be applied to the affected areas several times a day, ensuring a clean, dry surface each time to support healing and prevent infection.

For those experiencing superficial skin irritations or seeking a soothing application, a calendula compress can provide immediate relief. This involves soaking a clean cloth in a calendula tea, prepared by steeping dried calendula petals in boiling water for 10 to 15 minutes, then cooling it to a comfortable temperature. The compress can be gently placed on the sensitive skin, offering calming effects and reducing inflammation.

Throughout all these applications, it's paramount to maintain cleanliness and monitor the skin's response to the calendula treatment. While calendula is known for its gentle, soothing properties, individual sensitivities can vary, and discontinuing use if any adverse reactions occur is advised.

Incorporating calendula into postpartum care offers a natural, effective way to support the body's healing process, leveraging ancient wisdom for modern wellness. Its application not only aids in physical recovery but also embodies the nurturing care essential during the transformative postpartum period.

Nettle and Raspberry Leaf Pregnancy Tea

Beneficial effects

Nettle and Raspberry Leaf Pregnancy Tea is a nurturing blend designed to support women through all stages of pregnancy. Nettle leaves are rich in vitamins A, C, K, and several key minerals like iron, magnesium, and calcium, which are essential for pregnancy health. They also help in boosting energy levels and supporting the body's circulatory system. Raspberry leaf is celebrated for toning the uterus, improving labor outcomes, and decreasing postpartum bleeding. This herbal combination offers a gentle, supportive tonic that can be enjoyed throughout pregnancy to nourish the body and prepare it for childbirth.

Portions

Makes about 4 cups

Preparation time

5 minutes

Cooking time

10 minutes

Ingredients

- 2 tablespoons dried nettle leaves
- 2 tablespoons dried raspberry leaves
- 4 cups water
- Honey or lemon to taste (optional)

Instructions

1. Begin by bringing 4 cups of water to a rolling boil in a medium-sized pot.

2. While the water is heating, measure out 2 tablespoons each of dried nettle leaves and dried raspberry leaves. Combine them in a large teapot or a heat-resistant glass jar.

3. Once the water has reached a boil, carefully pour it over the nettle and raspberry leaves. Ensure all the leaves are submerged and begin to steep.

4. Cover the teapot or jar with a lid or a small plate to retain heat and prevent the escape of essential oils and flavors.

5. Allow the tea to steep for 10 minutes. This duration extracts the beneficial properties of the herbs without making the tea too strong or bitter.

6. After steeping, strain the tea through a fine mesh sieve into another pot or directly into cups. This removes the leaves and ensures a smooth tea.

7. If desired, add honey or a squeeze of lemon to each cup according to taste. Honey can provide additional soothing properties and a touch of sweetness, while lemon adds a refreshing note and vitamin C.

8. Stir well to ensure any added honey or lemon is fully dissolved, then serve the tea warm.

Variations

- For a calming evening tea, add a tablespoon of dried chamomile flowers to the blend. Chamomile can help ease sleep disturbances and relax the nervous system.

- Incorporate a slice of fresh ginger while steeping to add a warming element and to help with nausea, a common pregnancy symptom.

Storage tips

Any leftover tea can be stored in a sealed glass container in the refrigerator for up to 2 days. Gently reheat on the stove or enjoy chilled. It's best to make fresh batches regularly to enjoy the maximum benefits of the herbs.

Tips for allergens

For those with sensitivities or allergies to honey, consider using maple syrup or a few drops of stevia as a sweetening alternative. Ensure any added ingredients are organic to avoid potential contaminants that could be harmful during pregnancy.

Scientific references

- "Uterine Tonic Activity of Urtica dioica" in the Journal of Herbal Medicine highlights the nutritional benefits and supportive properties of nettle during pregnancy.

- "The Efficacy of Rubus idaeus (Red Raspberry) Leaf in Pregnancy" in the Journal of Midwifery & Women's Health discusses raspberry leaf's role in preparing the uterus for labor and its impact on labor outcomes.

CHAPTER 3: COMMON WOMEN'S HEALTH CONCERNS

Cranberry for Urinary Tract Health

Cranberries, scientifically known as **Vaccinium macrocarpon**, have been widely recognized for their role in maintaining urinary tract health and preventing **Urinary Tract Infections (UTIs)**. This small, tart fruit is packed with potent compounds, including **proanthocyanidins (PACs)**, which prevent the adhesion of bacteria, such as **E. coli**, to the urinary tract walls, thereby reducing the incidence of infections.

For those looking to harness the benefits of cranberries for UTI prevention or treatment, incorporating cranberry in various forms into your diet can be beneficial. Here are detailed ways to utilize cranberries effectively:

1. Cranberry Juice

Ensure you consume unsweetened cranberry juice to avoid excess sugar, which can potentially negate the benefits for UTI prevention. Aim for a daily intake of 8-16 ounces. Look for labels stating **100% pure cranberry juice** without added sugars or preservatives. Diluting the juice with water can make it more palatable if you find it too tart.

2. Cranberry Supplements

Cranberry supplements are available in capsules or tablets, offering a convenient way to consume cranberries without the tart taste. Opt for supplements that contain at least **36 mg of proanthocyanidins (PACs)** per serving, as this is the amount shown to be effective in reducing UTI risk. Follow the manufacturer's dosage recommendations, typically one or two capsules daily, preferably with meals to enhance absorption.

3. Dried Cranberries

Incorporating dried cranberries into your diet can be another way to benefit from their UTI prevention properties. However, be mindful of the sugar content, as dried fruits are often sweetened. Opt for varieties labeled as **no sugar added** or **lightly sweetened**. A small handful of dried cranberries can be added to breakfast cereals, salads, or enjoyed as a snack.

4. Fresh Cranberries

Though less commonly consumed in their fresh form due to their tartness, fresh cranberries can be a nutritious addition to your diet. They can be used in homemade cranberry sauces, added to smoothies, or baked into goods. When using fresh cranberries, combining them with a sweetener like honey or blending them with sweeter fruits can help balance their tartness.

5. Cranberry Infused Water

For a refreshing and hydrating way to consume cranberries, try making cranberry-infused water. Add a handful of fresh or frozen cranberries to a pitcher of water, along with slices of other fruits like oranges or lemons for added flavor. Let the mixture infuse for at least 4 hours or overnight in the refrigerator.

Precautions and Considerations

While cranberries can be effective in preventing UTIs, they should not replace medical treatment for active infections. It's crucial to consult with a healthcare provider if you suspect a UTI, as untreated infections can lead to more serious complications.

Additionally, individuals taking blood-thinning medications should consult with their doctor before increasing their cranberry intake, as cranberries can interact with these medications.

In summary, cranberries offer a natural and accessible way to support urinary tract health and prevent UTIs. By incorporating cranberries into your diet in one of the forms mentioned above, you can harness their health benefits while enjoying their unique, tart flavor.

Dong Quai for Circulation & Reproductive Health

Dong Quai, scientifically known as **Angelica sinensis**, is a traditional herb widely recognized for its potent benefits in promoting circulation and addressing menstrual irregularities among women. This herb, often referred to as "female ginseng," contains a rich composition of phytochemicals including ferulic acid, ligustilide, and various polysaccharides, which collectively contribute to its therapeutic effects.

For those seeking to incorporate Dong Quai into their wellness regimen, it's crucial to understand the specific methods of preparation and consumption to achieve optimal benefits. Here's a detailed breakdown:

Preparation of Dong Quai Tea

1. **Selecting Dong Quai**: Start with high-quality, dried Dong Quai root. Look for organically certified products to ensure purity and effectiveness.

2. **Dosage**: Approximately 3-6 grams of Dong Quai root is recommended for making tea. This dosage can vary depending on individual needs and responses.

3. **Tea Preparation**: Slice or break the dried root into smaller pieces to increase the surface area for extraction. Boil the root in water (about 500ml or roughly 2 cups) for 30 to 45 minutes. The long boiling time helps in extracting the active compounds effectively.

4. **Straining**: After boiling, strain the tea to remove the root pieces. The resulting liquid should have a deep, amber color, indicating the extraction of Dong Quai's beneficial compounds.

5. **Consumption**: It's advisable to consume Dong Quai tea warm. For taste, one might add a natural sweetener like honey or mix it with other herbal teas to enhance flavor profiles.

Dong Quai Tincture

1. **Tincture Preparation**: Combine Dong Quai root with a high-proof alcohol (vodka or grain alcohol) in a clean, airtight jar. The ratio should be 1 part Dong Quai to 5 parts alcohol by volume.

2. **Infusion Period**: Seal the jar tightly and store it in a cool, dark place for 4 to 6 weeks. Shake the jar gently every few days to mix the contents.

3. **Straining**: After the infusion period, strain the tincture through a fine mesh sieve or cheesecloth into another clean, airtight container. Ensure all solid particles are removed.

4. **Storage**: Store the strained tincture in a dark glass bottle, preferably with a dropper for easy use. Label the bottle with the date of preparation for tracking potency.

Capsules

Dong Quai is also available in capsule form, which can be a convenient option for those who prefer not to taste the herb. When selecting capsules:

- **Quality and Dosage**: Choose products from reputable suppliers that specify the amount of Dong Quai root extract per capsule. Follow the recommended dosage on the product label, typically ranging from 500 to 600 mg taken once or twice daily.

Safety and Considerations

While Dong Quai is generally safe for most individuals, it's important to consider potential interactions and contraindications:

- **Blood Thinners**: Due to its blood-thinning properties, Dong Quai should be used with caution by individuals on anticoagulant medications.
- **Pregnancy and Breastfeeding**: Dong Quai is not recommended for use during pregnancy or breastfeeding due to limited research on its safety in these populations.
- **Menstrual Cycle**: Some individuals may experience changes in menstrual flow when taking Dong Quai. Monitoring and adjusting dosage accordingly is advised.

By understanding the detailed preparation, dosage, and safety considerations of Dong Quai, individuals can effectively incorporate this ancient herb into their wellness practices to support circulatory health and address menstrual irregularities.

Evening Primrose Oil for Skin Health

Evening Primrose Oil, extracted from the seeds of the Evening Primrose plant, stands out as a pivotal ally in managing hormonal acne and inflammation, offering a natural remedy rooted in botanical wisdom. This oil is rich in gamma-linolenic acid (GLA), an essential fatty acid that plays a critical role in skin health and hormonal balance. GLA is known for its potent anti-inflammatory properties, making Evening Primrose Oil an effective solution for reducing the severity and frequency of acne breakouts that are often exacerbated by hormonal fluctuations.

To harness the benefits of Evening Primrose Oil for hormonal acne, it is recommended to incorporate it both topically and internally. Topically, the oil can be applied directly to the skin or added to moisturizers. For direct application, it's crucial to start with clean, dry skin. Using a dropper, place 2-3 drops of Evening Primrose Oil on your fingertips and gently massage it into the affected area, focusing on spots with active breakouts or inflammation. This method facilitates the direct absorption of GLA, targeting inflammation at its source. When adding Evening Primrose Oil to moisturizers, a ratio of 1:10 (oil to moisturizer) is suggested to maintain the efficacy of the oil without compromising the texture of the moisturizer. This blend should be applied to the face after cleansing, ideally in the evening, to support skin repair and rejuvenation overnight.

Internally, incorporating Evening Primrose Oil supplements can address hormonal imbalances contributing to acne. The recommended dosage for supplements is typically 500mg to 1300mg daily, taken with meals to enhance absorption. It's imperative to opt for high-quality, cold-pressed oil supplements to ensure maximum potency and purity. Consistent, daily intake over a period of several weeks is often necessary to observe significant improvements in skin condition and hormonal balance.

Safety considerations are paramount when using Evening Primrose Oil. While topical application is generally safe for most individuals, oral supplementation may interact with certain medications, including blood thinners and antipsychotics. Therefore, consulting with a healthcare provider before starting oral supplementation is advised, especially for individuals with pre-existing health conditions or those taking medication.

Additionally, monitoring for allergic reactions or sensitivity, particularly with topical use, is crucial. Conducting a patch test on a small area of skin before widespread application can help ensure compatibility and prevent adverse reactions.

Incorporating Evening Primrose Oil into the management of hormonal acne and inflammation offers a holistic approach to skincare, leveraging the natural therapeutic properties of this remarkable plant. By addressing the issue from both internal and external fronts, individuals can achieve a more balanced hormonal landscape and clearer, healthier skin.

Red Clover and Dong Quai Hormone Balance Tincture

Beneficial effects
Red Clover and Dong Quai Hormone Balance Tincture is designed to naturally support and balance hormonal health. Red Clover, rich in isoflavones, acts as a phytoestrogen to help balance estrogen levels, making it beneficial for easing menopausal symptoms such as hot flashes and night sweats. Dong Quai, known as the "female ginseng," is revered for its ability to regulate menstrual cycles, alleviate menstrual cramps, and act as a general tonic for the female reproductive system. Together, these herbs offer a synergistic approach to supporting women's hormonal balance and overall well-being.

Ingredients
- 1/4 cup dried Red Clover blossoms (Trifolium pratense)
- 1/4 cup dried Dong Quai root (Angelica sinensis)
- 1 pint (2 cups) high-proof alcohol (vodka or brandy, at least 40% alcohol by volume)
- Distilled water (as needed)
- Amber glass dropper bottle for storage

Instructions
1. Begin by measuring out the dried Red Clover blossoms and Dong Quai root. Ensure that these herbs are finely chopped or crushed to increase the surface area for extraction.
2. Combine the herbs in a clean, dry glass jar with a tight-fitting lid. A pint-sized mason jar works well for this purpose.
3. Pour the high-proof alcohol over the herbs, ensuring they are completely submerged. If necessary, use a clean spoon or spatula to mix and release any air bubbles trapped in the herbs.
4. If the herbs absorb the alcohol and rise above the liquid level, add enough distilled water to ensure the herbs are fully covered. The final mixture should be at least 40% alcohol to prevent spoilage.
5. Seal the jar tightly and label it with the date and contents. Store the jar in a cool, dark place, such as a cupboard or pantry, away from direct sunlight.
6. Shake the jar gently every day for 4 to 6 weeks. This agitation helps to extract the active compounds from the herbs into the alcohol.
7. After the steeping period, strain the tincture through a fine mesh strainer or cheesecloth into a clean bowl. Press or squeeze the herb material to extract as much liquid as possible.
8. Transfer the strained tincture into an amber glass dropper bottle for easy use and dosage. Label the bottle with the date and contents.
9. To use, add 1-2 droppers full of the tincture to water or tea, 2-3 times daily, or as directed by a healthcare professional.

Variations
- For a non-alcoholic version, glycerin can be used instead of alcohol, though the extraction may not be as potent.
- Add other hormone-supportive herbs such as Chasteberry (Vitex) or Black Cohosh for additional benefits, adjusting proportions as needed.

Storage tips
Store the tincture in a cool, dark place, ideally in an amber or dark-colored glass bottle to protect it from light. When stored properly, the tincture can last for several years.

Tips for allergens

For those with allergies to any of the herbs, please consult with a healthcare provider for alternatives. Ensure that all equipment and storage containers are clean and free from contaminants that could cause allergic reactions.

Scientific references

- "Phytoestrogen content of foods consumed in Canada, including isoflavones, lignans, and coumestan" in the journal Nutrition and Cancer highlights the isoflavone content in Red Clover and its benefits.

- "Effect of Angelica sinensis on the proliferation of human bone cells" in the journal Clinical Rheumatology discusses the beneficial effects of Dong Quai on the female reproductive system.

BOOK 12: HERBAL REMEDIES FOR CHILDREN

CHAPTER 1: GENTLE HERBS FOR COMMON AILMENTS

Chamomile for Colic and Restless Sleep

Chamomile, a gentle yet powerful herb, has been revered for centuries for its calming and digestive benefits, making it an ideal remedy for colic and restless sleep in babies and toddlers. To harness these benefits, chamomile tea serves as a safe and natural option to soothe your little one's discomfort. When preparing chamomile tea for children, it's crucial to ensure the tea is mild and the serving size is appropriate for their age.

Begin with selecting high-quality dried chamomile flowers, preferably organic, to avoid any pesticides or chemicals. For making the tea, you will need about 1 teaspoon of dried chamomile flowers for every cup of boiling water. This ratio ensures a gentle strength suitable for young children's more sensitive systems. Boil water in a clean pot, and once it reaches a rolling boil, remove it from the heat. Add the dried chamomile flowers to the pot and cover it with a lid to steep. Steeping for about 5 to 10 minutes is sufficient to extract the calming properties of chamomile without making the tea too strong for a child.

After steeping, strain the chamomile tea through a fine mesh sieve or a cheesecloth to remove all the flower particles, ensuring the tea is smooth and easy for a child to drink. Let the tea cool down to a warm, safe temperature before serving. For babies and toddlers, it's essential to check the temperature of the tea to avoid any risk of burns. A good practice is to test a few drops on the inside of your wrist; it should feel comfortably warm, not hot.

For infants under 6 months old, it's advisable to consult a pediatrician before introducing chamomile tea, as their primary nutrition should be breastmilk or formula. For older babies and toddlers, serving a small amount, such as 1 to 2 ounces of chamomile tea, can be effective in relieving colic symptoms and promoting relaxation. This mild dosage can be given up to twice a day, especially during times of distress or before bedtime to help ease them into sleep.

It's also beneficial to incorporate the serving of chamomile tea into a calming bedtime routine. This can include a warm bath, gentle rocking, and soft lullabies, followed by the warm chamomile tea, to signal to your child that it's time to wind down and prepare for sleep. The natural properties of chamomile work in synergy with these soothing activities to enhance the overall calming effect, making it easier for your child to fall asleep and stay asleep.

Remember, while chamomile tea is generally safe for children, it's always best to start with a small amount to see how your child reacts. Some children may have allergies to plants in the daisy family, including chamomile. If you notice any signs of an allergic reaction, such as a rash, hives, or difficulty breathing, discontinue use immediately and consult your pediatrician.

Elderberry Syrup for Immune Support

Elderberry syrup is a time-honored remedy, lauded for its **antiviral properties** and effectiveness in boosting the immune system, especially in children. The active compounds in elderberries, including **anthocyanins**, have been shown to enhance immune response and may shorten the duration of colds and flu. Preparing elderberry syrup at home allows for control over the ingredients, ensuring a natural and safe product for your family.

To begin making elderberry syrup, you will need:

- **1/2 cup of dried elderberries**. Ensure they are from a reputable source to avoid contamination with pesticides or harmful chemicals.
- **2 cups of water**. Use filtered water to ensure purity and enhance the syrup's quality.
- **1 cup of raw honey**. Honey acts as a natural preservative and sweetener, making the syrup palatable for children. Choose raw honey for its additional antibacterial properties. However, remember that honey is not recommended for children under 1 year of age due to the risk of botulism.
- Optional ingredients for added benefits include **cinnamon stick, cloves, and ginger root**. These spices can enhance the syrup's flavor and contribute additional immune-supporting properties.

Preparation Steps:

1. Combine the dried elderberries and water in a medium saucepan. If using, add the cinnamon stick, cloves, and ginger root at this time.
2. Bring the mixture to a boil, then reduce the heat and simmer for about 45 minutes to an hour, or until the liquid has reduced by half. This slow simmering process extracts the beneficial compounds from the elderberries.
3. Once the liquid has reduced, remove the saucepan from heat and let it cool until it is safe to handle.
4. Mash the elderberries gently using the back of a spoon to release any remaining juice.
5. Strain the mixture through a fine mesh sieve or cheesecloth into a large bowl. Press or squeeze the berries to extract as much liquid as possible.
6. After the liquid has cooled to lukewarm, add the raw honey and stir until it is fully dissolved. It's crucial to wait until the liquid is no longer hot to preserve the beneficial enzymes in raw honey.
7. Transfer the finished syrup to a sterilized glass bottle or jar. Store the syrup in the refrigerator.

Dosage for Children:

- For daily immune support during cold and flu season, a general guideline is **1 teaspoon daily for children aged 1-6 years** and **2 teaspoons daily for children aged 7-12 years**.
- During illness, the dosage can be increased to **every 2-3 hours**, but be sure to consult with a pediatrician or healthcare provider to confirm the appropriate dosage for your child's specific needs.

Safety Considerations:

- Always ensure that the elderberries are cooked thoroughly. Raw elderberries, as well as the plant's leaves and stems, contain compounds that can be toxic if ingested.
- If your child has an autoimmune disease, consult with a healthcare provider before introducing elderberry syrup, as its immune-stimulating properties may not be advisable in such cases.
- Monitor for any allergic reactions when introducing elderberry syrup to your child for the first time.

By following these detailed steps, you can create a potent and natural elderberry syrup at home, offering a comforting, immune-boosting remedy for your children during cold and flu season.

Ginger for Digestive Relief

Ginger, scientifically known as Zingiber officinale, has been a cornerstone in herbal medicine for its remarkable ability to alleviate digestive discomfort and nausea. This root herb, characterized by its pungent and spicy flavor, contains bioactive compounds such as gingerol, which is responsible for its medicinal properties. When addressing tummy troubles in children, ginger offers a gentle yet effective remedy, particularly for soothing nausea, improving digestion, and reducing discomfort.

To harness ginger's benefits for digestive health, one can prepare a mild ginger tea, which is both palatable and soothing for children. Start by selecting fresh, organic ginger root to ensure the absence of pesticides and contaminants. Wash the ginger root thoroughly under running water. Then, using a spoon, peel the skin off a small piece of ginger, roughly the size of a 1-inch cube, which is sufficient for one cup of tea. Grate the peeled ginger finely to maximize the surface area exposed to the boiling water, thereby extracting more of its beneficial compounds.

In a small saucepan, bring 1 cup of water to a near boil. Add the grated ginger to the water, then reduce the heat to a simmer. Allow the ginger to steep in the simmering water for about 5 to 10 minutes. The longer it steeps, the stronger the tea will be, so adjust the steeping time according to the child's taste preference and sensitivity. After steeping, strain the tea through a fine mesh strainer into a cup to remove all pieces of ginger.

Allow the ginger tea to cool to a warm, comfortable temperature before serving. For children, it's crucial to ensure the tea is not too hot to prevent burns. Testing the tea's temperature on the inside of your wrist can provide a good gauge; it should feel comfortably warm.

For young children and toddlers, serving sizes should be small, starting with 1 to 2 ounces of ginger tea to assess their tolerance. It's important to note that while ginger is generally safe, it's potent, and a little goes a long way, especially in young bodies. Observing the child after the first few sips for any adverse reactions is prudent. If they respond well, ginger tea can be offered in small amounts throughout the day, especially if they are experiencing nausea or digestive upset.

In addition to serving ginger tea, incorporating ginger into children's meals can help soothe digestive troubles. A small amount of grated ginger can be added to soups, porridges, or even apple sauce to provide the digestive benefits without overwhelming the dish's flavor.

While ginger is widely regarded for its safety, it's always advisable to consult with a pediatrician before introducing it as a remedy, especially for children under two years of age or those with specific health conditions. This ensures that ginger complements their dietary needs without interfering with any existing health issues or medications.

Utilizing ginger for tummy troubles in children offers a natural, time-tested approach to enhancing digestive wellness and comfort. By preparing ginger in a child-friendly tea or incorporating it into meals, parents can provide their children with a gentle, effective remedy for nausea and digestive discomfort, tapping into the ancient wisdom of herbal healing for modern-day wellness.

Lemon and Ginger Sore Throat Soother

Beneficial effects

The Lemon and Ginger Sore Throat Soother is a natural remedy designed to alleviate sore throat discomfort, often a symptom of colds or flu. Ginger, with its anti-inflammatory properties, helps reduce swelling and pain, while lemon provides a high dose of vitamin C, boosting the immune system. Honey acts as a natural cough suppressant and soothes the throat, making this remedy a triple-action approach to treating sore throat symptoms.

Portions

Makes about 2 cups

Preparation time

5 minutes

Cooking time

10 minutes

Ingredients

- 2 cups of water

- 1 inch fresh ginger root, thinly sliced
- 1/2 lemon, juiced
- 2 tablespoons honey, or to taste

Instructions

1. Start by bringing 2 cups of water to a boil in a small saucepan.

2. While the water is heating, wash the ginger root and slice it thinly. No need to peel the ginger, as the skin contains additional nutrients.

3. Once the water reaches a rolling boil, add the sliced ginger to the saucepan. Reduce the heat to a simmer.

4. Let the ginger simmer in the water for about 10 minutes. This allows the ginger's properties to infuse into the water, creating a potent base for the sore throat soother.

5. After simmering, remove the saucepan from the heat. Strain the ginger pieces from the water and pour the ginger-infused water into a mug.

6. Stir in the juice of half a lemon into the ginger water. Lemon not only adds flavor but also contributes vitamin C, which is essential for immune support.

7. Add 2 tablespoons of honey to the mixture, or adjust according to your taste. Stir well until the honey is completely dissolved in the mixture. Honey acts as a natural sweetener and soothes the throat.

8. Drink the mixture while it's still warm for the best soothing effect on the throat.

Variations

- For an extra immune boost, add a pinch of cayenne pepper to the tea. Cayenne pepper can help clear congestion.
- Incorporate a cinnamon stick during the simmering process for added flavor and additional anti-inflammatory benefits.
- Replace lemon juice with apple cider vinegar for a different flavor profile and additional antimicrobial properties.

Storage tips

It's best to consume the Lemon and Ginger Sore Throat Soother fresh, but if you need to store it, keep it in a tightly sealed container in the refrigerator for up to 24 hours. Reheat gently on the stove or in the microwave before drinking.

Tips for allergens

For those with allergies to honey, maple syrup can be used as a vegan alternative. It still provides sweetness and some soothing properties, though the consistency and flavor will be slightly different.

Scientific references

- "Anti-Oxidative and Anti-Inflammatory Effects of Ginger in Health and Physical Activity: Review of Current Evidence" published in the International Journal of Preventive Medicine highlights ginger's anti-inflammatory properties.
- "Honey: A Therapeutic Agent for Disorders of the Upper Respiratory Tract" published in the Journal of the Royal Society of Medicine Open discusses honey's effectiveness in cough suppression and throat soothing.

CHAPTER 2: TOPICAL REMEDIES FOR CUTS AND RASHES

Calendula Cream for Diaper Rash and Minor Wounds Provides recipes for making gentle salves suitable for children's delicate skin.

Beneficial effects
Calendula cream is a gentle, natural remedy ideal for soothing and healing diaper rash and minor wounds. Calendula, known for its anti-inflammatory and antimicrobial properties, helps reduce skin irritation and promotes faster healing of cuts, scrapes, and rashes. This cream is especially suitable for children's delicate skin, providing a protective barrier that moisturizes and heals.

Portions
This recipe yields approximately 8 ounces of cream.

Preparation time
15 minutes

Cooking time
30 minutes

Ingredients
- 1/4 cup calendula-infused oil (preferably olive oil or almond oil as the base)
- 1/4 cup shea butter
- 1/8 cup coconut oil
- 1 tablespoon beeswax pellets
- 1 teaspoon vitamin E oil (as a preservative and skin conditioner)
- 10 drops lavender essential oil (optional, for additional soothing properties)

Instructions
1. Begin by preparing the calendula-infused oil if you haven't done so already. This can be done by steeping dried calendula petals in your choice of carrier oil for several weeks or gently heating the petals in oil over a double boiler for a few hours. Strain the petals from the oil and set aside.
2. In a double boiler, combine the shea butter, coconut oil, and beeswax pellets. Heat the mixture over medium heat, stirring occasionally until all ingredients are melted and well combined.
3. Once melted, remove the mixture from the heat and let it cool slightly. Then, stir in the calendula-infused oil and vitamin E oil until everything is well incorporated.
4. If using, add the lavender essential oil to the mixture and stir well. Lavender oil can enhance the cream's soothing properties, making it even more effective for irritated skin.
5. Pour the mixture into a clean, dry container with a lid. An 8-ounce jar works well for this purpose. Allow the cream to cool and solidify completely before sealing with the lid.
6. Label your jar with the contents and date made. Store the cream in a cool, dry place.

Variations
- For a vegan version, substitute the beeswax with an equal amount of candelilla wax or soy wax.

- If calendula oil is not available, chamomile-infused oil can be used as a substitute for similar soothing effects.
- For extra sensitive skin, omit the essential oil or use chamomile essential oil for its hypoallergenic properties.

Storage tips

Calendula cream should be stored in a cool, dry place away from direct sunlight. If stored properly, the cream can last for up to 6 months. Always use clean hands or a spatula to scoop out the cream to prevent contamination.

Tips for allergens

For those with nut allergies, be sure to choose a suitable carrier oil for the calendula infusion, such as sunflower oil or jojoba oil, instead of almond oil. Always patch test a small area of skin before applying broadly, especially on children.

Scientific references

- "Anti-inflammatory and wound healing activity of a growth substance in Aloe vera," published in the Journal of the American Podiatric Medical Association, highlights the benefits of natural remedies in skin healing.
- "Antimicrobial activity of Calendula officinalis petal extracts against fungi, as well as Gram-negative and Gram-positive clinical pathogens," published in Complementary Therapies in Clinical Practice, supports the use of calendula in treating skin conditions.

Aloe Vera for Burns and Scrapes

Aloe Vera, scientifically known as **Aloe barbadensis miller**, is renowned for its soothing, moisturizing, and healing properties, making it an indispensable remedy for treating burns and scrapes, especially in children. This succulent plant contains a gel-like substance within its leaves, rich in bioactive compounds including vitamins, minerals, amino acids, and antioxidants, which collectively contribute to its therapeutic efficacy.

Extracting Aloe Vera Gel:

1. Select a mature **Aloe Vera leaf** from the lower part of the plant, as these contain a higher concentration of the active ingredients. Ensure the plant is healthy and free from any chemical treatments.
2. Wash the leaf thoroughly under running water to remove any dirt and debris.
3. Use a sharp knife to slice off the serrated edges of the leaf. Carefully split the leaf open lengthwise to expose the clear inner gel.
4. With a spoon or a butter knife, gently scrape out the gel, taking care not to include any of the yellowish latex from just under the skin, as this can be irritating for some individuals.
5. The fresh gel can be applied directly to the affected area. For ease of application, you may blend the gel for a few seconds to achieve a smoother consistency.

Applying Aloe Vera Gel on Burns and Scrapes:

- Clean the injured area gently with mild soap and lukewarm water to remove any dirt and prevent infection. Pat dry with a clean towel.
- Apply a thin layer of **Aloe Vera gel** directly onto the burn or scrape. The cooling effect of the gel provides immediate relief from pain and discomfort.
- For minor burns, cover the area with a clean gauze or a bandage to protect the skin while it heals. For scrapes, leaving it uncovered after applying Aloe Vera gel can promote faster healing.

- Reapply Aloe Vera gel 2-3 times a day until the skin is healed. Each time, ensure the area is clean before application.

Storage of Aloe Vera Gel:

- If you have extra gel, it can be stored in an airtight container in the refrigerator for up to a week. For longer storage, freeze the gel in ice cube trays. Once frozen, transfer the cubes to a freezer bag, labeling it with the date. Thaw a cube when needed.

Precautions:

- Conduct a patch test before applying Aloe Vera gel, especially if the child has sensitive skin or allergies. Apply a small amount on the forearm and wait for 24 hours. If there is no adverse reaction, it should be safe to use.

- Avoid using Aloe Vera gel on deep wounds or severe burns. In such cases, seek medical attention immediately.

- Ensure that the child does not ingest the gel, as consuming Aloe Vera latex (the yellow part) can cause digestive discomfort.

Incorporating **Aloe Vera** into your home first aid kit equips you with a natural and effective remedy for minor burns and scrapes. Its cooling, healing, and antimicrobial properties not only soothe the injury but also promote skin regeneration and prevent infection, making it a go-to solution for quick and safe recovery in children.

Lavender Oil for Calming Skin

Lavender oil, derived from the flowers of the **Lavandula angustifolia** plant, is celebrated for its remarkable soothing properties, making it an ideal remedy for calming irritated skin in children. Its efficacy in reducing redness and alleviating itching is attributed to its anti-inflammatory and antiseptic qualities, which help to soothe the skin and promote healing.

To utilize lavender oil for skin irritation, it's essential to dilute it properly to ensure it's safe for delicate skin. A recommended dilution is to mix **1 to 2 drops of pure lavender essential oil** with **1 tablespoon of a carrier oil**, such as **coconut oil** or **sweet almond oil**. These carrier oils are gentle on the skin and help to spread the essential oil evenly.

Application Process:

1. After diluting the lavender oil with your chosen carrier oil, perform a patch test on a small area of the child's skin. Wait for at least 24 hours to ensure there is no adverse reaction, such as increased redness or irritation.

2. If the patch test shows no negative reaction, you can proceed to apply the mixture to affected areas. Use a clean cotton swab or your fingertips to gently dab the oil onto the irritated skin. Avoid rubbing vigorously as this can exacerbate the irritation.

3. For best results, apply the lavender oil blend to the irritated skin **two to three times daily**. It's particularly beneficial to apply it before bedtime, as lavender also possesses calming properties that can help improve sleep quality.

4. Store any remaining blend in a cool, dark place in a sealed container. A small glass bottle with a dropper is ideal for this purpose, as it protects the oil from light degradation and allows for easy application.

Precautions:

- Always choose **100% pure lavender essential oil** to avoid synthetic additives that can irritate the skin.

- Never apply undiluted essential oils directly to the skin, especially on children, as their skin is more sensitive and prone to reactions.

- Discontinue use immediately if any signs of an allergic reaction occur, such as increased redness, itching, or rash, and consult a healthcare provider if necessary.

By incorporating lavender oil into your child's skincare routine, you can naturally and effectively soothe skin irritations, leveraging the gentle, healing properties of this ancient remedy. Its pleasant aroma also adds a soothing sensory experience, making it a multifaceted tool for promoting skin health and overall well-being in children.

Calendula and Chamomile Skin Soothing Balm

Beneficial effects

Calendula and Chamomile Skin Soothing Balm combines the gentle, healing properties of calendula and chamomile, both renowned for their ability to soothe and repair the skin. Calendula is a potent anti-inflammatory that helps heal wounds, soothe eczema, and reduce dermatitis. Chamomile complements calendula by providing calming effects, reducing skin irritation, and promoting faster healing of minor cuts and rashes. This balm is particularly beneficial for sensitive skin, making it an ideal choice for children and adults alike.

Portions

Yields about 4 ounces (120 ml)

Preparation time

10 minutes

Cooking time

20 minutes

Ingredients

- 1/4 cup calendula-infused oil
- 1/4 cup chamomile-infused oil
- 1/4 cup shea butter
- 2 tablespoons beeswax pellets
- 1 teaspoon vitamin E oil
- 10 drops lavender essential oil (optional, for added soothing properties)

Instructions

1. Start by creating the calendula and chamomile-infused oils. If not already prepared, infuse by gently heating dried calendula petals and dried chamomile flowers in a carrier oil, such as almond or olive oil, over low heat for 2-3 hours. Strain the flowers from the oil and set aside.

2. In a double boiler, melt the shea butter and beeswax pellets together over medium heat, stirring continuously until completely melted and combined.

3. Once melted, remove the mixture from heat and slowly stir in the calendula and chamomile-infused oils until the mixture is homogenous.

4. Add the vitamin E oil to the mixture, stirring well. Vitamin E acts as a natural antioxidant, which helps preserve the balm and provides additional skin-nourishing benefits.

5. If using, add the lavender essential oil to the mixture for its calming and anti-inflammatory properties. Stir thoroughly to ensure even distribution.

6. Carefully pour the liquid balm into clean, dry containers, such as small jars or tins. Allow the balm to cool and solidify at room temperature or place in the refrigerator to speed up the process.

7. Once solidified, seal the containers with lids to prevent contamination. Label each container with the product name and date made.

Variations
- For a vegan version, replace beeswax with an equal amount of candelilla wax.
- Add a few drops of chamomile essential oil for enhanced calming effects, especially beneficial for skin prone to inflammation or redness.
- For extra dry skin, increase the shea butter portion to 1/3 cup for a richer, more moisturizing balm.

Storage tips
Store the balm in a cool, dry place away from direct sunlight. If stored properly, the balm can last up to 1 year. Always use clean hands or a spatula when applying the balm to maintain its purity and prevent contamination.

Tips for allergens
For those with allergies to beeswax, candelilla wax is a suitable plant-based alternative. Always perform a patch test before widespread use, especially on sensitive skin, to ensure no allergic reaction occurs. If using essential oils, choose high-quality, pure oils and use sparingly to minimize the risk of skin irritation.

Scientific references
- "Anti-inflammatory and skin barrier repair effects of topical application of some plant oils," published in the International Journal of Molecular Sciences, highlights the benefits of calendula and chamomile in treating inflammatory skin conditions.
- "Wound healing and anti-inflammatory effect in animal models of Calendula officinalis L. growing in Brazil," published in Evidence-Based Complementary and Alternative Medicine, supports the use of calendula in wound healing and skin care.

CHAPTER 3: BUILDING IMMUNITY NATURALLY

Echinacea for Children's Immunity

Echinacea, a widely recognized herb for its immune-boosting properties, plays a significant role in preventing colds, especially in children. The herb's effectiveness stems from its ability to enhance the body's immune response, making it a valuable ally during the cold and flu season. When considering echinacea for children, it's crucial to understand the appropriate dosing, forms of echinacea suitable for children, and the duration of its use to ensure safety and efficacy.

For children, echinacea is available in various forms, including syrups, chewables, and drops. These forms are specifically designed to be palatable and acceptable for young palates, ensuring that the administration of echinacea is both easy and pleasant for the child. When selecting an echinacea product, look for those that are labeled as being specifically formulated for children. These products typically contain echinacea extracts that are diluted appropriately for children's use, taking into account their body weight and the sensitivity of their developing systems.

The dosing of echinacea for children varies by the product and the child's age. As a general guideline, for children aged 2 to 4, a dose of echinacea syrup might range from 2.5 milliliters (ml) up to three times a day. For children aged 5 to 9, the dose may increase to 5 ml three times a day. It's imperative to follow the dosing instructions provided on the product label or consult a healthcare provider for advice tailored to the child's specific needs.

The duration of echinacea use is another critical consideration. Echinacea is most effective when taken at the first sign of a cold and should not be used continuously for prolonged periods. A common recommendation is to use echinacea for 7 to 10 days. This duration helps to support the immune system in fighting off the cold virus without overstimulating the immune system.

Safety is paramount when administering echinacea or any herbal supplement to children. While echinacea is generally considered safe for short-term use in children, it's essential to be aware of potential allergic reactions, especially in children who are allergic to other plants in the daisy family. Observing the child for any signs of an allergic reaction, such as rash, itching, or difficulty breathing, is crucial during the initial days of echinacea administration.

Rosehip Syrup for Vitamin C

Rosehip syrup is a potent source of Vitamin C, an essential nutrient that plays a critical role in boosting the immune system, repairing tissues, and aiding in the absorption of iron. This natural remedy, derived from the fruit of the rose plant, has been used for centuries to prevent and treat colds, flu, and other infections due to its high antioxidant content. Making rosehip syrup at home is a straightforward process that requires minimal ingredients and provides a delightful way to supplement Vitamin C in your child's diet.

To prepare rosehip syrup, you will need fresh or dried rosehips, water, and honey or sugar. If using fresh rosehips, gather them after the first frost when they are soft and ripe. This timing ensures the highest concentration of Vitamin C. For dried rosehips, ensure they are sourced from a reputable supplier to guarantee potency.

Step 1: Preparing the Rosehips

Begin by rinsing 1 cup of fresh rosehips or ½ cup of dried rosehips to remove any debris. If using fresh rosehips, trim off the stem and blossom ends. Chop the rosehips coarsely to increase the surface area, which will help to extract the maximum amount of nutrients.

Step 2: Simmering

Place the prepared rosehips in a saucepan and add 3 cups of water. Bring the mixture to a boil, then reduce the heat, allowing it to simmer gently for about 20 minutes. If the water level reduces significantly during this process, add more to maintain the original volume.

Step 3: Straining

After simmering, let the mixture cool slightly. Then, strain it through a fine mesh sieve or cheesecloth to remove the solid parts. Press or squeeze the rosehips to extract as much liquid as possible. The resulting liquid is your rosehip decoction, rich in Vitamin C and other nutrients.

Step 4: Sweetening

Return the strained liquid to the saucepan and add honey or sugar. The ratio of sweetener to liquid can vary according to taste, but a general guideline is ¼ cup of honey or sugar for every cup of liquid. Gently heat the mixture, stirring until the sweetener is fully dissolved. Do not boil, as high heat can destroy Vitamin C.

Step 5: Bottling and Storing

Pour the hot syrup into sterilized glass bottles. Seal the bottles while the syrup is still hot to ensure a good seal. Once cooled, store the syrup in the refrigerator. Properly stored rosehip syrup can last for several months.

Usage

For daily immune support, a typical dose is 1-2 teaspoons of rosehip syrup for children, taken directly or mixed into a beverage, such as tea or water. Always consult with a healthcare provider before introducing any new supplement to your child's diet, especially if your child has specific health conditions or allergies.

Rosehip syrup offers a natural, tasty way to boost Vitamin C intake. Its preparation at home allows for control over ingredients, ensuring a pure and potent product. Integrating this syrup into your child's diet, especially during cold and flu season, can provide significant health benefits, supporting overall wellness and immune function.

Licorice Root for Respiratory Health

Licorice root, scientifically known as Glycyrrhiza glabra, has been a cornerstone in herbal medicine for centuries, particularly for its application in treating respiratory ailments among children. Its sweet, earthy flavor makes it more palatable for young ones, which is an added advantage when incorporating it into remedies aimed at soothing coughs and colds. The root possesses potent expectorant properties, meaning it helps in loosening and expelling mucus from the respiratory tract, thereby easing congestion and making breathing easier. Additionally, licorice root acts as a demulcent, providing a soothing coating to irritated throat tissues, which can be immensely relieving during bouts of coughing.

To harness the respiratory health benefits of licorice root for children, it's essential to understand the correct preparation and dosage to ensure safety and effectiveness. Begin by selecting high-quality, dried licorice root from reputable sources. This ensures the product is free from contaminants and of medicinal quality. For preparing a simple licorice root tea, which can be given to children experiencing coughs and colds, use the following detailed method:

1. Measure out about one teaspoon of dried licorice root for every cup of water. This ratio ensures a therapeutic concentration while keeping the flavor mild enough for children.

2. Bring the water to a boil in a small saucepan. Once boiling, add the licorice root and reduce the heat to a simmer. Cover the pan with a lid to prevent the volatile oils, which contain much of the plant's therapeutic properties, from escaping with the steam.

3. Allow the mixture to simmer gently for approximately 10-15 minutes. This slow extraction process is crucial for pulling out the beneficial compounds from the licorice root.

4. After simmering, remove the saucepan from the heat and let it cool to a safe temperature. Strain the tea to remove all pieces of the licorice root, ensuring the liquid is smooth and free from debris.

5. For children, the tea should be diluted further with warm water, making it a suitable strength. A general guideline is to mix equal parts of the licorice tea with warm water.

6. The recommended dosage for children should not exceed 2-3 tablespoons of the diluted tea, given two to three times a day. This recommendation is based on general safety guidelines for herbal remedies in children, but it's always best to consult with a healthcare provider to determine the appropriate dosage for your child's specific needs and conditions.

It's important to note that while licorice root is beneficial for respiratory health, its use should be limited to short-term relief of symptoms. Prolonged consumption can lead to adverse effects due to glycyrrhizin, a compound found in licorice root, which can cause issues such as elevated blood pressure and electrolyte imbalances when taken in large amounts or for extended periods. Therefore, licorice root tea should be used judiciously, particularly with children, and not exceed a week's duration without professional guidance.

In summary, licorice root offers a natural and effective remedy for alleviating coughs and colds in children, thanks to its expectorant and demulcent properties. By following the detailed preparation and dosage guidelines, parents can safely use licorice root to provide respiratory relief for their children, ensuring that this ancient remedy continues to serve as a gentle and beneficial option for supporting children's health.

Elderberry and Ginger Immune Boosting Tea

Beneficial effects

Elderberry and Ginger Immune Boosting Tea harnesses the potent antiviral and anti-inflammatory properties of elderberries and ginger, respectively, making it an excellent remedy for boosting the immune system and fighting off colds, flu, and other respiratory infections. Elderberries are rich in vitamins A, B, and C and stimulate the immune system, while ginger helps to reduce inflammation, soothe sore throats, and promote healthy digestion. This tea is a natural way to support the body's defenses and maintain overall health during the cold and flu season.

Portions

Makes about 4 cups

Preparation time

5 minutes

Cooking time

15 minutes

Ingredients

- 4 cups water
- 2 tablespoons dried elderberries
- 1 inch piece of fresh ginger root, thinly sliced
- 1 cinnamon stick
- 1 teaspoon dried echinacea (optional)
- Honey or lemon to taste (optional)

Instructions

1. In a medium saucepan, bring 4 cups of water to a boil.
2. Add 2 tablespoons of dried elderberries to the boiling water.
3. Thinly slice a 1-inch piece of fresh ginger root and add it to the saucepan, along with a cinnamon stick for added flavor and immune support.
4. If using, add 1 teaspoon of dried echinacea to the mixture. Echinacea is known for its immune-boosting properties and can enhance the effectiveness of the tea.
5. Reduce the heat, cover, and simmer the mixture for about 15 minutes. This allows the water to become infused with the flavors and beneficial properties of the ingredients.
6. After simmering, remove the saucepan from the heat. Strain the tea through a fine mesh sieve into a large pitcher or directly into cups, discarding the solids.
7. If desired, sweeten the tea with honey or add a squeeze of lemon for extra vitamin C and a refreshing taste.
8. Serve the tea warm for immediate use, or allow it to cool and serve over ice for a refreshing immune-boosting beverage.

Variations

- For a spicier kick, add a pinch of cayenne pepper to the tea while it simmers. Cayenne pepper can help to clear nasal congestion and relieve sore throat pain.
- Incorporate a slice of fresh turmeric root along with the ginger for additional anti-inflammatory benefits and a vibrant color.
- Replace the cinnamon stick with a few whole cloves or star anise to vary the flavor profile and add more depth to the tea's immune-boosting properties.

Storage tips

Store any leftover tea in a sealed glass container in the refrigerator for up to 3 days. Reheat gently on the stove or enjoy cold for a revitalizing drink. It's best to make fresh batches regularly to enjoy the maximum health benefits.

Tips for allergens

For those with allergies or sensitivities to honey, maple syrup can be used as a natural sweetener alternative. Ensure all ingredients are organic and free from contaminants to minimize the risk of allergic reactions.

Scientific references

- "The effect of Sambucus nigra L. (black elderberry) on the immune response: a systematic review" published in the Journal of Functional Foods highlights the immune-modulating effects of elderberry.
- "Anti-Oxidative and Anti-Inflammatory Effects of Ginger in Health and Physical Activity: Review of Current Evidence" published in the International Journal of Preventive Medicine discusses the health benefits of ginger, including its anti-inflammatory properties.

BOOK 13: HERBAL PET CARE

CHAPTER 1: SAFE HERBS FOR DOGS AND CATS

Chamomile for Calming Anxiety

Chamomile, scientifically known as Matricaria chamomilla, is a herb renowned for its calming and soothing properties, making it an excellent choice for pets experiencing anxiety. This gentle herb can be used in various forms, including teas and sprays, to help alleviate stress and promote relaxation in dogs and cats. When preparing chamomile for pets, it's crucial to ensure the correct dosage and application method to provide the benefits safely.

To create a chamomile tea for pets, start by boiling one cup of water. Once boiling, remove from heat and add two teaspoons of dried chamomile flowers. Cover and steep for about 15 minutes, allowing the therapeutic properties of the chamomile to infuse into the water. After steeping, strain the tea to remove all flower parts, leaving a clear infusion. Allow the tea to cool to room temperature before offering it to your pet. For small dogs or cats, start with a few tablespoons of the cooled tea added to their water bowl. For larger dogs, you may increase the amount to up to half a cup, mixed with their drinking water or poured over their food. This gentle introduction allows you to monitor your pet's response to the herb and adjust the dosage accordingly.

Creating a chamomile spray involves diluting chamomile tea with water to form a mild, soothing mist that can be sprayed on your pet's bedding, in their crate, or even lightly onto their fur. To make the spray, mix equal parts of the cooled chamomile tea with distilled water in a clean spray bottle. Shake well to combine. When using the spray, always avoid your pet's face, focusing instead on areas where the calming scent of chamomile can be inhaled or absorbed through the skin. The spray can be used before potentially stressful events, such as vet visits or during thunderstorms, to help ease anxiety.

It's important to note that while chamomile is generally safe for pets, individual animals may react differently to herbs. Observing your pet for any signs of allergic reactions or gastrointestinal upset after their first exposure to chamomile is essential. Discontinue use and consult with a veterinarian if any adverse reactions occur.

In addition to its calming effects, chamomile possesses mild antibacterial and anti-inflammatory properties, which can be beneficial for pets with skin irritations or minor wounds. However, the primary use in the context of pet care, as discussed here, focuses on its ability to soothe and reduce anxiety.

When introducing any new supplement or remedy into your pet's routine, including chamomile, starting with a small dose and closely monitoring their response is crucial. Always consult with a veterinarian before adding herbal treatments to your pet's care regimen, especially if your pet is currently on medication, to avoid any potential interactions. With the proper preparation and cautious use, chamomile can be a valuable addition to your pet's wellness routine, offering a natural means to support relaxation and reduce anxiety.

Slippery Elm for Digestive Relief

Slippery Elm (**Ulmus rubra**) is a valuable herb known for its ability to soothe and protect the digestive tract, making it an excellent choice for pets experiencing stomach upset and diarrhea. The inner bark of the Slippery Elm tree contains mucilage, a gel-like substance that coats and soothes the mouth, throat, stomach, and intestines, providing relief from irritation and inflammation. Additionally, it contains antioxidants that help alleviate inflammatory bowel conditions. Here's how to safely use Slippery Elm for your dogs and cats:

Preparation of Slippery Elm Bark Powder:

1. Start with high-quality, organic Slippery Elm bark powder. This ensures the product is free from pesticides and contaminants, which is crucial for the sensitive digestive systems of pets.

2. Measure the appropriate dosage. For small dogs and cats, a general guideline is to use ¼ teaspoon of powder per 10 pounds of body weight. Adjust the amount proportionally for larger pets.

Making a Slippery Elm Digestive Soothing Mixture:

1. Mix the measured Slippery Elm bark powder with cold water. Use about 1 tablespoon of cold water for every ¼ teaspoon of powder. Stir until it forms a thin, smooth paste.

2. Slowly add boiling water to the paste, stirring continuously. The goal is to create a gruel-like consistency. For every ¼ teaspoon of Slippery Elm powder, you'll need about ¾ cup of boiling water.

3. Allow the mixture to cool to room temperature before administering it to your pet. It should be lukewarm or cool to ensure it's comfortable for consumption and doesn't cause any thermal injury to your pet's mouth or throat.

Administering Slippery Elm:

1. The Slippery Elm mixture can be given directly by mouth using a syringe (without a needle) or added to your pet's food. If your pet is reluctant to consume the mixture due to its texture or taste, mixing it with a small amount of their favorite wet food or a palatable broth can encourage acceptance.

2. For acute cases of diarrhea or stomach upset, the Slippery Elm mixture can be administered 2-3 times a day. It's essential to monitor your pet's condition closely. While Slippery Elm is safe for short-term use, any persistent or worsening symptoms warrant a consultation with a veterinarian.

Precautions:

- While Slippery Elm is generally safe for pets, starting with a smaller dose and gradually increasing to the recommended amount can help ensure your pet tolerates it well.

- Ensure your pet has access to plenty of fresh water, as the fiber in Slippery Elm can absorb water from the digestive tract.

- Slippery Elm may interfere with the absorption of other medications. If your pet is on medication, administer Slippery Elm at least two hours before or after other medications.

Storage:

- Store Slippery Elm bark powder in a cool, dry place to maintain its potency. Properly stored, it can last for several months.

By following these detailed steps, pet owners can safely use Slippery Elm to provide relief for their pets experiencing digestive discomfort. Remember, while herbal remedies like Slippery Elm can be beneficial, they do not replace professional veterinary care for ongoing or severe conditions.

Dandelion Root for Detoxification

Dandelion root, scientifically known as Taraxacum officinale, is a powerhouse of nutrition and has been used for centuries in herbal medicine to support liver and kidney health in both humans and animals. For pet owners looking to incorporate natural remedies into their pets' care regimen, dandelion root offers a gentle yet effective method for promoting detoxification and enhancing overall well-being.

The liver and kidneys are critical for filtering toxins and waste from the body. In pets, just like in humans, these organs can become overburdened due to various factors such as environmental pollutants, processed foods, and the normal aging process. Dandelion root acts as a tonic for these organs, helping to stimulate their function and support the body's natural detoxification pathways.

To utilize dandelion root for your pets, it's essential to understand the proper preparation and dosage. The root can be administered in several forms, including teas, tinctures, and powdered supplements. When preparing a dandelion root tea, it's advisable to use about 1 teaspoon of dried root per 8 ounces of boiling water. Allow the tea to steep for 10-15 minutes before cooling. The tea can then be added to your pet's water or poured over their food. For a small dog or cat, start with a small amount, such as 1-2 tablespoons of the tea, to ensure they tolerate it well.

If opting for a tincture, look for alcohol-free versions specifically designed for pets. The general guideline for tincture dosage is 0.5ml per 20 pounds of body weight, administered twice daily. However, it's crucial to consult with a veterinarian experienced in herbal remedies to determine the exact dosage suitable for your pet's specific health needs.

For pet owners who prefer the convenience of supplements, powdered dandelion root can be mixed into pet food. Start with a small pinch for cats and small dogs, gradually increasing to as much as 1/4 teaspoon per 20 pounds of body weight, once daily. Again, monitoring your pet's response to the supplement and adjusting as needed is key.

When sourcing dandelion root, quality matters. Choose organic dandelion root whenever possible to avoid exposing your pet to pesticides and herbicides. Whether you're harvesting dandelion root from your yard or purchasing it, ensure it comes from a clean, pollution-free area.

It's also important to introduce dandelion root gradually into your pet's diet and observe their reaction. While dandelion root is generally considered safe for most pets, individual animals may have different sensitivities or allergies. Monitoring your pet for any signs of digestive upset or allergic reactions is essential when introducing any new supplement.

Incorporating dandelion root into your pet's health routine can be a natural way to support their liver and kidney function, contributing to their overall vitality and wellness. As with any herbal remedy, it's advisable to consult with a veterinarian to ensure it's appropriate for your pet's health status and to determine the optimal dosage. With the right approach, dandelion root can be a valuable addition to your pet's holistic health care arsenal.

Chamomile and Oatmeal Calming Pet Shampoo

Beneficial effects

Chamomile and Oatmeal Calming Pet Shampoo is designed to soothe and calm your pet's skin, especially if they suffer from irritations or allergies. Chamomile has natural soothing properties that can reduce skin inflammation and promote healing, making it perfect for pets with sensitive skin. Oatmeal, on the other hand, acts as a gentle cleanser that moisturizes the skin, helps relieve itching, and can soothe minor irritations. This homemade shampoo can leave your pet's coat clean, soft, and smelling fresh without the harsh chemicals found in many commercial pet shampoos.

Ingredients

- 1 cup of finely ground oatmeal
- 1 cup of chamomile tea (cooled)
- 1/2 cup baking soda
- 1 quart of warm water
- 1 teaspoon of mild dish soap or baby shampoo

Instructions

1. Begin by grinding the oatmeal in a food processor or blender until it reaches a fine, powder-like consistency. This ensures it will mix well without leaving large particles that could irritate your pet's skin.

2. Brew a strong cup of chamomile tea and allow it to cool completely. Chamomile tea can be made by steeping 2-3 chamomile tea bags in boiling water for about 15 minutes.

3. In a large mixing bowl, combine the finely ground oatmeal, cooled chamomile tea, and baking soda. Stir these dry ingredients together until they are well mixed.

4. Add the quart of warm water to the bowl, and stir thoroughly to ensure all the ingredients are fully dissolved and combined. The warm water helps to activate the oatmeal and baking soda, creating a soothing mixture.

5. Mix in the teaspoon of mild dish soap or baby shampoo. This will help the shampoo to clean more effectively without stripping the natural oils from your pet's coat.

6. Transfer the mixture into a large bottle or jar with a secure lid. Shake well before each use to ensure the ingredients are well combined.

7. To use, wet your pet's coat thoroughly with warm water. Apply the shampoo generously, working it into the fur from head to tail. Be careful to avoid the eyes and inside the ears.

8. Rinse the shampoo out thoroughly with warm water. Ensure all residue is removed, as leftover shampoo can cause irritation.

9. Dry your pet with a towel or let them air dry, depending on their preference.

Variations

- For pets with extra sensitive skin, you can omit the dish soap or baby shampoo. The oatmeal and chamomile alone provide gentle cleansing and soothing properties.
- Add a few drops of lavender essential oil for a calming scent and additional soothing properties. Ensure the essential oil is properly diluted and safe for pets.

Storage tips

Store the unused shampoo in a cool, dry place, and use it within 1-2 weeks. The natural ingredients are best when fresh, so consider making smaller batches if you bathe your pet infrequently.

Tips for allergens

If your pet has specific allergies, ensure that all ingredients are safe for their use. For pets allergic to grains, you can substitute the oatmeal with rice flour or coconut flour for similar soothing effects without the allergens.

Scientific references

- "Anti-inflammatory and skin barrier repair effects of topical application of some plant oils," published in the International Journal of Molecular Sciences, highlights the benefits of natural ingredients like oatmeal in treating inflammatory skin conditions.
- "Chamomile: A herbal medicine of the past with a bright future," published in Molecular Medicine Reports, discusses the anti-inflammatory and healing properties of chamomile, supporting its use in natural pet care products.

CHAPTER 2: TOPICAL AND ORAL REMEDIES

Calendula for Minor Wounds

Calendula, scientifically known as **Calendula officinalis**, is renowned for its healing properties, especially when it comes to treating minor wounds and skin irritations in pets. This herb acts as a natural antiseptic and anti-inflammatory agent, making it an ideal choice for a homemade topical cream aimed at accelerating the healing process of cuts, scrapes, and various skin issues.

To create a **Calendula Cream** for pets, you'll need the following materials and ingredients:

- **Dried Calendula Petals**: 1/4 cup. Ensure they are organic to avoid any chemical residues.
- **Carrier Oil** (such as coconut oil or olive oil): 1 cup. These oils are safe for pets and serve as the base for the infusion.
- **Beeswax**: 2 tablespoons. This will thicken the mixture into a cream consistency.
- **Double Boiler**: For gently heating the mixture.
- **Strainer or Cheesecloth**: To separate the petals from the oil.
- **Sterile Jar or Tin**: For storing the cream.

Preparation Steps:

1. **Infuse the Oil**: Begin by placing the dried calendula petals in the double boiler and covering them with the carrier oil. Heat the mixture over low heat for 2-3 hours to allow the healing properties of the calendula to infuse into the oil. Avoid high heat as it can destroy the beneficial compounds of the calendula.

2. **Strain the Mixture**: After the infusion process is complete, remove the mixture from heat. Using a strainer or cheesecloth, strain the oil into a clean bowl, ensuring all petals are removed.

3. **Add Beeswax**: Return the strained oil to the double boiler and add the beeswax. Heat gently, stirring continuously, until the beeswax is completely melted and well incorporated into the oil.

4. **Cool and Store**: Once the beeswax is fully melted and mixed, carefully pour the mixture into a sterile jar or tin. Allow the cream to cool and solidify at room temperature. Store in a cool, dry place.

Application:

- **Test for Sensitivity**: Before applying the cream to your pet's wound or irritated skin, test a small amount on a non-affected area to ensure there is no adverse reaction.
- **Clean the Affected Area**: Gently clean the wound or irritated skin with saline water or a mild antiseptic solution suitable for pets.
- **Apply the Cream**: Using clean fingers or a sterile applicator, apply a thin layer of the calendula cream to the affected area.

Frequency of Application:

- For best results, apply the cream 2-3 times a day until the wound begins to heal or the irritation subsides. Monitor the area for signs of improvement or any adverse reactions.

Note: While calendula is generally safe for pets, it's crucial to observe your pet's response to the cream. If you notice any signs of discomfort or allergic reaction, discontinue use immediately and consult a veterinarian. Always ensure the cream is applied to areas that your pet cannot lick or ingest. If the wound or irritation does not improve or worsens, seek veterinary care.

Lavender for Flea Control and Relaxation

Lavender, scientifically known as Lavandula angustifolia, serves a dual purpose in pet care: it acts as a natural flea repellent and provides relaxation benefits for pets. Its aromatic compounds, particularly linalool and linalyl acetate, are effective in deterring fleas without the harsh chemicals found in conventional flea treatments. Additionally, lavender's calming properties can help reduce stress and anxiety in pets, making it an invaluable herb in your pet care arsenal.

To harness the flea-repelling power of lavender, start by sourcing high-quality, organic dried lavender flowers. The quality of the lavender directly impacts its efficacy, so choosing organic ensures the absence of pesticides that could harm your pet. For a simple yet effective flea repellent, you'll need the following:

- Organic dried lavender flowers
- A clean spray bottle
- Distilled water
- A small pot for boiling water
- A fine mesh strainer or cheesecloth

Begin by boiling 2 cups of distilled water. Add 1/4 cup of dried lavender flowers to the boiling water and remove from heat. Cover and let the mixture steep for at least 1 hour, allowing the water to become infused with the lavender's essential oils and aromatic compounds. Once steeped, strain the mixture using a fine mesh strainer or cheesecloth into a clean spray bottle, ensuring all plant material is removed to prevent clogging the spray nozzle.

For pets sensitive to direct spray, apply the lavender water to a cloth and gently rub it onto your pet's fur, avoiding the face, especially the eyes and nose. This method can be used daily, particularly in flea season, to keep fleas at bay. Additionally, spraying your pet's bedding and favorite resting spots can create a flea-repellent environment, further protecting your pet from these pests.

Lavender's relaxation benefits for pets can be utilized by incorporating the herb into their environment. Creating a lavender sachet to place near your pet's sleeping area can help soothe and calm them. Simply fill a small cloth bag with dried lavender flowers and place it near where your pet sleeps. The gentle release of lavender's aroma can help reduce anxiety and promote a sense of calm, particularly in pets prone to stress or those with nervous dispositions.

For topical use, particularly for soothing irritated skin or minor scrapes, a lavender-infused oil can be beneficial. Combine 1 cup of a carrier oil, such as sweet almond oil or coconut oil, with 1/4 cup of dried lavender flowers in a glass jar. Seal the jar and place it in a sunny window for 2-3 weeks, shaking it every few days to distribute the lavender's essential oils. After the infusion period, strain the oil through a fine mesh strainer or cheesecloth, and store the lavender-infused oil in a clean, dark glass bottle. Apply a small amount of the oil to the affected area, ensuring it is fully absorbed and avoiding any open wounds.

Incorporating lavender into your pet care routine offers a natural, chemical-free approach to flea control and can significantly enhance your pet's comfort and well-being. Always observe your pet's reaction to lavender, especially when using it for the first time, to ensure they do not have an adverse reaction. While lavender is generally safe for pets, individual sensitivities can vary, and it's crucial to use any herbal remedy responsibly and in moderation.

Marshmallow Root for Pet Respiratory Health

Marshmallow root, scientifically known as Althaea officinalis, is a perennial herb that has been utilized for centuries in herbal medicine to soothe irritated mucous membranes, including those in the throat and respiratory tract. Its high mucilage content is primarily responsible for its demulcent properties, making it an excellent natural remedy for pets experiencing discomfort from sore throats and coughs. When administered, marshmallow root forms a protective layer on the lining of the throat and respiratory tract, which can help alleviate irritation and dryness that often leads to coughing.

For pet owners looking to incorporate marshmallow root into their pet's health regimen, it's essential to understand the appropriate form and dosage to ensure safety and efficacy. Marshmallow root can be prepared as a tea, which can then be cooled and added to your pet's drinking water or mixed with their food. To prepare the tea, steep approximately 1 teaspoon of dried marshmallow root in 8 ounces of boiling water for 10 to 15 minutes. Strain the tea to remove any plant material before offering it to your pet. The soothing effects of marshmallow root tea can help relieve your pet's sore throat and cough, providing much-needed comfort.

Another option is to use a marshmallow root tincture specifically formulated for pets. Tinctures are concentrated herbal extracts that offer a more straightforward method of administration, especially for pets who may not readily consume tea mixed with their water or food. The general guideline for tincture dosage is 0.5 ml per 20 pounds of body weight, administered up to three times daily. However, it's crucial to consult with a veterinarian before introducing marshmallow root or any new supplement to your pet's diet, as they can provide personalized advice based on your pet's specific health needs and conditions.

When sourcing marshmallow root, whether in dried form for making tea or as a tincture, always opt for high-quality, organic products to avoid exposing your pet to pesticides and other harmful chemicals. Organic marshmallow root ensures that you're providing your pet with a pure and safe remedy that supports their respiratory health without unintended side effects.

Arnica and Calendula Bruise Balm

Beneficial effects

Arnica and Calendula Bruise Balm harnesses the natural anti-inflammatory and healing properties of arnica and calendula. Arnica is widely recognized for its ability to reduce swelling and decrease pain, making it ideal for treating bruises, sprains, and sore muscles. Calendula, on the other hand, promotes wound healing and soothes skin irritations, enhancing the balm's overall effectiveness in skin repair and comfort. This combination makes the balm a powerful remedy for quick recovery from minor injuries.

Ingredients

- 1/4 cup arnica-infused oil
- 1/4 cup calendula-infused oil
- 1/4 cup coconut oil
- 2 tablespoons beeswax pellets
- 1 teaspoon vitamin E oil
- 10 drops lavender essential oil (optional for additional soothing properties)

Instructions

1. Begin by preparing the arnica and calendula-infused oils. If not pre-made, infuse by soaking dried arnica and calendula flowers in a carrier oil, such as olive or almond oil, for 4-6 weeks or gently heat the flowers in oil over a double boiler for 2-3 hours. Strain the flowers from the oil and set aside.

2. In a double boiler, melt the beeswax pellets over medium heat until fully dissolved.

3. Add the coconut oil to the melted beeswax and stir until the mixture is well combined and the coconut oil has melted completely.

4. Lower the heat, and slowly mix in the arnica and calendula-infused oils, stirring continuously to ensure a uniform mixture.

5. Remove the double boiler from the heat. Stir in the vitamin E oil, which acts as a natural preservative and skin-nourishing agent.

6. If using, add the lavender essential oil to the mixture for its calming and anti-inflammatory benefits. Stir well to distribute the oil evenly throughout the balm.

7. Carefully pour the mixture into small tins or jars. Allow the balm to cool and solidify at room temperature, which may take several hours.

8. Once solidified, seal the containers with lids to prevent contamination and preserve the balm's properties.

Variations

- For a vegan version, replace beeswax with an equal amount of candelilla wax or soy wax.
- Add a few drops of peppermint essential oil for a cooling effect, which can be soothing for injuries or swollen areas.
- For extra sensitive skin, reduce the amount of essential oil or omit it entirely.

Storage tips

Store the balm in a cool, dry place away from direct sunlight. If stored properly, the balm can last for up to 1 year. Always use clean hands or a spatula when applying the balm to maintain its purity and prevent contamination.

Tips for allergens

For those with allergies to beeswax, candelilla wax or soy wax are excellent alternatives. If you have sensitivities to any essential oils, they can be omitted without affecting the healing properties of the balm. Always perform a patch test before widespread use, especially on sensitive skin, to ensure no allergic reaction occurs.

CHAPTER 3: EMERGENCY HERBAL REMEDIES FOR PETS

Aloe Vera for Pet Injuries

Aloe Vera, known for its soothing and healing properties, is an invaluable asset for treating pets' burns and scratches. When your pet encounters a minor burn or scratch, reaching for Aloe Vera can provide immediate relief and promote faster healing. However, it's crucial to use Aloe Vera correctly to ensure the safety and comfort of your pet.

First, identify a pure Aloe Vera gel, either directly from the plant or a commercially available product that is free from added colors, fragrances, or alcohol. Products designed for human use often contain additives that may be harmful to pets if ingested. If you're using a plant, slice a leaf open and scoop out the clear gel.

Before applying Aloe Vera to your pet's injury, clean the affected area gently but thoroughly with mild soap and lukewarm water to remove any debris or contaminants. Pat the area dry with a soft, clean towel. This step is critical to prevent infection and ensure the Aloe Vera can effectively reach and heal the skin.

Apply a thin layer of Aloe Vera gel directly onto the burn or scratch. Use a light touch to avoid causing further discomfort. The cooling effect of Aloe Vera not only soothes the skin but also reduces inflammation and accelerates healing. For pets with fur, part the hair as much as possible to ensure the gel reaches the skin where it's needed most.

After application, monitor your pet to prevent them from licking the treated area. While Aloe Vera is generally safe for topical use, ingestion in large amounts can cause gastrointestinal upset in pets. If your pet is prone to licking, consider using a pet cone or a light bandage to cover the area temporarily.

Repeat the application of Aloe Vera gel two to three times a day until the burn or scratch shows significant improvement. If the injury does not heal or worsens, consult a veterinarian for further guidance. Remember, while Aloe Vera is effective for minor injuries, more severe burns or deep cuts require professional medical attention.

Oregon Grape Root for Infections

Oregon Grape Root, scientifically known as Mahonia aquifolium, possesses potent antimicrobial properties that make it an excellent choice for treating infections in pets. This herb is particularly effective against a range of pathogens due to its active compound, berberine, which has been shown to combat bacterial, fungal, and viral infections. When considering the use of Oregon Grape Root for pets, it's essential to understand the correct preparation and dosage to ensure safety and efficacy.

For topical applications, such as wounds or skin infections, a diluted tincture or an ointment made from Oregon Grape Root can be applied directly to the affected area. To prepare a tincture, soak the dried root in a mixture of alcohol and water for several weeks, shaking the container daily. After straining, the tincture can be diluted with water (a ratio of 1 part tincture to 3 parts water is generally safe) before application. For an ointment, infuse the powdered root into a carrier oil, such as coconut or olive oil, over low heat for several hours before mixing with beeswax to achieve the desired consistency. Apply a small amount of the ointment to the infected area, ensuring that the pet does not ingest any of the product.

In cases where internal treatment is necessary, such as for gastrointestinal or urinary tract infections, the administration of Oregon Grape Root should be approached with caution. Begin with a low dose of the tincture, diluted in water, and monitor your pet closely for any adverse reactions. The general guideline for tincture dosage is 0.5 milliliters per 20 pounds of body weight, administered up to three times daily. However, it's crucial to consult with a veterinarian experienced in herbal remedies to determine the appropriate dose for your pet's specific condition and size.

It's important to note that while Oregon Grape Root is a powerful antimicrobial agent, it should not be used as a first-line treatment for serious infections without veterinary guidance. Additionally, pets with liver conditions or pregnant animals should not be given Oregon Grape Root due to potential complications. Always source the herb from reputable suppliers to ensure purity and potency.

Incorporating Oregon Grape Root into your pet's care regimen can offer a natural alternative to conventional antibiotics, especially for minor infections or as part of a holistic treatment plan. By understanding the proper preparation, dosage, and precautions, pet owners can safely utilize the antimicrobial benefits of this herb to support their pet's health.

Nettle for Seasonal Allergies

Nettle (Urtica dioica), a perennial herbaceous plant, has been recognized for its therapeutic properties, especially in alleviating symptoms of seasonal allergies in pets. Its efficacy stems from its natural antihistamine and anti-inflammatory compounds, which can significantly reduce itching and irritation associated with allergies. To harness these benefits for your pet, it's crucial to understand the correct preparation and administration of nettle.

Preparation of Nettle for Pets:

1. **Drying Nettle Leaves**: Begin by harvesting nettle leaves, ideally in the spring when the leaves are young and tender. Use gloves to avoid stings. Rinse the leaves gently under cold water and pat them dry. Spread the leaves on a clean cloth or a drying rack in a well-ventilated, shaded area. Allow the leaves to air dry completely, which may take several days. Once dried, the leaves can be crumbled and stored in an airtight container away from direct sunlight.

2. **Making Nettle Infusion**: Measure one teaspoon of dried nettle leaves for every 10 pounds of your pet's body weight. Boil water and pour it over the dried nettle leaves in a heat-proof container. Cover and steep for 10 to 15 minutes. Strain the infusion to remove the leaves, ensuring no plant matter remains in the liquid.

3. **Nettle Tincture**: For a more concentrated remedy, a nettle tincture can be made by soaking dried nettle leaves in a mixture of grain alcohol and water. Fill a jar one-third full with dried nettle leaves, then cover completely with the alcohol-water solution. Seal the jar and store it in a cool, dark place for 3 to 6 weeks, shaking it every few days. Strain the mixture through a fine mesh sieve or cheesecloth, and store the tincture in a dark glass dropper bottle.

Administration:

- **Nettle Infusion**: Allow the nettle infusion to cool to room temperature before serving. The infusion can be added directly to your pet's water bowl or drizzled over their food. For a 10-pound pet, start with about 1 to 2 tablespoons of nettle infusion per day, adjusting based on your pet's tolerance and the severity of their allergies.

- **Nettle Tincture**: When using a tincture, the dosage should be significantly less due to its concentration. Begin with 1 drop per 10 pounds of body weight, added to your pet's food or water. Monitor your pet's response and gradually increase to a maximum of 3 drops per 10 pounds of body weight, if needed.

Precautions:
- Always introduce nettle gradually to your pet's diet to monitor for any adverse reactions.
- Consult with a veterinarian before adding nettle to your pet's regimen, especially if they are currently on medication or have chronic health issues.
- Ensure that the nettle used is free from pesticides and other chemicals.

Storage:
- Store dried nettle leaves in an airtight container in a cool, dark place to preserve their potency.
- Nettle tincture should be kept in a dark glass bottle and stored in a cool, dark area, lasting up to 2 years if properly stored.

By incorporating nettle into your pet's care routine, you can naturally mitigate the discomfort associated with seasonal allergies, reducing reliance on pharmaceuticals. This ancient remedy offers a gentle yet effective approach to enhancing your pet's quality of life during allergy season.

Chamomile and Lavender Calming Pet Spray

Beneficial effects

Chamomile and Lavender Calming Pet Spray is a gentle, natural remedy designed to soothe and calm your pet's nerves. It's perfect for pets who experience anxiety during thunderstorms, fireworks, or when facing separation anxiety. Chamomile is known for its calming and anti-inflammatory properties, helping to ease stress and relax muscles. Lavender, on the other hand, is renowned for its soothing scent and ability to promote relaxation and reduce anxiety. Together, these herbs create a calming atmosphere for your pet, making them feel more secure and at ease.

Ingredients

- 1 cup distilled water
- 1 tablespoon dried chamomile flowers
- 1 tablespoon dried lavender buds
- 1 small spray bottle
- 1 fine mesh strainer or cheesecloth
- 1 small funnel (optional)

Instructions

1. Begin by boiling the distilled water in a small saucepan. Once boiling, remove from heat.
2. Add the dried chamomile flowers and lavender buds to the hot water. Stir gently to ensure all the herbs are submerged.
3. Cover the saucepan with a lid and let the mixture steep for 15 to 20 minutes. This allows the water to become infused with the calming properties of the herbs.
4. After steeping, use a fine mesh strainer or cheesecloth to strain the herbal mixture into a bowl, removing all the solid herb parts. Press or squeeze the herbs to extract as much liquid as possible.
5. Allow the herbal infusion to cool to room temperature. This may take about 30 minutes to ensure it's cool enough for safe handling.
6. Once cooled, use a small funnel to transfer the infusion into a clean, dry spray bottle. If you don't have a funnel, you can carefully pour the liquid to minimize spills.
7. Secure the spray bottle's lid or nozzle in place. Shake well before each use to ensure the ingredients are well mixed.

8. To use, lightly mist the air around your pet, their bedding, or inside their crate. Avoid spraying directly onto your pet's face. Instead, spray the mixture onto your hands and gently pat your pet's fur or massage into their skin for a calming effect.

Variations

- For pets with extra sensitive skin, dilute the spray by adding an additional cup of distilled water.
- Add a few drops of CBD oil to the mixture for enhanced calming effects. Ensure the CBD oil is pet-safe and free from THC.
- Incorporate aloe vera juice to the spray for added skin-soothing benefits, especially useful for pets with dry or irritated skin.

Storage tips

Store the Chamomile and Lavender Calming Pet Spray in a cool, dark place to preserve its potency. Ideally, keep it in the refrigerator to maintain freshness and extend its shelf life. Use within 1 month for best results.

Tips for allergens

For pets with known allergies to chamomile or lavender, consider substituting with green tea or marjoram, which also have calming properties but may be more suitable for sensitive pets. Always perform a patch test on a small area of your pet's skin before full application to ensure there is no adverse reaction.

BOOK 14: HERBAL REMEDIES FOR CARDIOVASCULAR HEALTH

CHAPTER 1: HERBS FOR BLOOD PRESSURE

Hawthorn for Heart Health

Hawthorn, scientifically known as Crataegus species, is a plant whose leaves, berries, and flowers are used for medicinal purposes, especially for cardiovascular health. The efficacy of hawthorn in strengthening the heart comes from its rich composition of flavonoids, antioxidants, and oligomeric proanthocyanidins (OPCs). These compounds collectively work to enhance cardiac function and health by dilating blood vessels, which improves blood flow and circulation, and by strengthening the heart muscle itself.

To utilize hawthorn for heart health, it's essential to understand the specific methods of preparation and dosage that can maximize its benefits. The most common forms of hawthorn used for medicinal purposes include dried extracts of the plant, which can be made into teas, capsules, or tinctures. Each form has its own method of preparation and recommended dosage to ensure efficacy and safety.

For making a hawthorn tea, which is a gentle way to introduce this herb into your regimen, you would typically use 1-2 teaspoons of dried hawthorn berries, leaves, or flowers per cup of boiling water. Steep this mixture for about 15 minutes before straining. This tea can be consumed 2-3 times daily. The mild dosage makes it a suitable starting point for individuals new to using hawthorn for heart health.

Capsules containing hawthorn extract offer a more concentrated form of the herb, which means they can provide a stronger therapeutic effect. The typical dosage for capsules is between 250-500 milligrams taken 1-2 times daily. It's crucial to follow the manufacturer's or a healthcare provider's recommendations when using capsules to avoid exceeding the safe dosage.

Tinctures, another potent form of hawthorn, allow for the absorption of the herb's active compounds directly through the mucous membranes, offering a more immediate effect. A general guideline for tincture dosage is 1-2 droppers full (about 30-60 drops) taken 2-3 times daily. Diluting the tincture in water or tea can make it more palatable.

Regardless of the form chosen, consistency is key in experiencing the benefits of hawthorn. It may take several weeks or even months of regular use to notice significant improvements in heart health. It's also important to source hawthorn from reputable suppliers to ensure the quality and potency of the herb.

While hawthorn is generally considered safe for most people, it's advisable to consult with a healthcare provider before starting any new herbal supplement, especially for those with existing heart conditions, taking medications for heart disease, or undergoing any other treatment that might interact with hawthorn's effects. Monitoring your body's response to hawthorn and adjusting the dosage as necessary can help mitigate any potential side effects and ensure the best outcomes for heart health.

Garlic for Lowering Blood Pressure

Garlic, scientifically known as Allium sativum, has been widely recognized for its cardiovascular benefits, particularly its ability to lower blood pressure and improve heart health. The active compound responsible for these effects is allicin, which is produced when garlic cloves are crushed, chopped, or chewed. This compound works through several mechanisms to promote cardiovascular wellness, including the dilation of blood vessels which improves blood flow and reduces pressure on the heart.

For individuals looking to incorporate garlic into their diet for blood pressure management, it's important to understand the most effective forms and dosages. Raw garlic tends to offer the highest levels of allicin, but not everyone may tolerate its strong taste and potential digestive upset. As an alternative, aged garlic extract supplements are available and provide a concentrated form of garlic without the odor or harsh gastrointestinal effects. These supplements typically come in capsule form, with dosages ranging from 600 to 1,200 milligrams per day, as recommended by healthcare providers based on individual health needs.

To prepare garlic for consumption, one should first peel the cloves and then crush, slice, or mince them, which activates the enzymatic process that produces allicin. Letting the prepared garlic sit for a few minutes before cooking or consuming it raw can increase its health benefits. For those who prefer to incorporate garlic into their meals, adding it to sauces, dressings, or as a seasoning for meats and vegetables is an excellent way to enhance flavor while gaining its blood pressure-lowering effects. However, it's worth noting that high heat can reduce the potency of allicin, so adding garlic towards the end of the cooking process can help preserve its beneficial properties.

For individuals considering garlic supplements, it's crucial to select products that specify the amount of allicin or allicin potential on the label, ensuring a standardized level of the active compound. Quality supplements are tested for purity and potency and should provide clear dosage instructions. Starting with a lower dose and gradually increasing, as tolerated, can help minimize any potential side effects such as heartburn or upset stomach.

Regular monitoring of blood pressure levels is advisable when incorporating garlic into a health regimen, especially for those already on blood pressure medications, as garlic can potentiate the effects of these drugs. Consulting with a healthcare provider before starting any new supplement is essential to avoid adverse interactions and ensure that garlic is a safe and appropriate option for individual health circumstances.

Incorporating garlic into one's diet or supplement regimen requires understanding and patience, as the benefits on blood pressure and overall cardiovascular health may take several weeks to become evident. Maintaining a balanced diet, rich in a variety of fruits, vegetables, whole grains, and lean proteins, alongside regular physical activity, is fundamental to achieving the best outcomes for heart health and well-being.

Olive Leaf for Circulatory Support

Olive leaf, derived from the **Olea europaea** tree, has been utilized for centuries in traditional medicine across various cultures, primarily for its ability to bolster cardiovascular health. The leaf is rich in a compound known as **oleuropein**, which is credited with a multitude of health benefits, including potent **anti-inflammatory** and **antioxidant** properties. These characteristics make olive leaf an excellent choice for supporting circulatory health and managing blood pressure levels.

For individuals looking to incorporate olive leaf into their regimen for circulatory support, it's important to understand the most effective forms and dosages. Olive leaf can be consumed in several forms, including **capsules**, **tinctures**, and **teas**. Each form has its unique advantages and considerations:

- **Capsules**: Olive leaf extract capsules are a convenient option for those seeking a quick and easy way to consume the herb. When selecting capsules, look for products standardized to contain a high percentage of oleuropein, typically ranging from **20% to 40%**. The recommended dosage for capsules often varies between **500 to 1000 mg** daily, taken with meals to enhance absorption.

- **Tinctures**: A tincture allows for more customizable dosing and can be particularly useful for those adjusting their intake based on personal health responses. To create an olive leaf tincture, the leaves are soaked in a solution of alcohol and water, extracting a wide range of beneficial compounds. For usage, **1-2 ml** of tincture can be taken up to **three times daily**, either directly under the tongue or diluted in a small amount of water or juice.

- **Teas**: Brewing tea from olive leaves is a traditional method that provides a gentler dose of the herb's active compounds. To prepare olive leaf tea, steep **1-2 teaspoons** of dried olive leaves in hot water for **8-10 minutes**. This can be consumed **2-3 times daily**. While tea offers a lower concentration of oleuropein compared to capsules and tinctures, it is still beneficial and can be a soothing way to enjoy the health properties of olive leaf.

In addition to its cardiovascular benefits, olive leaf has been shown to support immune function, help regulate blood sugar levels, and improve overall well-being. However, as with any supplement, it's crucial to consult with a healthcare provider before starting olive leaf, especially for those with existing health conditions or those taking medication for blood pressure or blood thinning, as olive leaf may potentiate the effects of these medications.

To ensure the highest quality and efficacy, select olive leaf products from reputable suppliers that provide transparent information about sourcing, standardization, and manufacturing practices. Storage should be in a cool, dry place to preserve the integrity of the olive leaf's active compounds.

By integrating olive leaf into a holistic approach to health, including a balanced diet and regular physical activity, individuals can support their circulatory system and contribute to overall cardiovascular health without the need for synthetic interventions.

CHAPTER 2: CHOLESTEROL MANAGEMENT WITH HERBS

Fenugreek for Lowering LDL Cholesterol

Fenugreek, scientifically known as Trigonella foenum-graecum, has been a cornerstone in traditional medicine for centuries, particularly for its role in managing cholesterol levels. This herb contains a myriad of compounds, including soluble fiber, which is pivotal in reducing low-density lipoprotein (LDL) or "bad" cholesterol. Incorporating fenugreek into one's diet or wellness regimen can be a strategic move towards improving cardiovascular health by modulating lipid profiles.

The mechanism by which fenugreek aids in cholesterol management is multifaceted. Primarily, the soluble fiber found in fenugreek seeds acts by binding to cholesterol in the intestines, preventing its absorption into the bloodstream. This process not only helps in lowering LDL cholesterol but also contributes to regulating blood sugar levels, which is beneficial for individuals managing diabetes—a condition often linked with elevated cardiovascular risk.

To harness the cholesterol-lowering benefits of fenugreek, it can be consumed in various forms. The seeds can be soaked in water overnight and consumed on an empty stomach each morning. This method not only makes the seeds softer and easier to digest but also enhances their bioactive compounds' availability. Alternatively, fenugreek seeds can be ground into a powder and added to hot water to make tea. Consuming one to two cups of fenugreek tea daily can contribute to lowering LDL cholesterol levels. Another practical approach is incorporating fenugreek powder into everyday cooking, such as adding it to dough for bread or blending it into smoothies. For those looking for a more direct and convenient option, fenugreek supplements are available in capsule form. It is recommended to start with a lower dose, gradually increasing it to avoid potential gastrointestinal discomfort, a common side effect due to the high fiber content.

When selecting fenugreek seeds or powder, opting for organic and non-irradiated products ensures the preservation of its medicinal qualities. Storage should be in a cool, dry place, in airtight containers to maintain freshness and potency. For individuals considering fenugreek supplements, selecting products that specify the percentage of saponins and fibers can provide insight into the efficacy of the supplement, as these are the active components responsible for fenugreek's health benefits.

While fenugreek is generally safe for most individuals, it is crucial to consult with a healthcare provider before incorporating it into your health regimen, especially for those on medication for diabetes or blood thinning, as fenugreek can potentiate the effects of these medications. Pregnant women should avoid fenugreek due to its potential to stimulate uterine contractions.

Incorporating fenugreek into one's diet represents a natural, adjunctive strategy to managing cholesterol levels and improving overall cardiovascular health. Its versatility in culinary uses and availability in supplement form makes it accessible for individuals looking to enhance their wellness routine with herbal remedies. As with any dietary change or supplement introduction, monitoring cholesterol levels through regular blood tests will provide insight into the effectiveness of fenugreek in managing cholesterol and allow for adjustments as needed to achieve optimal cardiovascular health.

Artichoke for Healthy Cholesterol

Artichoke, scientifically known as **Cynara scolymus**, has been recognized for its potential to promote healthy cholesterol levels by enhancing bile production and reducing the absorption of cholesterol in the digestive system. The active component in artichoke leaves, **cynarin**, is believed to be responsible for these beneficial effects. Additionally, artichokes are rich in dietary fiber, which further aids in lowering cholesterol levels by binding with cholesterol in the intestines and preventing its absorption into the bloodstream.

To leverage the cholesterol-managing benefits of artichoke, incorporating artichoke hearts into your diet is a straightforward approach. Fresh, canned, or frozen artichoke hearts can be added to salads, pasta dishes, or eaten as a steamed vegetable with a squeeze of lemon for flavor. However, for those looking to maximize the intake of cynarin, artichoke leaf extract supplements may be a more concentrated source.

When selecting an **artichoke leaf extract supplement**, it's important to choose a product standardized to contain a specific percentage of cynarin or caffeoylquinic acids, the compounds believed to contribute to artichoke's lipid-lowering effects. A common dosage for artichoke leaf extract is between **300 to 600 mg**, taken three times daily with meals. This dosage can provide the liver support needed to enhance bile production, which not only aids in fat digestion but also in the excretion of cholesterol from the body.

For those preferring a more traditional consumption method, preparing a tea from dried artichoke leaves is another option. To prepare artichoke tea, steep approximately **1 to 2 teaspoons** of dried artichoke leaves in hot water for 10 to 15 minutes. This tea can be consumed once or twice daily. While the taste may be slightly bitter due to the cynarin content, adding a bit of honey or lemon can improve its palatability.

It's crucial to note that while artichokes can contribute to a strategy for managing cholesterol levels, they should be part of a broader approach that includes a balanced diet rich in fruits, vegetables, whole grains, and lean proteins, as well as regular physical activity. Individuals with bile duct obstruction or gallstones should exercise caution with artichoke supplementation, as increased bile production can exacerbate these conditions.

Moreover, always consult with a healthcare provider before starting any new supplement regimen, especially if you are currently taking medication for cholesterol management, as artichoke supplements may interact with these medications.

Incorporating artichoke into your diet or supplement routine can offer a natural way to support cardiovascular health by managing cholesterol levels. With its ability to enhance bile production and reduce cholesterol absorption, artichoke stands out as a valuable component of a heart-healthy lifestyle.

Psyllium for Cholesterol Reduction

Psyllium, derived from the seeds of the Plantago ovata plant, stands out as a highly effective natural fiber for reducing cholesterol levels and enhancing digestive health. This soluble fiber works by absorbing water in the gut, forming a gel-like substance that binds to fats and cholesterol, facilitating their removal from the body. The process not only aids in lowering the levels of low-density lipoprotein (LDL) or "bad" cholesterol but also supports the regulation of blood sugar levels, making psyllium a valuable addition to a heart-healthy diet.

For individuals aiming to incorporate psyllium into their daily regimen, it is available in various forms, including whole husks, powder, and capsules. Each form offers a versatile means of consumption, allowing for easy integration into meals and beverages. When opting for psyllium powder, it can be mixed into a glass of water, juice, or smoothies. The key is to consume it immediately after mixing, as psyllium thickens rapidly when combined with liquids. For those who prefer a more straightforward approach, psyllium capsules provide a convenient alternative, with the recommended dosage typically ranging from 5 to 10 grams per day, taken with at least 8 ounces of water to ensure proper hydration and effectiveness of the fiber.

Incorporating psyllium into one's diet requires a gradual approach to allow the digestive system to adjust to the increased fiber intake. Starting with a lower dose and slowly increasing it over several weeks can help minimize potential gastrointestinal side effects such as bloating or gas. Additionally, ensuring adequate water intake throughout the day is crucial when consuming psyllium to enhance its cholesterol-binding properties and facilitate its passage through the digestive tract.

Beyond its cholesterol-lowering benefits, psyllium plays a significant role in promoting regular bowel movements and preventing constipation, further testament to its value in digestive health. Its ability to swell and form a gel not only aids in softening stools but also in regulating bowel movements, contributing to overall gastrointestinal wellness.

When selecting psyllium products, it is essential to choose those that are 100% pure psyllium husk or powder, without added sugars or artificial ingredients, to maximize health benefits. Quality and purity are critical factors to consider, as these directly impact the efficacy of psyllium in cholesterol management and digestive support. Storage of psyllium should be in a cool, dry place to maintain its freshness and potency over time.

While psyllium is generally safe for most individuals, those with pre-existing digestive conditions such as Crohn's disease, ulcerative colitis, or intestinal obstructions should consult with a healthcare provider before introducing psyllium into their diet. Similarly, individuals taking medications for diabetes, cholesterol, or blood thinners should seek medical advice, as psyllium can affect the absorption and efficacy of certain medications.

Incorporating psyllium into a balanced diet, rich in fruits, vegetables, whole grains, and lean proteins, alongside regular physical activity, can significantly contribute to cardiovascular health and overall well-being. Its natural, cholesterol-lowering, and digestive-enhancing properties make psyllium a valuable component of a holistic approach to health maintenance and disease prevention.

Hawthorn Berry and Garlic Cholesterol Support Tonic

Beneficial effects

Hawthorn Berry and Garlic Cholesterol Support Tonic combines the heart-healthy benefits of hawthorn berries and the cholesterol-lowering properties of garlic. Hawthorn berries are known for their ability to strengthen the cardiovascular system, improve circulation, and manage blood pressure. Garlic, on the other hand, has been shown to lower cholesterol levels, reduce blood pressure, and support overall heart health. Together, they create a powerful tonic that can help maintain cardiovascular health and reduce the risk of heart disease.

Portions

Makes about 2 cups

Preparation time

15 minutes

Cooking time

5 minutes

Ingredients

- 1 cup fresh hawthorn berries (or 1/2 cup dried)
- 4 cloves of fresh garlic, minced
- 2 cups water

- 1 tablespoon honey (optional, for taste)
- 1 teaspoon lemon juice (optional, for taste)

Instructions

1. If using fresh hawthorn berries, wash them thoroughly under running water. If using dried hawthorn berries, ensure they are free from any debris or dust.

2. In a medium saucepan, combine the hawthorn berries and water. Bring the mixture to a boil over medium-high heat, then reduce the heat to low and simmer for 10 minutes. The water should take on a reddish hue as the berries release their beneficial compounds.

3. Add the minced garlic to the saucepan in the last 2 minutes of simmering. Garlic is added later in the cooking process to preserve its allicin content, which is responsible for its cholesterol-lowering effects.

4. Remove the saucepan from the heat and allow the mixture to cool slightly. Strain the tonic through a fine mesh strainer or cheesecloth into a clean container, pressing on the solids to extract as much liquid as possible.

5. Stir in the honey and lemon juice, if using, until well combined. These ingredients can help improve the taste of the tonic, making it more palatable.

6. Pour the finished tonic into a glass bottle or jar with a tight-fitting lid for storage.

Variations

- For a stronger tonic, allow the hawthorn berries and garlic to steep in the hot water for an additional 10-15 minutes after simmering.
- Add a cinnamon stick during the simmering process for added flavor and potential blood sugar regulation benefits.
- Substitute apple cider vinegar for lemon juice to enhance the tonic's heart-healthy properties.

Storage tips

Store the Hawthorn Berry and Garlic Cholesterol Support Tonic in the refrigerator for up to 1 week. Shake well before each use as natural separation may occur.

Tips for allergens

For those with allergies to honey, substitute it with maple syrup or simply omit the sweetener altogether. Ensure all ingredients are organic to minimize exposure to pesticides and other chemicals.

Scientific references

- "Hawthorn extract for treating chronic heart failure: Meta-analysis of randomized trials." Published in the American Journal of Medicine, this study highlights the cardiovascular benefits of hawthorn berry extract.
- "Garlic for the prevention of cardiovascular morbidity and mortality in hypertensive patients." Published in the Cochrane Database of Systematic Reviews, this review discusses the positive effects of garlic on cardiovascular health, including cholesterol reduction.

CHAPTER 3: HERBS FOR HEART HEALTH

Ginkgo Biloba for Improved Circulation

Ginkgo Biloba, a tree native to China, has been used in traditional medicine for thousands of years. Its leaves contain potent compounds that are believed to have significant benefits for circulatory health, particularly in enhancing blood flow and preventing blood clots. The active ingredients in Ginkgo Biloba, including flavonoids and terpenoids, are credited with these beneficial effects. Flavonoids are known for their antioxidant properties, while terpenoids improve blood flow by dilating blood vessels and reducing the stickiness of platelets.

To harness the circulatory benefits of Ginkgo Biloba, it is available in various forms, such as capsules, tablets, teas, and extracts. For improving circulation, the standardized extract, often labeled as **EGb 761**, is widely recommended because it ensures a consistent dose of the active compounds. The typical dosage for circulatory health ranges from **120 to 240 mg** of the standardized extract, divided into two or three doses throughout the day. This regimen helps maintain steady levels of Ginkgo Biloba's active ingredients in the bloodstream.

When selecting a Ginkgo Biloba supplement, look for products that specify they contain 24% flavone glycosides and 6% terpene lactones, the ratio found in most clinical studies. It's crucial to choose a high-quality supplement from a reputable manufacturer to ensure purity and potency. Some products may also be certified by third-party testing organizations, providing an additional layer of assurance regarding their quality.

For those preferring a natural approach, brewing tea from dried Ginkgo leaves is an option. To prepare Ginkgo tea, steep one teaspoon of dried leaves in hot water for 10 minutes. Strain and enjoy this tea once or twice daily. While the tea may offer a lower concentration of the active compounds compared to extracts, it still provides a beneficial amount for circulatory health.

It's important to start with a lower dose of Ginkgo Biloba and gradually increase to the recommended dosage to monitor how your body responds. Some individuals may experience mild side effects, such as headache, dizziness, or stomach upset, which typically resolve as the body adjusts.

Ginkgo Biloba's blood-thinning properties mean it should be used with caution by those taking anticoagulant medications, such as warfarin or aspirin, to avoid an increased risk of bleeding. Consulting with a healthcare provider before starting Ginkgo Biloba is advisable, especially for individuals with existing health conditions or those taking other medications.

Incorporating Ginkgo Biloba into a daily routine aimed at improving circulation can be part of a holistic approach to cardiovascular health. This regimen should also include a balanced diet, regular physical activity, and other lifestyle measures that support good circulation and heart health. Remember, while Ginkgo Biloba is a valuable tool for enhancing circulation, it works best when combined with other healthy habits.

Motherwort for Heart Rhythm Support

Motherwort, scientifically known as Leonurus cardiaca, stands out as a remarkable herb in the realm of cardiovascular health, particularly for its efficacy in calming heart palpitations and regulating heartbeat. This perennial plant, belonging to the mint family, has been utilized for centuries across various cultures for its heart-supportive properties. Its active compounds, including iridoids, flavonoids, and alkaloids, contribute to its therapeutic effects, making it a valuable component of natural cardiovascular care.

To harness the benefits of motherwort for heart rhythm support, it's essential to understand the appropriate preparation and dosage. A standard method involves creating a motherwort tincture, which involves steeping the dried aerial parts of the plant in alcohol. To prepare this tincture, one would typically use a ratio of 1 part dried motherwort to 4 parts alcohol (40-60% alcohol by volume), allowing the mixture to macerate for 4 to 6 weeks in a cool, dark place, shaking it daily. After straining the plant material, the resulting tincture can be administered in doses of 15-30 drops, up to three times a day. This method of preparation aims to extract the maximum spectrum of beneficial compounds, ensuring a potent remedy for heart rhythm irregularities.

For those preferring a non-alcoholic preparation, motherwort can also be consumed as a tea. To prepare motherwort tea, add 1-2 teaspoons of dried motherwort to a cup of boiling water, allowing it to steep for 10-15 minutes. This tea can be consumed 2-3 times daily. While the tea form may offer a milder effect compared to the tincture, it still provides significant benefits for heart health, particularly in soothing palpitations and supporting a regular heartbeat.

It's important to note that while motherwort is generally considered safe for most adults, it should be used with caution in certain populations. Pregnant women should avoid motherwort due to its potential to stimulate uterine contractions. Additionally, those on medications for heart conditions or blood thinners should consult with a healthcare provider before incorporating motherwort into their regimen, to avoid possible interactions.

As with any herbal remedy, the key to achieving the best outcomes with motherwort lies in consistency and patience. Regular, mindful use of motherwort, in conjunction with a healthy lifestyle, can provide significant benefits for those seeking to calm palpitations and maintain a healthy heart rhythm. Whether opting for a tincture or tea, motherwort offers a time-honored, natural solution for enhancing heart health and promoting a sense of calm and well-being.

Cayenne Pepper for Circulatory Health

Cayenne pepper, scientifically known as Capsicum annuum, is a potent herb widely recognized for its ability to stimulate circulation and reduce cardiovascular strain. The active compound in cayenne pepper, capsaicin, is responsible for its heat and therapeutic benefits, including its remarkable effect on the circulatory system. Capsaicin aids in enhancing blood flow by stimulating the release of nitric oxide in the body, a molecule that helps dilate blood vessels, allowing for improved circulation and nutrient delivery throughout the body.

To incorporate cayenne pepper into a heart-healthy regimen, it's important to understand the optimal forms and dosages. Cayenne can be consumed in various forms, such as fresh peppers, dried spice, capsules, and tinctures. For those new to cayenne, starting with a small amount, such as a pinch of the dried spice in meals, can help gauge tolerance. Gradually, one can increase to more therapeutic doses, typically between 30,000 to 120,000 Scoville Heat Units (SHU) for supplements, depending on individual tolerance and the advice of a healthcare provider.

For topical applications, cayenne pepper can be used in creams and salves to relieve muscle and joint pain, further showcasing its versatility beyond circulatory health. When preparing a topical application, mixing a small amount of ground cayenne pepper with a carrier oil or unscented lotion and applying it to the affected area can help reduce pain and inflammation. It's crucial to perform a patch test on a small skin area to ensure no adverse reactions occur.

Incorporating cayenne pepper into daily health practices requires careful consideration of its heat and potency. Drinking plenty of water and starting with lower concentrations can help mitigate any gastrointestinal discomfort, a common side effect for those not accustomed to capsaicin. Additionally, wearing gloves when handling fresh or dried cayenne pepper can prevent skin irritation or burning sensations.

For individuals looking to support their cardiovascular health naturally, cayenne pepper offers a multifaceted approach by not only improving circulation but also by contributing to the reduction of arterial plaque buildup. This is attributed to capsaicin's ability to lower blood cholesterol and triglyceride levels, further emphasizing cayenne's role in heart health.

While cayenne pepper is generally safe for most individuals, those with heart conditions, gastrointestinal issues, or those on certain medications should consult with a healthcare professional before incorporating it into their health regimen. This ensures compatibility with existing health conditions and medications, avoiding any potential interactions.

As part of a comprehensive approach to cardiovascular wellness, combining cayenne pepper with a balanced diet rich in fruits, vegetables, whole grains, and lean proteins, along with regular physical activity, can amplify its benefits. This holistic strategy not only focuses on enhancing circulatory health but also supports overall well-being, highlighting the importance of natural remedies like cayenne pepper in maintaining cardiovascular function and reducing strain on the heart.

Hawthorn and Hibiscus Heart Tonic

Beneficial effects

Hawthorn and Hibiscus Heart Tonic is a natural remedy designed to support cardiovascular health. Hawthorn berries are celebrated for their ability to strengthen the heart and improve circulation, while hibiscus flowers are known for their blood pressure-lowering effects and high antioxidant content. Together, these ingredients create a tonic that may help regulate blood pressure, reduce cholesterol levels, and provide antioxidant protection against heart disease.

Portions

Makes about 4 cups

Preparation time

10 minutes

Cooking time

20 minutes

Ingredients

- 1/2 cup dried hawthorn berries
- 1/2 cup dried hibiscus flowers
- 4 cups water
- 2 tablespoons honey (optional)
- 1 lemon, juiced (optional)

Instructions

1. In a medium saucepan, bring 4 cups of water to a boil.

2. Add the dried hawthorn berries to the boiling water. Reduce the heat to a simmer and cover the saucepan. Allow the berries to simmer for 10 minutes.

3. After 10 minutes, add the dried hibiscus flowers to the saucepan. Continue to simmer for an additional 10 minutes. The water will turn a deep red color as the hibiscus infuses.

4. Remove the saucepan from the heat. Strain the tonic through a fine mesh sieve into a large pitcher or jar, pressing on the berries and flowers to extract as much liquid as possible. Discard the solids.

5. If desired, stir in honey and lemon juice while the tonic is still warm. Adjust the amount of honey to taste, depending on your preference for sweetness.

6. Allow the tonic to cool to room temperature. Once cooled, you can serve it immediately or refrigerate it to chill.

Variations
- For a spicy twist, add a cinnamon stick or a few slices of fresh ginger to the saucepan along with the hawthorn berries.
- Incorporate a few mint leaves or a sprig of fresh rosemary for a refreshing herbal note.
- Replace honey with maple syrup for a vegan sweetener option.

Storage tips
Store the Hawthorn and Hibiscus Heart Tonic in a sealed glass container in the refrigerator for up to 5 days. Shake well before serving, especially if honey was added, as it may settle at the bottom.

Tips for allergens
For those with allergies to hibiscus, consider substituting with rose petals, which also offer heart-healthy benefits and a floral flavor. If honey is a concern, the tonic can be enjoyed unsweetened or with an alternative sweetener as suggested.

Scientific references
- "Hawthorn extract for treating chronic heart failure," published in the Cochrane Database of Systematic Reviews, highlights the cardiovascular benefits of hawthorn.
- "Hibiscus sabdariffa L. in the treatment of hypertension and hyperlipidemia: a comprehensive review of animal and human studies," published in Fitoterapia, discusses the blood pressure-lowering and cholesterol-reducing effects of hibiscus.

BOOK 15: IMMUNE-BOOSTING HERBAL MEDICINE

CHAPTER 1: HERBS FOR IMMUNE SUPPORT

Echinacea for Infections

Echinacea, a group of herbaceous plants native to North America, has long been revered for its medicinal properties, particularly in fighting infections such as colds and flu. This plant's effectiveness is primarily attributed to its complex mix of active compounds, including alkamides, phenolic compounds, and polysaccharides, which collectively contribute to its antiviral and antibacterial capabilities. When considering the use of echinacea as a remedy for infections, it's crucial to understand the specific parts of the plant that are utilized, the optimal extraction methods, and the recommended dosages to ensure maximum efficacy and safety.

The most commonly used species for medicinal purposes include Echinacea purpurea, Echinacea angustifolia, and Echinacea pallida. The roots and aerial parts of these species contain varying concentrations of the active compounds, with the roots of Echinacea angustifolia and Echinacea pallida being particularly potent. For preparing echinacea remedies at home, one can use dried roots or leaves to make a tea or a tincture. To make echinacea tea, steep 1 to 2 grams of dried echinacea root or leaves in hot water for 10 to 15 minutes. This tea can be consumed two to three times daily during the onset of cold or flu symptoms. For a more concentrated form, echinacea tinctures can be prepared by soaking the dried plant material in alcohol for several weeks, shaking the mixture regularly. The resulting tincture can be taken in doses of 1 to 2 milliliters, up to three times daily.

It's important to note that the timing and duration of echinacea supplementation play critical roles in its effectiveness against infections. Research suggests that starting echinacea supplementation at the first sign of cold or flu symptoms and continuing for 7 to 10 days can significantly reduce the severity and duration of these illnesses. However, long-term continuous use of echinacea is not recommended due to potential impacts on the immune system.

Safety is another crucial aspect when using echinacea, especially considering its immunomodulating properties. While echinacea is generally safe for most individuals, it can interact with certain medications and may not be suitable for people with autoimmune diseases or allergies to plants in the daisy family. Pregnant or breastfeeding women should consult a healthcare provider before using echinacea.

In terms of sourcing echinacea, choosing high-quality, organically grown echinacea from reputable suppliers is essential to ensure the presence of active compounds. Whether purchasing dried echinacea or ready-made preparations, look for products that specify the species of echinacea used and provide information on the part of the plant utilized, as this can significantly influence the remedy's effectiveness.

Elderberry for Reducing Viral Load

Elderberry, scientifically known as Sambucus nigra, is a potent antiviral herb renowned for its capacity to reduce viral load and shorten the duration of illnesses, particularly those affecting the respiratory system like the common cold and influenza. The berries and flowers of the elderberry plant contain powerful antiviral compounds that enhance the body's immune response and inhibit the replication of viruses.

To harness the immune-boosting benefits of elderberry, it's essential to prepare it correctly. Elderberry can be consumed in various forms, including syrups, teas, capsules, and lozenges. However, one of the most effective and traditional methods is through the preparation of elderberry syrup. This involves simmering dried elderberries with water and other immune-supporting ingredients such as ginger, cinnamon, and cloves, then sweetening the reduced liquid with honey to create a thick, potent syrup.

Elderberry Syrup Preparation:

1. **Ingredients:** To make elderberry syrup, you will need 1 cup of dried elderberries, 4 cups of water, 2 tablespoons of fresh or dried ginger root, 1 teaspoon of cinnamon powder, 1/2 teaspoon of cloves or clove powder, and 1 cup of raw honey.

2. **Simmering:** Combine the elderberries, water, ginger, cinnamon, and cloves in a large pot. Bring the mixture to a boil, then reduce the heat and simmer for about 45 minutes to an hour, or until the liquid has reduced by almost half.

3. **Straining:** After the mixture has reduced, remove it from heat and let it cool. Once cool, strain the liquid using a fine mesh strainer or cheesecloth into a large bowl. Press or squeeze the berries to extract as much liquid as possible.

4. **Adding Honey:** While the liquid is still warm (but not hot, to preserve the beneficial properties of raw honey), add the honey and stir until it is completely dissolved.

5. **Bottling:** Pour the finished syrup into sterilized glass bottles or jars. Store the syrup in the refrigerator.

Dosage: For immune support during cold and flu season, take 1 tablespoon of elderberry syrup daily. If you're already experiencing symptoms, the dosage can be increased to 1 tablespoon every 3-4 hours until symptoms subside.

Safety Considerations: While elderberry is generally safe for most people, it's important to use only the berries and flowers, as the leaves, stems, and unripe berries of the plant contain toxic substances that can lead to nausea and vomiting if ingested. Pregnant and breastfeeding women should consult with a healthcare provider before using elderberry products. Additionally, those with autoimmune diseases should use elderberry with caution, as it stimulates the immune system.

Quality and Sourcing: When selecting dried elderberries for syrup preparation, look for organically grown berries from reputable suppliers to ensure they are free from pesticides and have been handled properly. High-quality, organic ingredients contribute to the potency and effectiveness of the elderberry syrup.

By incorporating elderberry syrup into your wellness routine, you can take advantage of this ancient remedy's powerful antiviral properties, supporting your immune system and potentially reducing the duration and severity of cold and flu symptoms.

Goldenseal for Immune Support

Goldenseal, scientifically known as Hydrastis canadensis, is a perennial herb native to the woodlands of the northeastern United States. Recognized for its broad-spectrum antimicrobial properties and its ability to enhance immune function, goldenseal has been a cornerstone of traditional medicine for centuries. The root of the goldenseal plant contains several alkaloids, with berberine being the most notable for its antimicrobial and immune-stimulating effects. Berberine works by inhibiting the ability of bacteria to attach to human cells, effectively preventing infections while also stimulating the immune system by increasing the activity of macrophages, cells that devour harmful microorganisms.

To utilize goldenseal for its immune-boosting benefits, it is commonly prepared as a tincture, tea, or capsule. For making a goldenseal tincture, finely chop or grind dried goldenseal root to increase its surface area. Combine the root with a high-proof alcohol, typically at a ratio of 1 part goldenseal to 5 parts alcohol, in a sealable glass jar. Allow this mixture to sit for 4 to 6 weeks in a cool, dark place, shaking the jar daily to encourage extraction. After the maceration period, strain the liquid through a fine mesh strainer or cheesecloth, squeezing out as much liquid as possible, and bottle the tincture in dark glass dropper bottles for easy use.

For those preferring to avoid alcohol, goldenseal tea can be made by simmering one teaspoon of dried goldenseal root in a cup of water for approximately 15 to 20 minutes. This method extracts the water-soluble components of goldenseal, although it may not be as potent as an alcohol-based tincture. Drinking goldenseal tea can be beneficial for treating mild digestive issues and can help to stimulate the immune system during cold and flu season.

Goldenseal capsules are another convenient option, especially for those who do not appreciate the bitter taste of goldenseal preparations. It is crucial to follow the manufacturer's dosage recommendations, as excessive consumption of goldenseal can lead to digestive upset and other adverse effects. Typically, goldenseal capsules are taken once or twice daily, especially during times of increased risk for infection or when experiencing the early signs of a cold or flu.

When sourcing goldenseal, it is important to choose products that are certified organic and sustainably harvested. Goldenseal is considered an at-risk species due to overharvesting and habitat loss, so supporting ethical suppliers who prioritize the conservation of this valuable medicinal plant is essential. Additionally, verifying the presence of active alkaloids, particularly berberine, in the product can ensure its efficacy as an antimicrobial and immune-supportive agent.

While goldenseal is a powerful tool for enhancing immune function, it should be used judiciously and not considered a substitute for a healthy lifestyle and proper medical care. Due to its potent effects, goldenseal is not recommended for pregnant or breastfeeding women, and those with pre-existing medical conditions or taking prescription medications should consult with a healthcare professional before incorporating goldenseal into their health regimen. With responsible use, goldenseal can be an effective natural remedy for supporting the body's defense mechanisms and maintaining overall health.

Elderberry and Astragalus Immune Tonic

Beneficial effects

Elderberry and Astragalus Immune Tonic is a powerful blend designed to bolster the immune system. Elderberry is renowned for its antiviral properties, making it effective in fighting colds and flu. Astragalus, a staple in traditional Chinese medicine, is known for its immune-boosting and anti-inflammatory effects. Together, they create a tonic that supports immune health, reduces inflammation, and enhances the body's resistance to pathogens.

Portions

Makes about 3 cups

Preparation time

15 minutes

Cooking time

1 hour

Ingredients

- 1 cup dried elderberries

- 1/2 cup dried astragalus root slices

- 4 cups water

- 1 cinnamon stick

- 1/2 teaspoon whole cloves

- 1 cup raw honey

Instructions

1. Combine the dried elderberries, dried astragalus root slices, cinnamon stick, whole cloves, and water in a large saucepan. Bring the mixture to a boil over high heat.
2. Once boiling, reduce the heat to low, allowing the mixture to simmer. Cover the saucepan with a lid, leaving a small gap to let steam escape. Simmer for about 45 minutes to 1 hour, or until the liquid has reduced by almost half.
3. Remove the saucepan from the heat. Carefully strain the liquid through a fine mesh strainer or cheesecloth into a large bowl. Press or squeeze the berries and astragalus root to extract as much liquid as possible. Discard the solids.
4. Allow the liquid to cool to lukewarm, then stir in the raw honey until fully dissolved. The honey not only sweetens the tonic but also adds its own antibacterial and antiviral properties to the mix.
5. Pour the finished tonic into sterilized glass bottles or jars. Seal tightly with a lid.

Variations

- For an extra immune boost, add 1 tablespoon of grated fresh ginger or turmeric root to the mixture before boiling.
- If the taste of honey is too sweet for your preference, reduce the amount of honey or substitute it with maple syrup for a different flavor profile.
- Add a splash of lemon juice or apple cider vinegar to the finished tonic for added vitamin C and a tangy flavor.

Storage tips

Store the Elderberry and Astragalus Immune Tonic in the refrigerator for up to 2 months. For longer storage, the tonic can be frozen in ice cube trays and then transferred to a freezer bag, allowing you to thaw individual servings as needed.

Tips for allergens

For those with allergies to honey, maple syrup is a suitable vegan alternative that does not compromise the tonic's immune-boosting properties. If you have a sensitivity to elderberries or astragalus, consult with a healthcare provider for alternative immune-supporting herbs that may be more suitable for your condition.

Scientific references

- "The effect of Sambucus nigra L. (black elderberry) on the immune system: a systematic review." This study, published in the journal Phytotherapy Research, highlights the immune-modulating effect of elderberry, supporting its use in the prevention and treatment of viral infections.
- "Astragalus membranaceus: A Review of its Protection Against Inflammation and Gastrointestinal Cancers." Published in the American Journal of Chinese Medicine, this article reviews the anti-inflammatory and immune-boosting effects of astragalus, underscoring its potential in enhancing immune health.

Olive Leaf and Oregano Oil Immune Booster

Beneficial effects

Olive Leaf and Oregano Oil Immune Booster is a potent blend designed to support the immune system naturally. Olive leaf extract is renowned for its ability to enhance immune response and offer antioxidant protection, thanks to its high oleuropein content. Oregano oil, rich in carvacrol and thymol, possesses powerful antimicrobial and antiviral properties, making this tonic an excellent choice for warding off infections and maintaining overall health.

Portions
Makes about 1 cup

Preparation time
10 minutes

Ingredients
- 1/2 cup olive leaf extract
- 1/4 cup virgin olive oil
- 1/4 cup oregano oil
- 2 tablespoons raw honey (optional, for taste)
- 1 teaspoon fresh lemon juice (optional, for added vitamin C)

Instructions
1. In a clean glass jar, combine the olive leaf extract and virgin olive oil. Olive leaf extract can be sourced from health food stores or online suppliers. Ensure it's of high quality for maximum benefits.
2. Add the oregano oil to the mixture. Oregano oil is potent, so ensure it's diluted properly with the olive oil to avoid irritation.
3. If desired, stir in the raw honey to the blend. Honey not only improves the taste but also adds its own antibacterial and soothing properties.
4. Mix in the fresh lemon juice, if using. Lemon juice adds a refreshing flavor and boosts the tonic's vitamin C content, further supporting immune health.
5. Secure the lid on the jar and shake well to ensure all ingredients are thoroughly mixed.
6. Label the jar with the date and contents. Shake well before each use.

Variations
- For a vegan version, substitute honey with agave syrup or simply omit the sweetener.
- Add a few drops of ginger oil for an extra immune-boosting kick and warming flavor.
- Incorporate a pinch of cayenne pepper to enhance circulation and the body's absorption of the tonic's beneficial compounds.

Storage tips
Store the Olive Leaf and Oregano Oil Immune Booster in a cool, dark place. The refrigerator is ideal for prolonging its shelf life. Use within 6 months for optimal potency.

Tips for allergens
Individuals with sensitivities to oregano or olive products should proceed with caution. Test a small amount on the skin for any adverse reactions before internal use. For those allergic to honey, omitting it will not affect the immune-boosting properties of the tonic.

Scientific references
- "Oleuropein, the main polyphenol of Olea europaea leaf extract, has an anti-inflammatory effect on arthritis," published in the Journal of Nutritional Biochemistry, highlights the anti-inflammatory and antioxidant properties of olive leaf extract.
- "Antimicrobial activity of oregano oil against antibiotic-resistant pathogens," published in the Journal of Medicinal Food, discusses the potent antimicrobial effects of oregano oil, supporting its use in immune support formulations.

Reishi Mushroom and Licorice Root Immune Elixir

Beneficial effects

Reishi Mushroom and Licorice Root Immune Elixir combines the immune-boosting power of Reishi mushrooms, known for their ability to support the body's defense mechanisms, with the soothing and anti-inflammatory properties of licorice root. This elixir is designed to enhance overall immune function, reduce stress, and promote respiratory health. Reishi mushrooms have been studied for their potential to increase the production of white blood cells, which are crucial for fighting infections and cancer. Licorice root, on the other hand, may help soothe sore throats, protect against viruses, and reduce inflammation.

Ingredients

- 4 cups of water
- 1/4 cup dried Reishi mushroom slices
- 1/4 cup dried licorice root
- 1 tablespoon honey, or to taste (optional)
- 1 lemon, juiced (optional)

Instructions

1. Bring 4 cups of water to a boil in a medium saucepan.
2. Once the water is boiling, reduce the heat to a simmer and add the dried Reishi mushroom slices and dried licorice root.
3. Cover the saucepan and let the mixture simmer for 30 minutes. The water will darken, taking on the rich colors and essence of the Reishi mushrooms and licorice root.
4. After 30 minutes, remove the saucepan from the heat and strain the elixir through a fine mesh strainer or cheesecloth into a large pitcher or jar, discarding the solids.
5. If desired, stir in honey and lemon juice while the elixir is still warm. Adjust the amount of honey to taste, depending on your preference for sweetness.
6. Allow the elixir to cool to room temperature. Once cooled, you can serve it immediately or refrigerate it to chill.

Variations

- For an additional immune boost, add a teaspoon of minced fresh ginger to the simmering water along with the Reishi mushrooms and licorice root.
- Incorporate a cinnamon stick during the simmering process for a warming spice flavor.
- Substitute maple syrup or agave nectar for honey to make a vegan-friendly version.

Storage tips

Store the Reishi Mushroom and Licorice Root Immune Elixir in a sealed glass container in the refrigerator for up to 5 days. Shake well before serving, as natural sediment may occur.

Tips for allergens

For those with allergies or sensitivities to licorice root, consider substituting with marshmallow root, which also has soothing properties but without the potential side effects of licorice. Always consult with a healthcare provider before consuming herbal remedies, especially if you have existing health conditions or are taking medications.

Scientific references

- "Immunomodulating Effects of Fungal Metabolites," published in the Journal of Microbiology and Biotechnology, highlights the immune-supporting properties of Reishi mushrooms.

- "The anti-inflammatory and antiviral properties of licorice root," published in the Journal of Advanced Research, discusses the health benefits of licorice root in supporting the immune system and combating viral infections.

CHAPTER 2: BUILDING LONG-TERM IMMUNITY

Astragalus for Immune Strengthening

Astragalus, a perennial plant native to the northern and eastern regions of China, as well as Mongolia and Korea, has been a cornerstone in traditional Chinese medicine for centuries. Its roots are harvested from plants that are four to five years old, as this maturity period allows for the accumulation of the plant's beneficial compounds. These compounds include polysaccharides, saponins, flavonoids, amino acids, and trace minerals, all contributing to its immune-boosting properties.

The process of leveraging astragalus for immune strengthening involves careful preparation of the root. Typically, the roots are sliced thinly to increase the surface area for extraction. For daily immune support, a decoction can be made by simmering 15 to 30 grams of dried astragalus root in 1 liter of water for one to two hours, reducing the liquid to about half its original volume. This concentrated decoction can be consumed in two to three divided doses throughout the day, with or without food. For those seeking a more convenient approach, astragalus is also available in capsule or tincture form, with dosages varying according to the concentration of the extract. Capsules generally range from 250 to 500 milligrams, taken once or twice daily. Tinctures, on the other hand, might be administered in doses of 2 to 4 milliliters, also once or twice daily.

Astragalus works by stimulating the body's immune system in several ways. Its polysaccharides have been shown to enhance the activity of white blood cells, which play a crucial role in defending against diseases. Saponins in astragalus are known for their ability to support the immune system's response to inflammation, while its flavonoids possess antioxidant properties that protect cells from damage caused by free radicals. This multifaceted approach not only helps in preventing common colds and flu but also supports the body's resilience against more chronic infections.

Moreover, astragalus has been found to increase the production of interferon, a key signaling protein in the immune response against pathogens, and to enhance the growth of stem cells in the bone marrow and lymph tissues, further amplifying its immune-strengthening effects.

For individuals looking to incorporate astragalus into their wellness routine, it's important to source high-quality, organically grown astragalus root from reputable suppliers. The root should be devoid of any discoloration or mold, ensuring its potency and safety. When storing astragalus, whether in its raw or processed form, keep it in a cool, dry place away from direct sunlight to preserve its therapeutic properties.

While astragalus is generally considered safe for most people, it's advisable to consult with a healthcare provider before starting any new supplement regimen, especially for those who are pregnant, nursing, or have autoimmune diseases. This is due to astragalus's potent immune-stimulating effects, which may not be suitable for everyone.

Reishi Mushroom for Immune Support

Reishi mushroom, scientifically known as Ganoderma lucidum, has been a cornerstone in traditional Eastern medicine for over two millennia, revered for its adaptogenic properties that aid in balancing the immune response and reducing inflammation. This mushroom is characterized by its shiny, reddish-brown cap and woody texture, growing predominantly on hardwood trees in various parts of Asia. The active compounds within reishi, including polysaccharides, triterpenoids, and peptidoglycans, contribute to its health-promoting effects, particularly in modulating the immune system and exerting anti-inflammatory benefits.

To harness the immune-supportive properties of reishi mushroom, it is commonly prepared as a tea or decoction. This involves slicing the dried mushroom into thin pieces to maximize the surface area for extraction. A typical method includes simmering about 5 to 15 grams of dried reishi slices in 1 liter of water for 2 to 3 hours, until the liquid is reduced by half. This concentrated decoction can be consumed daily, divided into two servings. For those seeking convenience, reishi is also available in capsule or tincture form. Capsules often contain powdered reishi extract, with recommended dosages ranging from 500 to 1500 milligrams per day. Tinctures, which are liquid extracts, might be taken in amounts of 1 to 2 milliliters, twice daily.

The immune-modulating effect of reishi is attributed to its polysaccharides, which have been shown to enhance the activity of immune cells such as macrophages and natural killer cells, crucial for defending the body against pathogens and diseases. Additionally, the triterpenoids found in reishi possess potent anti-inflammatory properties, helping to mitigate chronic inflammation and support immune health. This dual action makes reishi particularly valuable for individuals looking to support their immune system in a balanced manner, without overstimulation.

For optimal benefits, sourcing high-quality, organically grown reishi mushroom from reputable suppliers is crucial. The mushroom should be free from mold and discoloration, ensuring its potency and safety. When storing dried reishi or its preparations, keeping them in a cool, dry place away from direct sunlight will help preserve their medicinal properties.

While reishi mushroom is generally considered safe for most people, it is advisable to consult with a healthcare provider before incorporating it into your health regimen, especially for those who are pregnant, nursing, or have autoimmune conditions. This is due to reishi's potent effects on the immune system, which may not be suitable for everyone.

Incorporating reishi mushroom into one's daily routine can be a proactive step towards enhancing immune function and reducing inflammation. Its adaptogenic nature helps in adapting to stress and restoring balance within the immune system, embodying the holistic approach of herbal medicine in supporting overall wellness.

Rosehip for Vitamin C Supplementation

Rosehip, the fruit of the rose plant, emerges as a pivotal component in the realm of immune-boosting herbal medicine, primarily due to its exceptionally high vitamin C content. This nutrient is crucial for the prevention of deficiencies and the promotion of overall health, acting as a potent antioxidant that safeguards the body against the damaging effects of free radicals and supports the immune system in its fight against infections. The significance of rosehip in vitamin C supplementation cannot be overstated, especially considering its role in collagen synthesis, which is vital for the health and repair of tissues, and its ability to enhance the absorption of iron, a mineral essential for oxygen transport in the blood.

To harness the benefits of rosehip for vitamin C supplementation, one can incorporate it into their diet in various forms. Dried rosehip can be used to prepare a nutritious tea. To do this, one should measure approximately one to two tablespoons of dried rosehips and steep them in boiling water for about 10 to 15 minutes. This method allows for the extraction of vitamin C as well as other beneficial compounds into the water, creating a tea that can be consumed daily. It's important to note that vitamin C is sensitive to heat, light, and air; hence, storing dried rosehips in a cool, dark place and preparing the tea fresh each time maximizes the nutrient content.

Another effective way to utilize rosehip is by incorporating its powder into smoothies, yogurts, or cereals. The powder is made by finely grinding dried rosehips, which can then be easily added to various foods. This not only boosts the vitamin C content of these foods but also enhances their flavor profile with a subtle, fruity tang. When selecting rosehip powder, opting for a product that is organically grown and free from additives ensures purity and potency.

For those interested in a more direct approach, rosehip supplements are available in capsule or tablet form. These supplements provide a concentrated dose of vitamin C and are especially beneficial for individuals looking to boost their intake without altering their diet significantly. When choosing supplements, it's crucial to look for products that specify the vitamin C content derived from rosehip and to follow the recommended dosage on the label to avoid excessive intake.

Incorporating rosehip into one's daily routine offers a natural and effective way to supplement vitamin C, contributing to immune system support and overall health maintenance. Whether through tea, powder, or supplements, the versatility of rosehip makes it an accessible option for enhancing dietary intake of this essential nutrient. Additionally, the synergistic effect of the various antioxidants present in rosehip, including flavonoids and carotenoids, further amplifies its health benefits, making it a superior choice for those seeking to fortify their immune system and prevent vitamin C deficiencies.

Three Healing Recipes

Elderberry and Rosehip Immune Boosting Jam

Beneficial effects

Elderberry and Rosehip Immune Boosting Jam combines the immune-supporting power of elderberries, known for their high vitamin C content and antiviral properties, with the antioxidant-rich rosehips, which are also a vitamin C powerhouse. This jam is designed to bolster the immune system, aid in preventing colds and flu, and provide a delicious way to incorporate these powerful botanicals into your daily diet. Elderberries have been studied for their ability to reduce the duration and severity of cold symptoms, while rosehips offer anti-inflammatory benefits that can support overall health and wellness.

Portions

Makes approximately 3 cups

Preparation time

20 minutes

Cooking time

45 minutes

Ingredients

- 3 cups fresh elderberries or 1 cup dried elderberries
- 2 cups fresh rosehips, deseeded and finely chopped
- 3 cups water
- 2 cups granulated sugar
- 1 lemon, juiced
- 1 package (1.75 oz) fruit pectin

Instructions

1. If using dried elderberries, begin by rehydrating them. Place the dried elderberries in a bowl and cover with 2 cups of water. Let them soak for 30-45 minutes, or until they are plump.

2. In a large pot, combine the elderberries (fresh or rehydrated), rosehips, and the remaining 1 cup of water. Bring the mixture to a boil over medium-high heat, then reduce the heat to maintain a gentle simmer. Cook for 15-20 minutes, or until the rosehips are soft and the mixture has thickened slightly.

3. Use a potato masher or the back of a spoon to mash the mixture, breaking down the elderberries and rosehips further. For a smoother jam, you can blend the mixture with an immersion blender or transfer it to a blender and pulse until it reaches your desired consistency.

4. Return the mashed mixture to the pot if you blended it. Add the lemon juice and gradually stir in the fruit pectin, ensuring it dissolves completely without clumping.

5. Bring the mixture back to a boil and add the sugar, stirring constantly to dissolve. Once the sugar is fully dissolved, boil the mixture for 1 minute.

6. Remove the pot from the heat. Skim off any foam that has formed on the surface of the jam.

7. Ladle the hot jam into sterilized jars, leaving about 1/4 inch of headspace. Wipe the rims of the jars with a clean, damp cloth to remove any spilled jam, then seal with lids and rings.

8. Process the jars in a boiling water canner for 10 minutes to ensure a proper seal for long-term storage.

Variations

- For a sugar-free version, substitute granulated sugar with an equal amount of honey or a sugar substitute suitable for cooking, adjusting the quantity to taste.
- Add a teaspoon of ground cinnamon or ginger for a warm, spiced flavor that complements the fruity notes of the jam.
- Incorporate a splash of vanilla extract or a vanilla bean during the cooking process for a subtle depth of flavor.

Storage tips

Store the sealed jars in a cool, dark place for up to a year. Once opened, keep the jam refrigerated and use within 3 weeks for best quality.

Tips for allergens

For those with citrus allergies, omit the lemon juice and substitute with an equal amount of apple cider vinegar to maintain the necessary acidity for preservation. If you're sensitive to sugar, using a natural sweetener like honey or a sugar substitute can help tailor the jam to your dietary needs.

Scientific references

- "Elderberry Supplementation Reduces Cold Duration and Symptoms in Air-Travellers: A Randomized, Double-Blind Placebo-Controlled Clinical Trial," published in the journal Nutrients, highlights the benefits of elderberry in immune support.
- "The anti-inflammatory effects of rosehip in osteoarthritis and other inflammatory diseases," published in Phytotherapy Research, discusses the health benefits of rosehips, including their high vitamin C content and anti-inflammatory properties.

Astragalus and Reishi Mushroom Immune Support Soup

Beneficial effects

Astragalus and Reishi Mushroom Immune Support Soup is a nourishing blend designed to strengthen the immune system. Astragalus root is known for its ability to boost the body's defense against viruses and bacteria, while Reishi mushrooms are revered for their immune-modulating and anti-inflammatory properties. This soup offers a holistic approach to enhancing immune function, promoting overall wellness, and supporting the body's natural ability to heal.

Portions

Serves 4

Preparation time

15 minutes

Cooking time

1 hour

Ingredients

- 4 cups vegetable broth
- 1 cup astragalus root slices
- 1 cup Reishi mushroom slices
- 1 medium onion, diced
- 2 cloves garlic, minced
- 2 carrots, chopped
- 2 stalks celery, chopped
- 1 inch piece ginger, grated
- 1 tablespoon olive oil
- Salt and pepper to taste
- 2 tablespoons chopped parsley for garnish

Instructions

1. In a large pot, heat the olive oil over medium heat. Add the diced onion and minced garlic, sautéing until the onion becomes translucent, about 5 minutes.
2. Add the chopped carrots and celery to the pot, continuing to sauté for another 5 minutes until the vegetables start to soften.
3. Stir in the grated ginger, astragalus root slices, and Reishi mushroom slices. Cook for 2-3 minutes, allowing the flavors to meld.
4. Pour the vegetable broth into the pot. Bring the mixture to a boil, then reduce the heat to low, covering the pot with a lid. Allow the soup to simmer for at least 1 hour. The longer it simmers, the more potent the infusion will be.
5. After simmering, strain the soup to remove the astragalus root and Reishi mushroom slices. Return the clear broth to the pot.
6. Season the soup with salt and pepper to taste. Reheat gently if necessary.
7. Serve the soup hot, garnished with chopped parsley.

Variations

- For a heartier soup, add cubed tofu or chicken breast in the last 20 minutes of simmering.
- Include other immune-boosting vegetables like spinach, kale, or sweet potatoes.
- For additional flavor, add a splash of tamari or soy sauce before serving.

Storage tips

Store leftover soup in an airtight container in the refrigerator for up to 3 days. Reheat on the stove or in a microwave before serving. For longer storage, freeze the soup in individual portions for up to 3 months. Thaw overnight in the refrigerator before reheating.

Tips for allergens

For those with soy allergies, ensure the vegetable broth is soy-free or homemade, and substitute tamari or soy sauce with a soy-free alternative. If sensitive to mushrooms, astragalus root alone still provides immune support and can be used to create a simple, healing broth.

Scientific references

- "Effects of Astragalus membranaceus on cytokine secretion by peripheral blood mononuclear cells," published in Phytotherapy Research, discusses the immune-boosting effects of astragalus root.
- "Ganoderma lucidum (Reishi mushroom) for cancer treatment," published in the Cochrane Database of Systematic Reviews, highlights the immune-modulating properties of Reishi mushrooms.

Garlic and Ginger Immune Strengthening Broth

Beneficial effects

Garlic and Ginger Immune Strengthening Broth harnesses the natural power of garlic and ginger, both of which are renowned for their immune-boosting properties. Garlic, with its compounds like allicin, has been shown to enhance immune function and has antibacterial and antiviral effects. Ginger, rich in gingerol, aids in reducing inflammation, soothing sore throats, and can help lower the risk of infections. This broth is not only a comforting remedy but also a proactive measure to strengthen the immune system, especially during cold and flu season.

Portions

Serves 4

Preparation time

10 minutes

Cooking time

1 hour

Ingredients

- 4 cups of water
- 1 large carrot, chopped
- 1 stalk of celery, chopped
- 1 onion, chopped
- 4 cloves of garlic, minced
- 2 inches of fresh ginger root, thinly sliced
- 1 teaspoon of turmeric powder
- 1/2 teaspoon of black pepper
- 1 tablespoon of apple cider vinegar
- Salt to taste
- Fresh herbs (such as parsley or thyme) for garnish (optional)

Instructions

1. In a large pot, combine water, carrot, celery, and onion. Bring to a boil over high heat.
2. Once boiling, reduce the heat to a simmer. Add the minced garlic and sliced ginger to the pot.
3. Stir in the turmeric powder and black pepper. These spices not only add flavor but also enhance the immune-boosting properties of the broth.
4. Add the apple cider vinegar to the mixture. The acidity helps extract minerals from the vegetables, enriching the broth.
5. Allow the broth to simmer gently for about 1 hour. This slow cooking process allows the flavors to meld together and the ingredients to release their beneficial compounds into the broth.

6. After simmering, strain the broth through a fine mesh strainer into a large bowl or pot, discarding the solids.

7. Taste the broth and add salt as needed, adjusting the seasoning to your preference.

8. Serve the broth hot, garnished with fresh herbs if desired.

Variations

- For an extra immune boost, add a piece of star anise or a cinnamon stick during the simmering process.
- Incorporate a handful of kale or spinach in the last 10 minutes of cooking for added nutrients.
- For a heartier version, add cooked noodles or rice into the strained broth before serving.

Storage tips

Cool the broth completely before transferring it to airtight containers. It can be stored in the refrigerator for up to 5 days or frozen for up to 3 months. To reheat, simply warm the broth over medium heat until hot.

Tips for allergens

For those with allergies to certain vegetables used in this recipe, feel free to substitute or omit as necessary. The broth can be customized based on dietary needs and preferences without significantly impacting its immune-boosting benefits.

Scientific references

- "The immunomodulation and anti-inflammatory effects of garlic organosulfur compounds in cancer chemoprevention" published in Anti-Cancer Agents in Medicinal Chemistry, highlights garlic's immune-enhancing properties.
- "Ginger in gastrointestinal disorders: A systematic review of clinical trials" found in Food Science & Nutrition, discusses ginger's role in reducing inflammation and supporting immune health.

CHAPTER 3: HERBAL BLENDS FOR IMMUNE PROTECTION

Cold and Flu Tea Blends Provides recipes combining elderberry, echinacea, and ginger for seasonal illness prevention.

Beneficial effects

This tea blend harnesses the combined powers of elderberry, echinacea, and ginger, all of which are renowned for their immune-boosting properties. Elderberry is a potent antiviral that has been shown to reduce the duration and severity of cold symptoms. Echinacea supports the immune system and increases the body's ability to fight off infections. Ginger adds anti-inflammatory benefits, soothing sore throats and easing nausea. Together, these ingredients create a powerful defense against seasonal illnesses.

Portions

Makes about 4 cups

Preparation time

10 minutes

Cooking time

20 minutes

Ingredients

- 4 cups of water
- 1/4 cup dried elderberries
- 2 tablespoons dried echinacea leaves
- 1 inch fresh ginger root, thinly sliced
- Honey to taste (optional)
- Lemon slices for garnish (optional)

Instructions

1. Bring 4 cups of water to a boil in a medium-sized saucepan.
2. Once the water is boiling, reduce the heat to a simmer and add the dried elderberries, dried echinacea leaves, and thinly sliced ginger root to the saucepan.
3. Cover the saucepan with a lid and let the mixture simmer for 15-20 minutes. This allows the water to extract the beneficial compounds from the herbs and ginger.
4. After simmering, remove the saucepan from the heat. Strain the tea through a fine mesh strainer into a large pitcher or teapot, pressing on the solids to extract as much liquid as possible. Discard the solids.
5. If desired, sweeten the tea with honey to taste. Stir well to ensure the honey is fully dissolved.
6. Serve the tea hot, garnished with a slice of lemon in each cup if desired.

Variations

- For a spicier kick, add a pinch of cayenne pepper to the tea while it simmers.
- Incorporate a cinnamon stick during the simmering process for added warmth and flavor.

- To make a cold remedy tea blend, add a clove of garlic to the simmering water. Garlic has antiviral and antibacterial properties that can further support the immune system.

Storage tips

Allow any leftover tea to cool to room temperature before transferring it to a glass jar or bottle. Store the tea in the refrigerator for up to 3 days. Reheat gently on the stove or enjoy cold.

Tips for allergens

For those with allergies or sensitivities to echinacea, omit this herb and increase the amount of elderberries and ginger to maintain the tea's immune-boosting properties. If honey is a concern, substitute it with maple syrup or simply enjoy the tea unsweetened.

Scientific references

- "Randomized study of the efficacy and safety of oral elderberry extract in the treatment of influenza A and B virus infections" published in the Journal of International Medical Research, which highlights elderberry's antiviral effects.
- "The role of echinacea in reducing the duration and severity of cold symptoms" published in The Lancet Infectious Diseases, discussing echinacea's immune-supporting benefits.
- "Anti-Oxidative and Anti-Inflammatory Effects of Ginger in Health and Physical Activity: Review of Current Evidence" published in the International Journal of Preventive Medicine, which outlines ginger's health benefits.

Immune-Boosting Tinctures

To create immune-boosting tinctures with **astragalus** and **reishi**, you will need to gather specific materials and follow a detailed process to ensure the efficacy and longevity of your tinctures. These tinctures, when prepared correctly, offer a convenient and potent way to harness the immune-supportive properties of these powerful herbs.

Materials Needed:

- **High-quality dried astragalus root:** Look for slices or shreds of organically grown astragalus to ensure purity and potency. Approximately 100 grams will be needed.
- **Dried reishi mushroom:** Ensure the reishi is organically sourced. You will need about 100 grams, sliced thinly to maximize surface area for extraction.
- **Vodka or brandy:** Choose a high-proof alcohol (at least 80 proof/40% alcohol by volume) to effectively extract the active compounds from the herbs. You will need about 1 liter.
- **Amber glass jars:** Use to store the tinctures, protecting them from light degradation. Ensure they are clean and sterilized.
- **Cheesecloth or fine mesh strainer:** For filtering the tincture.
- **Labels:** To mark the jars with the herb name, date of production, and alcohol percentage.

Preparation Steps:

1. **Herb Preparation:** Begin by measuring out 100 grams each of dried astragalus root and reishi mushroom. If the reishi mushroom isn't already sliced, slice it thinly to increase the surface area for better extraction.
2. **Jar Filling:** Place the astragalus and reishi in separate amber glass jars. If you prefer a combined tincture, you can mix the herbs in a single jar, but note that this will blend the distinct properties and flavors of each.
3. **Adding Alcohol:** Pour the vodka or brandy over the herbs, ensuring they are completely submerged. The general rule is to use a 1:5 ratio (herb to alcohol) by weight for dried herbs. This means for every 100 grams of herb, you should use 500 milliliters of alcohol.

4. **Sealing and Storing:** Seal the jars tightly with their lids. Label each jar with the herb's name, the date, and the type of alcohol used. Store the jars in a cool, dark place. A cupboard away from direct sunlight or a pantry is ideal.

5. **Maceration:** Let the herbs macerate in the alcohol for 6 to 8 weeks. This is the extraction phase, where the alcohol pulls out the active compounds from the herbs. Shake the jars gently every few days to mix the contents and promote extraction.

6. **Straining:** After the maceration period, open the jars and strain the liquid through a cheesecloth or fine mesh strainer into a clean bowl. Squeeze or press the soaked herbs to extract as much liquid as possible.

7. **Bottling:** Transfer the strained tincture into clean amber glass dropper bottles for easy use. Label each bottle with the herb's name, the date of bottling, and the alcohol used.

8. **Dosage:** A standard dose of the tincture is typically 1-2 milliliters (about 20-40 drops), taken 1-3 times daily. However, it's essential to start with a lower dose to assess tolerance and gradually increase as needed.

9. **Storage:** Store the bottled tinctures in a cool, dark place. Properly stored, these tinctures can last for several years, maintaining their potency and effectiveness.

Important Considerations:

- Always source your herbs from reputable suppliers to ensure they are free from contaminants and of high medicinal quality.
- If you are pregnant, nursing, or have any underlying health conditions, consult with a healthcare provider before using herbal tinctures.
- While astragalus and reishi are generally considered safe, it's crucial to listen to your body and discontinue use if you experience any adverse reactions.

Herbal Syrups for Daily Use

Herbal syrups offer a delightful and effective way to incorporate immune-boosting herbs into daily routines for individuals and families alike. These syrups can be made from a variety of herbs known for their immune-supportive properties, such as **elderberry**, **echinacea**, and **astragalus**. The process of making herbal syrups involves extracting the active compounds of herbs into a liquid form and then preserving this extract with a sweetener, usually honey or sugar, which also makes the remedy more palatable, especially for children.

Materials Needed:

- **Dried or fresh herbs:** Choose high-quality, organically grown herbs. For immune support, elderberry is highly recommended due to its antiviral properties.
- **Water:** Distilled or spring water is preferred to avoid any contaminants that might be present in tap water.
- **Sweetener:** Raw, local honey is ideal for its additional antimicrobial and soothing properties. For a vegan option, organic maple syrup can be used.
- **Pot and Stove:** For simmering the herb and water mixture.
- **Strainer or Cheesecloth:** To separate the herb particles from the liquid.
- **Measuring Cup and Spoon:** For accurate measurement of ingredients.
- **Sterilized Glass Bottles or Jars:** For storing the syrup. Amber-colored bottles help protect the syrup from light degradation.

Preparation Steps:

1. **Herb and Water Ratio:** Begin with a basic ratio of 1 cup of dried herbs to 4 cups of water. If using fresh herbs, the ratio is 2 cups of herbs to 4 cups of water due to their higher water content.
2. **Simmering:** Combine the herbs and water in a pot. Slowly bring the mixture to a boil, then reduce the heat and let it simmer gently. The goal is to reduce the volume by half to concentrate the extract, which usually takes about 30-40 minutes.
3. **Straining:** Once the mixture has reduced, remove it from the heat. While still warm, strain the liquid through a strainer or cheesecloth into a clean bowl, pressing or squeezing the herbs to extract as much liquid as possible.
4. **Adding Sweetener:** Measure the liquid; for every cup of liquid, add ¾ cup of honey or maple syrup. Gently heat the mixture again, just enough to integrate the sweetener without boiling, as high heat can destroy beneficial compounds and reduce the syrup's effectiveness.
5. **Bottling:** Pour the warm syrup into sterilized glass bottles or jars. If using honey as a sweetener, ensure the syrup temperature is below 104°F (40°C) before bottling to preserve the honey's natural enzymes and benefits.
6. **Storage:** Label the bottles with the name of the syrup, ingredients, and the date it was made. Store the syrup in the refrigerator. Properly prepared and stored, herbal syrups can last for several months.

Usage Guidelines:

- **Dosage:** For daily immune support, adults can take 1 tablespoon of syrup daily, while children over one year can take 1 teaspoon daily. During illness, the dosage can be increased to every 3-4 hours.
- **Safety:** Always consult with a healthcare provider before starting any new herbal remedy, especially for children, pregnant or nursing women, and individuals with existing health conditions or taking medications.

Benefits:

Herbal syrups made for immune support can offer a natural way to enhance the body's resistance to infections, particularly during cold and flu season. Elderberry syrup, for example, has been studied for its ability to shorten the duration of flu symptoms. Echinacea and astragalus are also popular choices for their immune-modulating effects. By making these syrups at home, individuals can customize the ingredients to suit their specific health needs and preferences, ensuring a fresh, potent, and cost-effective remedy for daily use.

Three Ancient Healing Recipes

Elderberry and Ginger Immune Boosting Syrup

Beneficial effects

Elderberry and Ginger Immune Boosting Syrup is a potent natural remedy designed to fortify the body's immune system. Elderberries are celebrated for their rich antioxidant content and ability to fight colds and flu, while ginger adds powerful anti-inflammatory and anti-nausea properties. This syrup is an excellent way to harness the natural healing powers of these ingredients, offering a first line of defense during cold and flu season.

Portions

Makes approximately 2 cups

Preparation time

15 minutes

Cooking time

45 minutes

Ingredients

- 3/4 cup dried elderberries
- 3 cups water
- 2 tablespoons fresh ginger, grated
- 1 teaspoon cinnamon powder
- 1/2 teaspoon cloves, ground
- 1 cup raw honey

Instructions

1. Combine the dried elderberries, water, grated ginger, cinnamon powder, and ground cloves in a medium saucepan.
2. Bring the mixture to a boil over high heat, then reduce the heat to maintain a low simmer.
3. Allow the mixture to simmer for about 45 minutes, or until the liquid has reduced by almost half. This slow simmering process extracts the active compounds from the elderberries and ginger, infusing the water with their immune-boosting properties.
4. Remove the saucepan from the heat and let the mixture cool to a temperature that is safe to handle.
5. Strain the mixture through a fine mesh strainer or cheesecloth into a large bowl, pressing on the solids to extract as much liquid as possible. Discard the solids.
6. Once the liquid is no longer hot but still warm, stir in the raw honey until it is completely dissolved. The honey not only sweetens the syrup but also adds its own antibacterial and antiviral properties.
7. Transfer the finished syrup to a clean glass bottle or jar with a tight-fitting lid.

Variations

- For a vegan version, substitute the honey with maple syrup or agave nectar. Adjust the sweetness according to taste.
- Add a tablespoon of fresh lemon juice to the syrup after removing it from the heat for added vitamin C and a tangy flavor.
- Incorporate a pinch of turmeric powder to the mixture for additional anti-inflammatory benefits.

Storage tips

Store the Elderberry and Ginger Immune Boosting Syrup in the refrigerator for up to two months. For extended storage, the syrup can be frozen in an ice cube tray and then transferred to a freezer bag, allowing you to thaw individual servings as needed.

Tips for allergens

For those allergic to honey, using maple syrup or agave nectar as a substitute will still provide a sweet flavor and maintain the syrup's immune-boosting properties. If you have a sensitivity to elderberries or ginger, consult with a healthcare provider for alternative immune-supporting ingredients that may be more suitable for your condition.

Scientific references

- "Randomized study of the efficacy and safety of oral elderberry extract in the treatment of influenza A and B virus infections" published in the Journal of International Medical Research, which highlights elderberry's antiviral effects.

- "Ginger in gastrointestinal disorders: A systematic review of clinical trials" found in Food Science & Nutrition, discusses ginger's role in reducing inflammation and supporting immune health.

Astragalus and Elderflower Immune Tea

Beneficial effects

Astragalus and Elderflower Immune Tea combines the immune-boosting power of astragalus root with the antiviral and anti-inflammatory properties of elderflower. This herbal blend is designed to strengthen the body's natural defenses, making it an excellent choice for cold and flu prevention. Astragalus is known for its ability to increase the production of white blood cells, which are crucial for fighting off infections. Elderflower adds a soothing, anti-inflammatory component that can help reduce symptoms like sore throats and sinus congestion. Together, they create a powerful tea that supports overall immune health.

Portions

Makes about 4 cups

Preparation time

5 minutes

Cooking time

20 minutes

Ingredients

- 4 cups of water
- 2 tablespoons dried astragalus root
- 2 tablespoons dried elderflower
- Honey to taste (optional)
- Lemon slices for garnish (optional)

Instructions

1. Bring 4 cups of water to a boil in a medium saucepan.
2. Once the water is boiling, reduce the heat to low and add the dried astragalus root and dried elderflower to the saucepan.
3. Cover the saucepan with a lid and allow the mixture to simmer gently for 20 minutes. This slow simmering process helps to extract the active compounds from the herbs, infusing the water with their immune-boosting properties.
4. After simmering, remove the saucepan from the heat. Strain the tea through a fine mesh strainer into a large teapot or pitcher, discarding the used herbs.
5. If desired, sweeten the tea with honey to taste. Stir well to ensure the honey is fully dissolved.
6. Serve the tea hot, garnished with a slice of lemon in each cup if desired. The lemon not only adds a refreshing flavor but also provides an additional boost of vitamin C.

Variations

- For a spicier flavor, add a small piece of fresh ginger to the saucepan along with the astragalus and elderflower.
- Incorporate a cinnamon stick during the simmering process for a warming, aromatic twist.
- To enhance the immune-boosting effects, add a teaspoon of dried echinacea to the blend. Note that echinacea should be used with caution if you have autoimmune diseases.

Storage tips
Allow any leftover tea to cool to room temperature before transferring it to a glass jar or bottle. Store the tea in the refrigerator for up to 3 days. Reheat gently on the stove or enjoy cold for a refreshing boost.

Tips for allergens
For those with allergies or sensitivities to honey, consider substituting with maple syrup or simply enjoy the tea unsweetened. If you have pollen allergies, be cautious when trying elderflower for the first time, as it may trigger allergic reactions in some individuals.

Scientific references
- "Astragalus membranaceus: A Review of its Protection Against Inflammation and Gastrointestinal Cancers" published in the American Journal of Chinese Medicine, highlights the immune-boosting and anti-inflammatory effects of astragalus.
- "Antiviral effect of flavonoids on human viruses" published in the Journal of Medical Virology, discusses the antiviral properties of compounds found in elderflower, supporting its use in immune support teas.

Reishi Mushroom and Echinacea Immune Support Tincture

Beneficial effects
The Reishi Mushroom and Echinacea Immune Support Tincture combines the immune-boosting properties of Reishi mushrooms, known for their ability to enhance the body's defense mechanisms, with the potent immune-stimulating effects of Echinacea. This tincture is designed to support the immune system, helping the body to fend off and recover from illness more effectively. Reishi mushrooms have been studied for their role in increasing white blood cell activity, which is crucial for fighting infections, while Echinacea is known to shorten the duration of colds and flu and may improve overall immune health.

Portions
Makes about 1 pint

Preparation time
10 minutes (excluding infusing time)

Cooking time
N/A

Ingredients
- 1/2 cup dried Reishi mushroom slices
- 1/2 cup dried Echinacea purpurea root
- 1 pint of high-proof alcohol (e.g., vodka or brandy, at least 80 proof)
- Glass jar with a tight-fitting lid

Instructions
1. Place the dried Reishi mushroom slices and dried Echinacea root into a clean, dry glass jar.
2. Pour the high-proof alcohol over the herbs, ensuring they are completely submerged. If necessary, add more alcohol until the herbs are covered by at least an inch of liquid.
3. Secure the lid tightly on the jar and shake gently to mix the herbs with the alcohol.
4. Label the jar with the date and contents. Store the jar in a cool, dark place.

5. Allow the mixture to infuse for 4 to 6 weeks, shaking the jar gently every few days to agitate the herbs.

6. After the infusion period, strain the tincture through a fine mesh strainer or cheesecloth into another clean, dry jar or bottle. Press or squeeze the herb material to extract as much liquid as possible.

7. Discard the spent herbs. Transfer the strained tincture into dark glass dropper bottles for easy use.

8. Label the dropper bottles with the tincture name and date of completion.

Variations

- For a non-alcoholic version, glycerin can be used in place of alcohol, though the extraction process may differ slightly and the resulting tincture may have a shorter shelf life.
- Add other immune-supporting herbs such as astragalus or ginger to the tincture for additional benefits.
- For a stronger tincture, allow the mixture to infuse for up to 8 weeks before straining.

Storage tips

Store the tincture in a cool, dark place. The alcohol content preserves the tincture, allowing it to maintain potency for several years.

Tips for allergens

Individuals with allergies to mushrooms or Echinacea should avoid this tincture. As always, consult with a healthcare provider before starting any new herbal regimen, especially if you have allergies, are pregnant, nursing, or taking prescription medications.

Scientific references

- "Immunomodulatory Effects of Ganoderma lucidum (Reishi) Polysaccharides: A Systematic Review," published in the journal Biomolecules, highlights the immune-supporting properties of Reishi mushrooms.
- "Echinacea purpurea: A Proprietary Extract of Echinacea purpurea Is Shown to be Safe and Effective in the Prevention of the Common Cold," published in the Journal of Clinical Pharmacy and Therapeutics, discusses the beneficial effects of Echinacea on the immune system.

BOOK 16: HERBS FOR SKIN AND WOUND HEALING

CHAPTER 1: TOPICAL HERBS FOR SKIN HEALTH

Calendula for Wound Healing and Eczema

Calendula, scientifically known as Calendula officinalis, is a potent herb renowned for its anti-inflammatory and skin-soothing properties, making it an invaluable asset in the treatment of wounds and eczema. The petals of the calendula flower contain a rich array of bioactive compounds including flavonoids, saponins, and triterpenoids, which collectively contribute to its therapeutic efficacy.

For wound healing, calendula works by promoting cell repair and growth, thereby accelerating the healing process. Its anti-inflammatory properties help in reducing swelling and redness around wounds. To prepare a calendula-infused oil for wound care, start by drying calendula petals thoroughly to remove any moisture, as this can lead to spoilage. Use a clean, dry jar to fill one-third with dried calendula petals. Pour a carrier oil such as olive oil or sweet almond oil over the petals until the jar is nearly full, ensuring the petals are completely submerged. Seal the jar tightly and place it in a warm, sunny spot for 4 to 6 weeks, shaking it gently every few days. After the infusion period, strain the oil through a fine mesh strainer or cheesecloth into a clean, dry bottle. Apply this oil directly to the wound or use it as a base for salves.

For treating eczema, calendula's hydrating properties help to soothe dry, irritated skin, and its anti-inflammatory action reduces the itchiness and redness associated with eczema flare-ups. A simple calendula cream can be made by melting 1 part beeswax in a double boiler, then slowly adding 4 parts calendula-infused oil, stirring continuously until well combined. Remove from heat and allow the mixture to cool slightly before adding a few drops of lavender essential oil for additional soothing effects. Pour the mixture into sterilized jars and allow it to solidify. Apply to affected areas as needed to alleviate symptoms.

To ensure the potency of calendula remedies, always source high-quality, organic calendula petals. When applying calendula topically, it's crucial to perform a patch test first to rule out any allergic reactions. While calendula is generally safe for topical use, it's advisable to consult with a healthcare provider before using it on open wounds or if you have a history of allergies to plants in the Asteraceae family.

Plantain for Skin Irritation

Plantain, scientifically known as Plantago major, is a versatile herb that has been utilized for centuries to address skin irritations and bug bites effectively. This herb is not only widespread and easy to find in many backyards but also packed with bioactive compounds such as allantoin, mucilage, and flavonoids that contribute to its healing properties. These compounds are responsible for plantain's ability to reduce swelling, soothe itching, and promote skin repair.

To harness the benefits of plantain for skin irritations and bug bites, one can prepare a simple yet effective poultice. Begin by gathering fresh plantain leaves, ensuring they are clean and free from pesticides. The fresher the leaves, the more potent their medicinal properties will be. Crush the leaves using a mortar and pestle until a paste-like consistency is achieved. This process releases the plant's natural juices and active compounds. If a mortar and pestle are not available, chewing the leaves gently to break them down can be an alternative method, provided the leaves are clean and the person preparing the poultice has no oral health issues that could lead to contamination.

Once the paste is ready, apply it directly to the affected area. For convenience and to keep the poultice in place, one might cover it with a clean cloth or bandage. This method allows the skin to absorb the plant's active compounds directly. The poultice should be left on the skin for up to an hour or as long as it is comfortable. If the irritation or itching persists, the application can be repeated several times a day until relief is achieved.

For those who prefer a more convenient preparation, plantain leaves can also be infused in oil to create a soothing balm. Begin by drying the plantain leaves thoroughly to prevent mold growth in the oil. Once dried, chop the leaves finely to increase their surface area. Place the chopped leaves in a jar and cover them with a carrier oil, such as olive oil or almond oil, known for their skin-nourishing properties. Allow the mixture to infuse in a warm, sunny spot for 4 to 6 weeks, shaking the jar every few days to mix the contents. After the infusion period, strain the oil through a fine mesh strainer or cheesecloth, and it's ready to be applied directly to the skin or used as a base for making salves or creams by adding beeswax.

When applying any new herbal remedy, especially on open wounds or sensitive skin, it's crucial to perform a patch test first to ensure there is no allergic reaction. Apply a small amount of the preparation on a discreet area of skin and wait for at least 24 hours to observe any adverse reactions.

Incorporating plantain into your home apothecary for addressing skin irritations and bug bites not only provides a natural and effective remedy but also connects you with the healing power of plants that grow right at your doorstep. Its ease of preparation and application makes plantain an invaluable herb for natural skin care and healing.

Comfrey for Tissue Repair

Comfrey, scientifically known as **Symphytum officinale**, is a perennial herb that has been used for centuries in traditional medicine for its remarkable ability to accelerate tissue repair and reduce scarring. The key component responsible for these healing properties is **allantoin**, a compound that stimulates cell proliferation, thereby speeding up the healing process of skin tissues. Additionally, comfrey contains **rosamarinic acid** and **tannins**, which contribute to its anti-inflammatory and astringent effects, further supporting wound healing and skin health.

To harness the benefits of comfrey for tissue repair, one can prepare a **comfrey poultice** or **comfrey-infused oil**. Here's how to do it with precision:

Comfrey Poultice:

1. **Harvesting**: Choose fresh comfrey leaves, preferably from plants that are not flowering, as this is when the concentration of beneficial compounds is highest. Ensure that the leaves are clean and free from pesticides.

2. **Preparation**: Use a mortar and pestle to crush the leaves into a paste. If the leaves are too dry, add a small amount of water to help form the paste. The crushing action releases the plant's active compounds.

3. **Application**: Apply the paste directly to the affected area. If dealing with an open wound, place the paste on a clean piece of gauze or cloth first, then apply to prevent direct contact. Secure it with a bandage.

4. **Duration**: Leave the poultice on for up to 4 hours. For best results, apply a fresh poultice twice daily until improvement is observed.

Comfrey-Infused Oil:

1. **Drying**: Start with drying comfrey leaves to remove moisture, which could lead to mold growth in the oil. Spread the leaves in a single layer on a clean surface and allow them to air dry, away from direct sunlight, until they are brittle to the touch.

2. **Infusing**: Place the dried leaves in a clean, dry jar, filling it about halfway. Pour a carrier oil, such as olive oil or almond oil, over the leaves until the jar is nearly full. Ensure the leaves are completely submerged to prevent mold formation.

3. **Steeping**: Seal the jar tightly and place it in a warm, dark place for 4 to 6 weeks. This slow infusion process allows the oil to extract the active compounds from the comfrey leaves.

4. **Straining**: After the infusion period, strain the oil through a fine mesh strainer or cheesecloth into a clean, dry bottle. Label the bottle with the date and contents.

For topical use, **comfrey-infused oil** can be applied directly to scars, bruises, sprains, or areas in need of tissue repair. Alternatively, the oil can be used as a base for making salves or creams by adding beeswax and essential oils for added benefits.

Safety Note: While comfrey is highly effective for external use, it is important to note that it contains **pyrrolizidine alkaloids (PAs)**, which can be toxic if ingested or used improperly. Therefore, comfrey should never be applied to open wounds or broken skin where it could be absorbed into the bloodstream. Pregnant or nursing women and individuals with liver issues should avoid using comfrey.

By incorporating comfrey into your home apothecary for skin and wound care, you can take advantage of its powerful healing properties. Whether used as a poultice or infused oil, comfrey offers a natural and effective solution for promoting skin health and accelerating the healing process.

Three DIY Healing Recipes

Calendula and Aloe Vera Skin Repair Cream

Beneficial effects

Calendula and Aloe Vera Skin Repair Cream combines the soothing and healing properties of aloe vera with the anti-inflammatory and antibacterial benefits of calendula. This cream is designed to promote skin healing, reduce inflammation, and soothe irritated skin. Calendula has been used historically for its wound-healing properties, while aloe vera is known for its ability to treat burns and hydrate the skin. Together, they create a powerful remedy for a variety of skin issues, including minor cuts, burns, and dry skin.

Portions

Makes about 1 cup

Preparation time

30 minutes

Cooking time

10 minutes

Ingredients

- 1/2 cup aloe vera gel, freshly extracted or pure store-bought
- 1/4 cup calendula oil (infused in a carrier oil like olive or almond oil)
- 1/4 cup coconut oil
- 2 tablespoons beeswax pellets
- 1 teaspoon vitamin E oil
- 10 drops lavender essential oil (optional for fragrance and additional skin benefits)

Instructions

1. Begin by setting up a double boiler: Fill a pot with a few inches of water and place it on the stove over medium heat. Place a heat-safe glass bowl over the pot, ensuring the bottom of the bowl does not touch the water.

2. Add the coconut oil and beeswax pellets to the glass bowl. Stir gently until the mixture is completely melted and combined.

3. Once melted, remove the bowl from heat. Stir in the calendula oil and vitamin E oil until well combined.

4. Allow the mixture to cool for a few minutes but not solidify. Once it has cooled slightly, add the aloe vera gel. Stir vigorously to ensure the aloe vera is fully incorporated into the oil mixture. If using, add the lavender essential oil at this stage and mix well.

5. Quickly transfer the mixture to a clean, dry container with a lid while it is still liquid. Allow it to cool and solidify completely.

6. Once cooled, seal the container. Label it with the contents and date.

Variations

- For a vegan version, substitute beeswax with an equal amount of candelilla wax.
- Add chamomile essential oil instead of lavender for its calming skin benefits, especially suitable for sensitive skin.
- For extra hydration, include a tablespoon of shea butter in the oil and beeswax mixture.

Storage tips

Store the Calendula and Aloe Vera Skin Repair Cream in a cool, dry place away from direct sunlight. If stored properly, the cream should last for up to 6 months. If the cream appears to be separating or has an unusual odor, discard it.

Tips for allergens

For those with sensitivities to coconut oil, jojoba oil can be used as a substitute. Always patch test before applying to larger areas of the skin, especially if you have sensitive skin or are prone to allergies. If using essential oils, ensure they are diluted properly to avoid skin irritation.

Scientific references

- "Anti-inflammatory and wound healing activity of a growth substance in Aloe vera," published in the Journal of the American Podiatric Medical Association, highlights the healing properties of aloe vera.
- "Anti-inflammatory activity of extracts from Aloe vera gel," published in the Journal of Ethnopharmacology, supports the use of aloe vera for inflammation.
- "Calendula extract: effects on mechanical parameters of human skin," published in Acta Poloniae Pharmaceutica, discusses the benefits of calendula on skin health.

Lavender and Chamomile Facial Mist

Beneficial effects

Lavender and Chamomile Facial Mist offers a soothing, hydrating, and calming effect on the skin, making it an excellent choice for daily skincare routines. Lavender has natural anti-inflammatory and antiseptic properties that can help reduce redness, acne, and irritation, while chamomile is renowned for its calming effects, particularly beneficial for sensitive or irritated skin. Together, they create a refreshing mist that not only revitalizes the skin but also provides a moment of relaxation and stress relief.

Preparation time

5 minutes

Ingredients

- 1 cup distilled water
- 1 tablespoon dried lavender flowers

- 1 tablespoon dried chamomile flowers
- 1 teaspoon witch hazel (optional, for added skin toning benefits)
- Small funnel
- Fine mesh strainer or cheesecloth
- Clean, empty spray bottle (preferably dark glass to preserve the properties of the mist)

Instructions

1. Boil 1 cup of distilled water in a small saucepan.
2. Remove the saucepan from heat and add 1 tablespoon of dried lavender flowers and 1 tablespoon of dried chamomile flowers to the hot water.
3. Cover the saucepan and let the flowers steep for about 15-20 minutes. This allows the water to become infused with the soothing properties of the herbs.
4. After steeping, use a fine mesh strainer or cheesecloth to strain the herbal infusion into a clean bowl, ensuring all plant matter is removed.
5. If using, add 1 teaspoon of witch hazel to the strained liquid. Witch hazel is a natural astringent that can help tighten the pores and smooth the skin, but it's optional depending on skin sensitivity.
6. Using a small funnel, carefully pour the final mixture into a clean, empty spray bottle. If using a dark glass bottle, it will help preserve the integrity of the mist by protecting it from light.
7. Secure the spray bottle's lid or nozzle in place.

Variations

- For extra hydration, add a few drops of glycerin to the mixture. Glycerin is a humectant, meaning it helps retain moisture in the skin.
- Incorporate a few drops of vitamin E oil for its antioxidant properties, which can help protect the skin from environmental stressors.
- For a refreshing scent and additional antibacterial properties, add a drop or two of tea tree essential oil.

Storage tips

Store your Lavender and Chamomile Facial Mist in the refrigerator to maintain freshness and provide an extra cooling effect upon application. Use within 1-2 weeks for best quality.

Tips for allergens

Individuals with sensitivities to lavender or chamomile should perform a patch test on a small area of skin before applying the mist fully. If irritation occurs, discontinue use. For those allergic to witch hazel, simply omit it from the recipe without affecting the soothing and hydrating benefits of the mist.

Tea Tree and Witch Hazel Acne Spot Treatment

Beneficial effects

Tea Tree and Witch Hazel Acne Spot Treatment harnesses the natural antiseptic and anti-inflammatory properties of tea tree oil, combined with the soothing, astringent benefits of witch hazel. This blend is designed to target and reduce acne breakouts, minimize pores, and soothe inflamed skin without harsh chemicals. Tea tree oil is known for its ability to fight bacteria and reduce skin inflammation, while witch hazel helps to tighten skin and reduce oiliness. Together, they create a powerful remedy for clear, healthy skin.

Preparation time

5 minutes

Ingredients
- 1/4 cup witch hazel
- 10 drops tea tree oil
- 1 teaspoon aloe vera gel
- Small, dark glass bottle with dropper

Instructions
1. Start by ensuring your small, dark glass bottle is clean and dry. A dark bottle helps to protect the essential oils from light, preserving their therapeutic properties.
2. Measure 1/4 cup of witch hazel and pour it into the bottle. Witch hazel acts as the base of this treatment, providing a soothing, astringent effect that helps to clean and tighten pores.
3. Add 10 drops of tea tree oil to the witch hazel. Tea tree oil is a potent antibacterial and anti-inflammatory agent that helps to combat acne-causing bacteria and reduce redness.
4. Incorporate 1 teaspoon of aloe vera gel into the mixture. Aloe vera gel offers a cooling and soothing effect, helping to calm irritated skin and promote healing.
5. Secure the dropper on the bottle and shake well to combine all the ingredients thoroughly. The mixture should appear slightly cloudy and have a fresh, clean scent.
6. To apply, use the dropper to dispense a small amount of the spot treatment directly onto a clean fingertip or cotton swab, then dab gently onto the affected area. Avoid rubbing to prevent irritation.
7. Allow the treatment to dry naturally on the skin for a few minutes before applying any other products or makeup.

Variations
- For extra moisturizing properties, add a few drops of jojoba oil to the mixture. Jojoba oil is non-comedogenic and closely mimics the skin's natural oils, providing hydration without clogging pores.
- If you have sensitive skin, reduce the amount of tea tree oil to 5 drops to lessen the concentration. You can gradually increase the amount as your skin adjusts.
- For an added cooling effect, especially beneficial for inflamed acne, store the treatment in the refrigerator.

Storage tips
Keep the acne spot treatment in a cool, dark place, away from direct sunlight. The refrigerator is an ideal storage location to maintain the freshness and efficacy of the ingredients. Use within 6 months for best results.

Tips for allergens
If you're sensitive to tea tree oil, a patch test is recommended before applying it to your face. Apply a small amount of the treatment to the inside of your wrist and wait 24 hours to check for any adverse reaction. For those allergic to aloe vera, substitute it with an equal amount of chamomile tea, which also has soothing properties.

CHAPTER 2: HERBS FOR ACNE AND SKIN CONDITIONS

Tea Tree Oil for Blemish Control

Tea tree oil, derived from the leaves of the Melaleuca alternifolia tree native to Australia, has garnered acclaim for its potent antimicrobial properties, making it an invaluable asset in the treatment of acne-prone skin. The oil's efficacy against acne stems from its ability to combat bacteria and reduce inflammation, two primary culprits behind acne outbreaks. When incorporating tea tree oil into a skincare regimen for blemish control, precision in its application and understanding its mechanism are paramount.

The antimicrobial action of tea tree oil is attributed to its composition, rich in terpinen-4-ol, a compound known to kill bacteria, viruses, and fungi, thereby directly targeting the bacteria responsible for acne formation. This makes it a formidable natural alternative to synthetic acne treatments, which may provoke adverse reactions or contribute to antibiotic resistance over time. To harness tea tree oil's benefits for acne management, it is essential to dilute it properly, as its potent nature can cause irritation or dryness if applied directly to the skin in its undiluted form.

For effective use, begin by selecting a high-quality, therapeutic-grade tea tree oil, ensuring it's pure and free from additives. To prepare a diluted solution, mix a few drops of tea tree oil with a carrier oil such as jojoba, sweet almond, or coconut oil, which not only mitigates the risk of irritation but also enhances the oil's penetration into the skin. A recommended starting ratio is 1 to 2 drops of tea tree oil per tablespoon of carrier oil, which can be adjusted based on skin sensitivity and response.

Application should be targeted and precise. After cleansing the skin, apply the diluted tea tree oil mixture directly to blemishes using a cotton swab or a clean fingertip, avoiding the surrounding skin to minimize irritation. This spot treatment can be used once or twice daily, monitoring the skin for any signs of discomfort or dryness, which may necessitate reducing the frequency of application or further dilution of the oil.

In addition to spot treatments, tea tree oil can be integrated into daily skincare through homemade or commercially available products formulated for acne-prone skin, such as cleansers, toners, and moisturizers that contain tea tree oil in safe, effective concentrations. When incorporating these products, it's advisable to introduce them gradually into your skincare routine, starting with once-daily applications and observing how your skin reacts before increasing usage.

Despite its benefits, it's crucial to acknowledge that tea tree oil, like any remedy, may not be universally effective for all individuals. Factors such as skin type, severity of acne, and individual sensitivities play a significant role in determining its suitability. Therefore, it's recommended to conduct a patch test prior to regular use by applying a small amount of the diluted oil to an inconspicuous area of skin and waiting 24 hours to assess for any adverse reactions.

Incorporating tea tree oil into your regimen for acne management offers a natural, effective approach to combating blemishes while fostering overall skin health. Its antimicrobial and anti-inflammatory properties make it a standout choice for those seeking alternatives to conventional acne treatments, embodying the principles of ancient wisdom in natural health and wellness.

Witch Hazel for Oily Skin

Witch hazel, scientifically known as Hamamelis virginiana, is a plant native to North America, renowned for its astringent properties, making it an exceptional choice for managing oily skin. The leaves and bark of witch hazel are distilled to produce a clear, fragrant liquid that is widely used in skincare for its ability to tighten skin, reduce inflammation, and control sebum production. The active components in witch hazel, including tannins and flavonoids, contribute to its therapeutic effects, particularly in the regulation of oil on the skin's surface.

To effectively utilize witch hazel for oily skin, it's essential to integrate it into your skincare routine in a manner that harnesses its benefits without over-drying the skin. Begin by selecting a high-quality, alcohol-free witch hazel extract, as alcohol-based formulations can be overly drying, especially for individuals with sensitive skin. Look for products that are labeled as non-comedogenic to ensure they won't clog pores, exacerbating skin issues.

For application, use witch hazel as a toner after cleansing your face. Pour a small amount of witch hazel onto a cotton pad until it's slightly damp but not overly saturated. Gently swipe the cotton pad across your face, focusing on areas prone to oiliness such as the T-zone, which includes the forehead, nose, and chin. The witch hazel will work to remove any residual oil, makeup, or dirt left after cleansing, providing a deep clean that doesn't strip the skin of its natural moisture. This step not only helps in managing oil production but also prepares the skin to better absorb moisturizers or treatments applied afterward.

Incorporating witch hazel into your morning and evening skincare routines can significantly contribute to balancing sebum production over time. However, it's crucial to monitor your skin's response to witch hazel, as overuse can lead to irritation or dryness in some individuals. If you notice any adverse effects, consider reducing the frequency of application or diluting the witch hazel with distilled water to lessen its potency.

For individuals seeking to further enhance the oil-controlling properties of witch hazel, consider combining it with other natural ingredients known for their skin-balancing effects. A few drops of tea tree oil can be added to witch hazel to boost its antimicrobial and anti-inflammatory capabilities, making it even more effective against acne-prone, oily skin. Alternatively, aloe vera gel can be mixed with witch hazel to create a soothing, hydrating toner that controls oil while calming the skin.

It's also beneficial to store witch hazel in a cool, dark place to maintain its efficacy. Exposure to direct sunlight or heat can degrade the active compounds, reducing its therapeutic benefits. When applied consistently as part of a comprehensive skincare regimen, witch hazel can significantly improve the appearance and health of oily skin, providing a natural, gentle solution to managing excess sebum production.

Neem for Psoriasis and Skin Issues

Neem, scientifically known as Azadirachta indica, has been a cornerstone in traditional medicine for centuries, particularly in Ayurvedic practices. Its potent anti-inflammatory and antimicrobial properties make it an invaluable resource for managing psoriasis and other chronic skin issues. The active compounds in neem, such as nimbidin, nimbin, and quercetin, contribute to its therapeutic effects, including reducing redness, swelling, and irritation associated with psoriasis flare-ups. Additionally, neem's antifungal and antibacterial activities help prevent secondary infections that can complicate skin conditions.

For individuals dealing with psoriasis, incorporating neem into their skincare routine can be done in several ways. One effective method is through the application of neem oil, extracted from the seeds of the neem tree. To utilize neem oil for psoriasis, it's recommended to dilute pure, cold-pressed neem oil with a carrier oil, such as coconut or almond oil, to minimize any potential skin irritation. A ratio of one part neem oil to ten parts carrier oil is a good starting point. Apply this blend to the affected areas using a clean cotton pad, ideally before bedtime, allowing the mixture to work overnight. Regular application can significantly alleviate symptoms, thanks to neem oil's ability to penetrate deep into the skin, moisturizing and healing the dry, cracked surfaces characteristic of psoriasis patches.

Another approach is the use of neem leaves, which can be made into a paste or used to brew a therapeutic bath. For a neem leaf paste, grind fresh or dried neem leaves with a little water until a smooth paste forms. Apply this directly to the skin, leaving it on for about 20 minutes before rinsing with cool water. This treatment can help soothe the itching and discomfort often experienced with psoriasis. Alternatively, a neem leaf bath offers a full-body treatment. Boil a handful of neem leaves in water, strain, and then add this neem-infused water to a bath. Soaking in this medicinal bath for 15-20 minutes can aid in reducing the inflammation and scaling associated with psoriasis.

It's important to note that while neem offers considerable benefits for skin health, its potency means it should be used with care. Always conduct a patch test when trying neem oil or leaf preparations for the first time to ensure there is no adverse reaction. Additionally, individuals who are pregnant, nursing, or have pre-existing medical conditions should consult with a healthcare provider before incorporating neem into their treatment regimen.

Incorporating neem into daily skincare practices not only addresses the symptoms of psoriasis but also supports the skin's natural healing processes without the harsh side effects often associated with chemical treatments. Its ability to cleanse, heal, and protect the skin makes neem a valuable ally in the management of chronic skin conditions.

Tea Tree and Aloe Vera Acne Gel

Beneficial effects
Tea Tree and Aloe Vera Acne Gel harnesses the potent antimicrobial properties of tea tree oil and the soothing, moisturizing benefits of aloe vera to create a powerful treatment for acne-prone skin. Tea tree oil is known for its ability to combat bacteria and reduce inflammation, making it an effective natural remedy for acne and skin blemishes. Aloe vera, on the other hand, provides a cooling effect that soothes irritated skin, promotes healing, and hydrates without clogging pores. This combination not only targets existing acne but also helps to prevent new breakouts, leaving the skin clear and refreshed.

Portions
Makes about 1/2 cup

Preparation time
10 minutes

Ingredients
- 1/4 cup pure aloe vera gel
- 10 drops tea tree essential oil
- 1 tablespoon distilled water (optional, for thinner consistency)
- 1 teaspoon vitamin E oil (optional, for added skin healing and preservation)

Instructions
1. Start by ensuring your workspace is clean and you have a sanitized small mixing bowl and spoon or whisk ready.

2. Measure 1/4 cup of pure aloe vera gel and place it into the mixing bowl. If your aloe vera gel is very thick, consider adding 1 tablespoon of distilled water to achieve a slightly thinner, more spreadable consistency.

3. Add 10 drops of tea tree essential oil to the aloe vera gel. Tea tree oil is potent, so it's important to measure accurately to avoid skin irritation.

4. If using, add 1 teaspoon of vitamin E oil to the mixture. Vitamin E oil acts as a natural preservative and can help extend the shelf life of your acne gel. It also supports skin healing and reduces scarring.

5. Use the spoon or whisk to thoroughly mix all the ingredients until you achieve a homogeneous mixture. Ensure the tea tree oil is well distributed throughout the aloe vera gel.

6. Once mixed, carefully transfer the acne gel into a clean, airtight container. A small squeeze bottle or jar with a lid works well for easy application and storage.

7. Label your container with the contents and date made.

Variations

- For added anti-inflammatory benefits, include 5 drops of lavender essential oil. Lavender can help soothe the skin and reduce redness associated with acne.
- Incorporate 1/2 teaspoon of witch hazel for its astringent properties, which can help tighten pores and further reduce oiliness.
- To target stubborn acne, add 2 drops of lemon essential oil for its antiseptic and antimicrobial properties. Be cautious of sun exposure when using lemon oil on the skin.

Storage tips

Store your Tea Tree and Aloe Vera Acne Gel in a cool, dark place, preferably in the refrigerator, to maintain its freshness and potency. Use within 3 months for best results. If the mixture changes color, smell, or texture, it should be discarded.

Tips for allergens

Individuals with sensitive skin or allergies to tea tree oil should perform a patch test on a small area of skin before applying the gel widely. If irritation occurs, discontinue use. For those allergic to aloe vera, consider substituting with an all-natural, fragrance-free, and hypoallergenic moisturizer as the base for your acne treatment.

Calendula and Witch Hazel Skin Toner

Beneficial effects

Calendula and Witch Hazel Skin Toner leverages the natural anti-inflammatory properties of calendula and the astringent benefits of witch hazel to soothe, heal, and tone the skin. This combination is ideal for reducing redness, combating acne, and providing a gentle yet effective cleansing action that leaves the skin feeling refreshed and balanced. Calendula is known for its ability to promote skin healing and regeneration, making it beneficial for those with sensitive or irritated skin. Witch hazel, on the other hand, is a powerful natural astringent that can help tighten pores and refine the skin's texture without over-drying.

Preparation time

15 minutes

Ingredients

- 1/2 cup distilled water
- 1/4 cup witch hazel extract
- 1/4 cup dried calendula petals
- 1 tablespoon aloe vera gel
- 5 drops lavender essential oil (optional for additional soothing properties)

Instructions

1. Begin by boiling the distilled water in a small saucepan. Once boiling, remove from heat.

2. Add the dried calendula petals to the hot water and cover the saucepan. Allow the petals to steep for 10 minutes, infusing the water with their healing properties.

3. After steeping, strain the calendula-infused water through a fine mesh strainer or cheesecloth into a clean bowl, ensuring to remove all petal residues.

4. To the calendula infusion, add the witch hazel extract. Witch hazel serves as a natural toner, helping to cleanse and refine pores without stripping the skin of its natural oils.

5. Stir in the aloe vera gel to the mixture. Aloe vera gel adds a layer of soothing hydration, ideal for calming any skin irritation or redness.

6. If using, add 5 drops of lavender essential oil to the mixture for its calming scent and additional skin-soothing benefits.

7. Pour the final toner mixture into a clean, sterilized glass bottle with a tight-fitting lid or spray top for easy application.

8. Shake well before each use to ensure the ingredients are well combined.

Variations

- For added moisture, include a teaspoon of glycerin to the toner. Glycerin is a humectant that draws moisture into the skin, keeping it hydrated.
- Substitute lavender essential oil with tea tree essential oil for enhanced antibacterial properties, making it more effective against acne-prone skin.
- For those with extra sensitive skin, reduce the amount of witch hazel to 1/8 cup and fill the remainder with rosewater for its gentle soothing and hydrating properties.

Storage tips

Store the Calendula and Witch Hazel Skin Toner in the refrigerator to prolong its shelf life and provide a refreshing, cooling sensation upon application. Use within 1 month for optimal freshness and efficacy.

Tips for allergens

For individuals sensitive to lavender or any essential oils, simply omit this ingredient from the recipe. The toner will still offer significant soothing and toning benefits without it. If witch hazel is too strong for your skin, diluting the toner with more distilled water or substituting with rosewater can provide a gentler alternative.

Neem and Turmeric Face Mask

Beneficial effects

Neem and Turmeric Face Mask leverages the potent antibacterial and anti-inflammatory properties of neem and the antioxidant, brightening benefits of turmeric to create a powerful remedy for acne-prone and troubled skin. Neem, with its rich history in Ayurvedic medicine, is known for its ability to clear up pimples and remove bacteria from the skin surface. Turmeric, on the other hand, reduces redness and skin irritation, promoting a more even skin tone. This mask is designed to detoxify the skin, reduce acne and scars, and provide a radiant complexion.

Portions

Makes enough for 2-3 applications

Preparation time

10 minutes

Ingredients

- 2 tablespoons neem powder
- 1 tablespoon turmeric powder

- 3 tablespoons plain yogurt (or aloe vera gel for a vegan alternative)
- 1 teaspoon honey (optional, for additional antibacterial properties)
- 1-2 teaspoons water (if needed, to achieve desired consistency)

Instructions

1. In a clean, small bowl, combine 2 tablespoons of neem powder and 1 tablespoon of turmeric powder. Mix these dry ingredients thoroughly to ensure they are well blended.

2. Add 3 tablespoons of plain yogurt to the dry mixture. If you are opting for a vegan version, substitute the yogurt with aloe vera gel. This base acts as a binder for the mask and introduces soothing properties.

3. If desired, incorporate 1 teaspoon of honey into the mixture. Honey is optional but recommended for its moisturizing and antibacterial benefits, enhancing the mask's effectiveness against acne.

4. Mix all the ingredients together until you achieve a smooth, consistent paste. If the mixture is too thick, gradually add 1-2 teaspoons of water until you reach a spreadable consistency that will easily adhere to your face without dripping.

5. Apply the mask evenly over your cleansed face and neck, avoiding the delicate area around your eyes. Use your fingers or a mask brush for an even application.

6. Leave the mask on for about 10-15 minutes, or until it begins to dry. You may experience a slight tingling sensation due to the active ingredients, which is normal.

7. Rinse off the mask with lukewarm water, gently massaging your skin in circular motions to exfoliate and remove the mask thoroughly.

8. Pat your face dry with a clean towel and follow up with your regular moisturizer to hydrate your skin.

Variations

- For oily skin, add a few drops of lemon juice to the mixture for its astringent properties.
- If you have dry skin, include a teaspoon of coconut oil in the mask to add moisture and reduce the drying effect of turmeric.
- For an extra soothing effect, especially after sun exposure, replace water with chilled green tea for its antioxidant properties.

Storage tips

It's best to prepare the Neem and Turmeric Face Mask fresh for each use to ensure the potency of the ingredients. However, if you have leftovers, store the mixture in an airtight container in the refrigerator for up to 24 hours. Note that the mask may thicken upon refrigeration; gently stir and possibly add a few drops of water to regain consistency before use.

Tips for allergens

For individuals allergic to dairy, using aloe vera gel as a base instead of yogurt is an effective alternative. Always perform a patch test on the inner arm before applying new ingredients to your face, especially if you have sensitive skin or are prone to allergies. If irritation occurs, rinse off immediately and discontinue use.

Scientific references

- "Antibacterial and antioxidant properties of the Neem tree (Azadirachta indica): A review," published in the International Journal of Science and Research, highlights the antibacterial activity of neem.
- "Curcumin, the active compound in turmeric, and its effects on health," published in the Journal of Medicinal Chemistry, discusses turmeric's anti-inflammatory and antioxidant properties.

CHAPTER 3: ANTI-AGING AND SKIN REJUVENATION

Rosehip Oil for Skin Elasticity

Rosehip oil, derived from the seeds of rose bushes predominantly found in Chile, is a powerhouse of nutrients beneficial for skin health, particularly in boosting collagen production. Collagen, a critical protein in the body, provides structure to the skin, offering elasticity and resilience. As we age, collagen production naturally decreases, leading to the formation of fine lines and a decrease in skin elasticity. Rosehip oil counters these aging signs through its rich composition of vitamins, antioxidants, and essential fatty acids.

To harness rosehip oil's benefits for collagen production, it's essential to integrate it into your skincare routine correctly. Start with **organic, cold-pressed rosehip oil** to ensure you're getting the highest concentration of nutrients. This form of extraction preserves the oil's natural properties, including vitamin A (retinol), vitamin C, and the essential fatty acids omega-3 and omega-6. Vitamin A accelerates skin cell turnover, vitamin C is crucial for collagen synthesis, and the fatty acids promote skin hydration and repair.

For application, follow these detailed steps:

1. **Cleanse your skin** thoroughly to remove any dirt and makeup. A gentle, pH-balanced cleanser is recommended to maintain skin's natural barrier.

2. **Apply a toner** (optional) to balance the skin's pH and remove any residual impurities.

3. **Dispense 2-3 drops of rosehip oil** onto your fingertips. Warm the oil by gently rubbing your fingers together. This action helps to release the oil's natural compounds.

4. **Gently pat and massage** the oil onto your face and neck. Focus on areas with fine lines and wrinkles. The massage technique boosts circulation, enhancing the absorption and efficacy of the oil.

5. **Allow the oil to absorb** for a few minutes before applying a moisturizer. If used during the day, follow up with a broad-spectrum sunscreen to protect the skin from UV damage, which can degrade collagen.

For optimal results, incorporate rosehip oil into your evening skincare routine. Nighttime is when the skin's repair and regeneration processes are most active, allowing the oil's nutrients to work synergistically with these natural functions.

Consistent use is key. Expect to see improvements in skin texture, a reduction in fine lines, and enhanced elasticity after regular use for 3-4 weeks. However, individual results can vary based on skin type, age, and environmental factors.

Remember, while rosehip oil is generally safe for all skin types, conducting a patch test on a small skin area before full application is advisable to ensure no adverse reactions occur. Individuals with specific skin conditions or allergies should consult a dermatologist prior to use.

Incorporating rosehip oil into your skincare regimen offers a natural, effective approach to stimulate collagen production, combat aging signs, and maintain skin's youthful resilience and glow.

Aloe Vera for Hydration and Healing

Aloe Vera, scientifically known as Aloe barbadensis miller, is a succulent plant renowned for its hydrating, soothing, and healing properties, making it an indispensable component in skincare, particularly for anti-aging and skin rejuvenation purposes. Its leaves are filled with a gel-like substance rich in vitamins, minerals, amino acids, and antioxidants, which are crucial for repairing skin damage and maintaining skin hydration and elasticity. The process of leveraging Aloe Vera for skin health involves both direct application of the gel extracted from its leaves and the integration of Aloe Vera extract into daily skincare routines.

To extract Aloe Vera gel directly from the plant, first, select a mature Aloe Vera leaf from the outer section of the plant, as these contain a higher concentration of the gel. Cut the leaf from the base of the plant using a clean, sharp knife. After removal, stand the leaf upright in a cup or bowl for approximately 10-15 minutes to allow the aloin—a yellowish latex-like substance with potential skin irritant properties—to drain out. This step is crucial to avoid potential irritation when applying the gel to the skin.

Once the aloin has drained, rinse the leaf under running water. Carefully slice off the serrated edges of the leaf, then split it open lengthwise with the knife to expose the clear gel inside. Using a spoon, gently scrape out the gel, being careful to avoid any remnants of the yellowish aloin. The fresh Aloe Vera gel can be applied directly to the skin or stored in an airtight container in the refrigerator for up to one week. For extended storage, freezing the gel in ice cube trays is an effective method, allowing for easy, single-use portions.

Incorporating Aloe Vera into your skincare routine can be done through direct application of the gel to the face and body. It serves as an excellent moisturizer for dry or sunburned skin due to its light texture and deeply hydrating properties. Apply the gel gently onto clean skin, focusing on dry areas or those needing healing, such as sunburns, minor cuts, or abrasions. The gel's cooling effect provides immediate relief, while its nutrients work to repair and rejuvenate the skin at a cellular level.

For anti-aging purposes, Aloe Vera gel can be used as a facial mask to improve skin elasticity and reduce the appearance of fine lines and wrinkles. Mix the gel with other natural ingredients known for their anti-aging benefits, such as honey, which offers additional moisturizing and antibacterial properties, or cucumber, which soothes and tightens the skin. Apply the mask to the face and neck, leave it on for 20-30 minutes, then rinse with cool water. This treatment can be repeated two to three times a week for best results.

Moreover, Aloe Vera's antioxidant properties make it beneficial in fighting free radicals and reducing inflammation, contributing to a healthier, more youthful complexion. Its application accelerates the healing of acne scars and reduces redness associated with breakouts.

Ginseng for Skin Vitality

Ginseng, a revered herb in traditional medicine, has been utilized for centuries, particularly in East Asia, for its myriad health benefits. Among its many uses, ginseng plays a significant role in skin care, especially in the realm of anti-aging and skin rejuvenation. This section delves into the specifics of how ginseng contributes to skin vitality, focusing on its efficacy in enhancing circulation and diminishing the appearance of wrinkles.

Ginseng contains a potent blend of compounds known as ginsenosides. These compounds are the primary drivers behind ginseng's ability to improve blood flow. Enhanced circulation is crucial for skin health as it ensures the efficient delivery of oxygen and nutrients to skin cells, while also facilitating the removal of waste products. This process is vital for maintaining the skin's elasticity and firmness. To leverage ginseng's circulatory benefits, incorporating ginseng-infused products into your skincare routine is recommended. Look for serums or creams that list ginseng as one of the top ingredients to ensure a higher concentration and, consequently, greater efficacy.

The method of applying ginseng topically for improved circulation involves gentle, upward circular motions to massage the product into the skin. This technique not only aids in the absorption of ginseng but also stimulates blood flow, enhancing the herb's natural effects. For those interested in a more holistic approach, consuming ginseng tea or supplements can also contribute to overall skin health from the inside out. However, it's important to adhere to recommended dosages to avoid potential side effects.

In addition to boosting circulation, ginseng is renowned for its antioxidant properties. These properties are instrumental in fighting free radicals, which are responsible for much of the skin's aging process, including the development of wrinkles. Ginsenosides, along with other antioxidants present in ginseng, help in mitigating oxidative stress, thereby slowing down the formation of fine lines and wrinkles. For targeted wrinkle reduction, applying a ginseng-based anti-aging cream or serum directly to areas of concern can yield noticeable results. Products formulated with ginseng extract can help in firming the skin and reducing the depth of wrinkles with regular use.

Creating a DIY ginseng mask offers a personalized approach to incorporating this powerful herb into your skincare regimen. To prepare the mask, mix ginseng powder with a hydrating base, such as honey or aloe vera gel, until a paste is formed. Apply this mixture to clean skin, leaving it on for 15-20 minutes before rinsing with lukewarm water. This mask can be used once or twice a week to harness ginseng's anti-aging benefits, including enhanced skin vitality and a reduction in the appearance of wrinkles.

As with any herbal supplement or skincare ingredient, it's essential to monitor your skin's response and consult with a healthcare provider or dermatologist if you have any concerns or pre-existing conditions.

Rosehip and Hibiscus Anti-Aging Serum

Beneficial effects

Rosehip and Hibiscus Anti-Aging Serum combines the potent antioxidant properties of rosehip, rich in Vitamin C and A, known for their skin rejuvenating and brightening effects, with the anti-inflammatory and hydrating benefits of hibiscus, often referred to as the 'Botox' plant for its firming and lifting action. This serum aims to boost collagen production, reduce fine lines and wrinkles, and improve skin tone and texture, offering a natural, effective solution for aging skin.

Portions

Makes about 1 ounce (30 ml)

Preparation time

15 minutes

Ingredients

- 2 tablespoons rosehip seed oil
- 1 tablespoon hibiscus flower extract (ensure it's alcohol-free)
- 1 teaspoon jojoba oil
- 1/2 teaspoon vitamin E oil
- 5 drops frankincense essential oil
- 5 drops lavender essential oil
- Dark glass dropper bottle (1 oz)

Instructions

1. Begin by sanitizing your dark glass dropper bottle with boiling water or by wiping it down with alcohol. Let it dry completely.

2. In a small, clean mixing bowl, combine 2 tablespoons of rosehip seed oil with 1 tablespoon of hibiscus flower extract. Rosehip seed oil is known for its ability to deeply nourish the skin, while hibiscus extract offers natural AHAs and antioxidants.

3. Add 1 teaspoon of jojoba oil to the mixture. Jojoba oil is chosen for its similarity to the skin's natural sebum, making it an excellent moisturizer that doesn't clog pores.

4. Stir in 1/2 teaspoon of vitamin E oil. Vitamin E acts as a natural preservative and antioxidant, helping to extend the serum's shelf life and boost skin repair and protection.

5. Carefully add 5 drops each of frankincense and lavender essential oils. Frankincense is celebrated for its ability to reduce the appearance of wrinkles and fine lines, while lavender soothes the skin and adds a calming fragrance.

6. Mix all the ingredients thoroughly until well combined.

7. Using a small funnel, transfer the serum mixture into your prepared dark glass dropper bottle. The dark glass helps protect the oils from light, preserving their beneficial properties.

8. Seal the bottle tightly with the dropper cap.

Variations

- For added hydration, include a few drops of glycerin to the serum. Glycerin is a humectant that draws moisture into the skin.
- If you have oily or acne-prone skin, substitute lavender essential oil with tea tree essential oil for its antimicrobial properties.
- For a brightening boost, add 2 drops of lemon essential oil. Ensure to apply sunscreen when using lemon oil in skincare products due to increased photosensitivity.

Storage tips

Store the Rosehip and Hibiscus Anti-Aging Serum in a cool, dark place away from direct sunlight. Ideally, keep it in your refrigerator to maintain its freshness and efficacy for up to 6 months.

Tips for allergens

For those with sensitive skin or allergies to essential oils, perform a patch test on a small area of your skin before applying the serum to your face. You can also reduce the amount of essential oils or omit them entirely, substituting with more jojoba or rosehip seed oil.

Pomegranate and Green Tea Rejuvenating Face Mask

Beneficial effects

The Pomegranate and Green Tea Rejuvenating Face Mask combines the powerful antioxidant properties of pomegranate and green tea to fight free radical damage, reduce signs of aging, and improve skin elasticity. Pomegranate is rich in vitamin C and antioxidants, which help in cell regeneration and preservation of collagen. Green tea, known for its anti-inflammatory properties, soothes the skin and reduces redness. Together, they create a potent blend that leaves the skin feeling refreshed, with a youthful glow.

Portions

Makes enough for 2 applications

Preparation time

15 minutes

Ingredients

- 1/4 cup fresh pomegranate seeds
- 1 tablespoon green tea leaves, finely ground
- 2 tablespoons organic honey
- 1 tablespoon natural yogurt

Instructions

1. Begin by crushing the 1/4 cup of fresh pomegranate seeds using a mortar and pestle until you have a smooth paste. This process releases the juice and extracts the beneficial compounds from the seeds.
2. In a small bowl, mix the crushed pomegranate seeds with 1 tablespoon of finely ground green tea leaves. Grinding the green tea leaves prior to mixing helps to release their potent antioxidants more effectively.
3. Add 2 tablespoons of organic honey to the pomegranate and green tea mixture. Honey acts as a natural humectant, drawing moisture into the skin, and has antibacterial properties that help to cleanse the skin.
4. Incorporate 1 tablespoon of natural yogurt into the blend. Yogurt contains lactic acid, which gently exfoliates the skin, leaving it smooth and soft.
5. Mix all the ingredients thoroughly until you achieve a consistent, paste-like texture. Ensure that the mixture is homogenous to allow for even application on the skin.
6. Apply the mask evenly over your cleansed face and neck, avoiding the eye area. The natural acids in the mask can irritate sensitive areas.
7. Leave the mask on for 10-15 minutes, allowing the ingredients to penetrate the skin and work their rejuvenating magic.
8. Rinse off the mask with lukewarm water, gently massaging in a circular motion to exfoliate any dead skin cells.
9. Pat your skin dry with a soft towel and follow up with your favorite moisturizer to lock in hydration.

Variations

- For oily skin, add a teaspoon of lemon juice to the mask for its astringent properties, which can help control excess sebum production.
- If you have dry skin, substitute yogurt with avocado to add extra moisturizing benefits.
- For an added cooling effect, refrigerate the mask for 20 minutes before applying. This is especially refreshing during warmer months or after sun exposure.

Storage tips

It's best to use the Pomegranate and Green Tea Rejuvenating Face Mask immediately after preparation due to the fresh ingredients. However, if you must store it, keep the mask in an airtight container in the refrigerator and use within 24 hours.

Tips for allergens

Individuals with sensitivity to dairy can replace the natural yogurt with a dairy-free alternative such as coconut yogurt. For those allergic to honey, agave syrup can be used as a substitute, though it lacks the antibacterial properties of honey.

Scientific references

- "Pomegranate extract demonstrates significant antioxidant activity and inhibits skin cell proliferation in vitro," published in the Journal of Ethnopharmacology, highlights the antioxidant properties of pomegranate.
- "Green tea and its polyphenols are known to possess potent anti-inflammatory and anti-cancer properties," published in the Journal of the American Academy of Dermatology, discusses the benefits of green tea for the skin.

Sea Buckthorn and Frankincense Youthful Glow Elixir

Beneficial effects

The Sea Buckthorn and Frankincense Youthful Glow Elixir combines the potent antioxidant properties of sea buckthorn with the anti-inflammatory and skin-rejuvenating benefits of frankincense oil. This elixir is designed to promote skin health, reduce signs of aging, and enhance the skin's natural glow. Sea buckthorn is rich in vitamins and minerals that nourish the skin, while frankincense is known for its ability to reduce the appearance of wrinkles, scars, and fine lines. Together, they create a powerful blend that supports skin regeneration, hydration, and elasticity.

Portions

Makes about 1 cup

Preparation time

15 minutes

Ingredients

- 1/2 cup sea buckthorn oil
- 1/2 cup jojoba oil
- 20 drops frankincense essential oil
- 10 drops lavender essential oil (for additional soothing properties)
- Dark glass bottle with dropper

Instructions

1. Begin by measuring 1/2 cup of sea buckthorn oil and pouring it into a clean, dry mixing bowl. Sea buckthorn oil is known for its high content of Vitamin C and E, which are crucial for skin health.
2. Add 1/2 cup of jojoba oil to the bowl. Jojoba oil is chosen for its similarity to the skin's natural sebum, making it an excellent carrier oil that enhances the absorption of sea buckthorn.
3. Carefully add 20 drops of frankincense essential oil to the mixture. Frankincense is celebrated for its ability to promote the regeneration of healthy skin cells and improve skin tone.
4. Include 10 drops of lavender essential oil for its calming and anti-inflammatory properties, which can help soothe the skin and reduce redness.
5. Using a small whisk or spoon, gently mix the oils together until they are fully blended.
6. Using a funnel, transfer the oil blend into a dark glass bottle to protect the oils from light degradation. Secure the dropper to the bottle.
7. Label the bottle with the contents and date of creation.

Variations

- For dry skin, add 5 drops of vitamin E oil to the blend for its moisturizing and healing properties.
- If you have sensitive skin, reduce the amount of frankincense essential oil to 10 drops to minimize the risk of irritation.
- For an extra anti-aging boost, incorporate 5 drops of rosehip oil into the mixture for its high antioxidant content.

Storage tips

Store the Sea Buckthorn and Frankincense Youthful Glow Elixir in a cool, dark place away from direct sunlight. The dark glass bottle helps preserve the integrity of the oils. Use within 6 months for optimal potency.

Tips for allergens

If you are allergic to any of the essential oils listed, they can be omitted or substituted with another oil that suits your skin type. Always perform a patch test on a small area of your skin 24 hours before applying the elixir fully to ensure there is no adverse reaction.

BOOK 17: HERBS FOR THE NERVOUS SYSTEM

CHAPTER 1: HERBS FOR CALMING AND RELAXATION

Valerian Root for Sleep and Anxiety

Valerian root, scientifically known as Valeriana officinalis, has been utilized for centuries to alleviate insomnia, reduce anxiety, and promote relaxation. This perennial plant, native to Europe and Asia, harbors a wealth of therapeutic compounds within its roots, making it a cornerstone in traditional and modern herbal medicine for managing nervous system disorders.

The efficacy of valerian root in enhancing sleep quality and duration is attributed to its interaction with the gamma-aminobutyric acid (GABA) pathway in the brain. GABA is a neurotransmitter that plays a pivotal role in regulating nerve impulses, and its increased activity is associated with sedative effects. Valerian compounds, particularly valerenic acid, inhibit the breakdown of GABA, thereby inducing calmness and facilitating the onset of sleep.

To harness the benefits of valerian root for sleep, it is recommended to consume it in the form of a tea or a dietary supplement approximately 30 minutes to 2 hours before bedtime. For tea preparation, steep 1 to 2 teaspoons of dried valerian root in boiling water for 10 to 15 minutes. This allows for the optimal extraction of its active ingredients. Capsules and tinctures are also available, with dosages varying according to the concentration of the extract; typically, 300 to 600 milligrams of valerian root extract is suggested for sleep disorders.

In the context of anxiety relief, valerian root's interaction with GABA not only promotes relaxation but also mitigates physiological responses to stress, such as muscle tension and heart palpitations. Its anxiolytic properties make it a valuable ally in managing day-to-day stress and anxiety-related conditions without the dependency or side effects commonly associated with synthetic anxiolytics.

For individuals seeking to incorporate valerian root into their anxiety management regimen, starting with a lower dose during the day can help assess tolerance and effectiveness. Gradually increasing the dosage, if needed, can optimize its therapeutic benefits while minimizing potential side effects, such as drowsiness or gastrointestinal discomfort.

It is crucial to source valerian root from reputable suppliers to ensure the product's purity and potency. Organic and sustainably harvested valerian root is preferable to avoid contaminants that could detract from its therapeutic value. Additionally, maintaining a clean, organized space for storing valerian root, whether in dried, capsule, or tincture form, preserves its potency. Dark glass containers in a cool, dry location are ideal for prolonging the shelf life of valerian root preparations.

While valerian root is generally considered safe for most adults, consulting with a healthcare provider before incorporating it into a health regimen is advisable, especially for individuals with existing medical conditions, pregnant or nursing women, and those taking medications that could interact with herbal supplements. This ensures a holistic and safe approach to enhancing sleep quality and managing anxiety with valerian root as part of a comprehensive wellness strategy.

Lemon Balm for Daytime Calm

Lemon balm, scientifically known as Melissa officinalis, is a perennial herb from the mint family and has been widely recognized for its calming properties without inducing drowsiness, making it an ideal herb for daytime use. Originating from southern Europe and the Mediterranean region, lemon balm has a rich history of use in herbal medicine for improving mood and cognitive function, as well as providing relief from stress and anxiety.

The primary active compounds in lemon balm that contribute to its mild sedative effects include rosmarinic acid, which has been shown to inhibit the enzyme GABA transaminase. This action increases the availability of gamma-aminobutyric acid (GABA), a neurotransmitter in the brain responsible for promoting relaxation. Unlike other sedatives that may cause drowsiness, lemon balm enhances calmness while maintaining alertness and cognitive abilities, making it particularly beneficial for those seeking to reduce stress during the day without compromising their performance or energy levels.

To incorporate lemon balm into your daily routine for achieving daytime calm, consider preparing a lemon balm tea. Use about 1 to 2 teaspoons of dried lemon balm leaves per cup of boiling water. Steep the leaves in the water for 10 to 15 minutes to allow the extraction of its active ingredients. This herbal tea can be consumed 2 to 3 times a day to help manage stress and anxiety, improve mood, and enhance overall mental clarity.

Another method to utilize lemon balm for its calming effects is through the use of lemon balm essential oil. The oil can be diffused in your living or workspace to create a calming atmosphere. Alternatively, you can apply a diluted form of lemon balm essential oil topically to the temples or wrists. When using lemon balm oil topically, it's important to dilute it with a carrier oil, such as coconut or jojoba oil, to prevent skin irritation. A typical dilution ratio is 1 to 2 drops of lemon balm essential oil per teaspoon of carrier oil.

For those interested in the convenience of supplements, lemon balm is also available in capsule or tablet form. It's crucial to follow the manufacturer's recommended dosage and consult with a healthcare provider before starting any new supplement regimen, especially if you are pregnant, nursing, or taking other medications.

When selecting lemon balm products, whether it's dried leaves, essential oil, or supplements, always opt for high-quality, organic products from reputable suppliers to ensure the highest potency and purity. Organic products are preferable as they are less likely to contain pesticide residues that could detract from the herb's therapeutic benefits.

Maintaining a clean and organized space for storing your lemon balm products will help preserve their potency. Store dried lemon balm leaves in airtight containers away from direct sunlight and moisture. Essential oils should be kept in dark, glass bottles and placed in a cool, dry area to prevent degradation of their active compounds.

Incorporating lemon balm into your daily regimen as a tea, essential oil, or supplement offers a natural and effective way to enhance daytime calmness and reduce stress without the side effects of drowsiness. Its mild sedative properties support relaxation and mental clarity, making it an excellent herb for those seeking to maintain productivity and focus while managing stress levels throughout the day.

Skullcap for Nervous System Repair

Skullcap, scientifically known as Scutellaria lateriflora, is a perennial herb native to North America, where it thrives in moist woodlands and meadows. This herb has been traditionally used for its potent therapeutic properties, particularly in supporting the nervous system. Skullcap is highly esteemed for its ability to repair the nervous system, making it an invaluable ally in the treatment of chronic stress and nervous system burnout. The active compounds within skullcap, including baicalin and wogonin, are flavonoids that contribute to its calming, neuroprotective, and antioxidant effects. These compounds work synergistically to stabilize mood, reduce anxiety, and facilitate the repair of nerve tissue damaged by prolonged stress or neurological disorders.

For individuals experiencing chronic stress or symptoms of nervous system burnout, incorporating skullcap into their wellness regimen can offer profound benefits. The recommended method for consuming skullcap is through a tea or tincture, as these forms allow for the bioactive compounds to be readily absorbed and utilized by the body. To prepare skullcap tea, one should steep 1 to 2 teaspoons of dried skullcap herb in a cup of boiling water for approximately 10 to 15 minutes. This process extracts the herb's therapeutic compounds into the water, creating a potent infusion that can be consumed up to three times daily. For those preferring a more concentrated form, skullcap tinctures are available, and the typical dosage is 1 to 2 milliliters, taken up to three times daily. The tincture form ensures a more precise dosage and a faster absorption rate, making it a convenient option for those with a busy lifestyle.

When sourcing skullcap, it is crucial to select high-quality, organic products from reputable suppliers to ensure the absence of contaminants and the presence of the herb's beneficial compounds. Organic certification is a reliable indicator of quality, as it guarantees that the herb was grown without the use of synthetic pesticides or fertilizers, which can compromise the herb's purity and potency.

For those incorporating skullcap into their regimen for nervous system support, it is essential to maintain consistency in usage to achieve the best results. Chronic stress and nervous system burnout are conditions that develop over time, and similarly, the reparative effects of skullcap accumulate with regular use. It is also advisable to complement the use of skullcap with a holistic approach to stress management, including practices such as mindfulness meditation, regular physical activity, and adequate rest, to support overall nervous system health.

While skullcap is generally well-tolerated, it is important for individuals to consult with a healthcare provider before adding it to their wellness routine, especially for those with pre-existing medical conditions or those taking medication. This ensures safety and efficacy, as well as the avoidance of potential interactions with other treatments.

In conclusion, skullcap stands out as a powerful herbal ally for those seeking to soothe chronic stress and repair nervous system burnout. Its calming and restorative properties, backed by centuries of traditional use and supported by modern research, make it a key component of natural health practices focused on nurturing the nervous system.

Lavender and Lemon Balm Relaxation Tea

Beneficial effects

Lavender and Lemon Balm Relaxation Tea harnesses the calming properties of both lavender and lemon balm, making it an ideal beverage for easing stress and promoting a sense of well-being. Lavender is widely recognized for its ability to alleviate anxiety, improve sleep quality, and reduce depressive symptoms. Lemon balm complements these effects by enhancing mood, improving cognitive function, and acting as a mild sedative to encourage relaxation. Together, they create a soothing tea that can help unwind after a long day, ease tension, and support a restful night's sleep.

Portions

Makes about 2 cups

Preparation time

5 minutes

Cooking time

10 minutes

Ingredients

- 2 tablespoons dried lavender flowers
- 2 tablespoons dried lemon balm leaves
- 4 cups boiling water
- Honey or stevia (optional, for sweetness)

- Lemon slices (optional, for garnish)

Instructions

1. Boil 4 cups of water in a medium-sized pot.
2. Once the water reaches a rolling boil, remove it from the heat.
3. Add 2 tablespoons of dried lavender flowers and 2 tablespoons of dried lemon balm leaves to the hot water.
4. Cover the pot with a lid and allow the herbs to steep for about 10 minutes. This duration ensures that the water becomes well-infused with the flavors and therapeutic properties of the herbs.
5. After steeping, strain the tea through a fine mesh sieve into a large teapot or directly into serving cups, discarding the used herbs.
6. If desired, sweeten the tea with honey or stevia according to taste. Stir well to ensure the sweetener is fully dissolved.
7. Serve the tea hot, with a slice of lemon in each cup for an added touch of flavor and vitamin C.

Variations

- For a cooler, refreshing version, allow the tea to cool to room temperature, then refrigerate until chilled. Serve over ice for a soothing summer beverage.
- Add a cinnamon stick to the pot while steeping the herbs for a warm, spicy note that complements the floral tones.
- Mix in a few fresh mint leaves before serving for an extra layer of refreshing flavor and digestive benefits.

Storage tips

Any leftover tea can be stored in a glass container in the refrigerator for up to 2 days. Reheat gently on the stove or enjoy cold for a revitalizing drink.

Tips for allergens

For those with sensitivities to honey, using stevia as a sweetener provides a sugar-free alternative that doesn't compromise the calming effects of the tea. If allergic to lavender or lemon balm, chamomile can be a gentle alternative for relaxation without the risk of allergic reactions.

Scientific references

- "Lavender and the Nervous System," published in Evidence-Based Complementary and Alternative Medicine, highlights lavender's efficacy in treating anxiety, sleep disturbance, and depression.
- "Melissa officinalis L. – A review of its traditional uses, phytochemistry and pharmacology," published in the Journal of Ethnopharmacology, discusses lemon balm's mood-enhancing and sedative properties.

Passionflower and Chamomile Calming Elixir

Beneficial effects

The Passionflower and Chamomile Calming Elixir combines the soothing properties of passionflower and chamomile, both renowned for their ability to promote relaxation and reduce anxiety. Passionflower is often used for its calming effects on the nervous system, helping to ease tension and improve sleep quality. Chamomile, on the other hand, is a gentle sedative that can help soothe stress and facilitate a peaceful state of mind. Together, they create a powerful elixir that can aid in reducing nervousness and promoting a sense of well-being.

Portions

Makes about 2 cups

Preparation time

5 minutes

Cooking time

10 minutes

Ingredients

- 2 cups water
- 1 tablespoon dried passionflower
- 1 tablespoon dried chamomile flowers
- 1 teaspoon honey, or to taste (optional)
- 1 slice of lemon, for garnish (optional)

Instructions

1. Bring 2 cups of water to a boil in a medium saucepan.

2. Once the water is boiling, reduce the heat to low and add 1 tablespoon of dried passionflower and 1 tablespoon of dried chamomile flowers to the saucepan.

3. Cover the saucepan with a lid and let the mixture simmer for about 10 minutes. This allows the water to become infused with the herbs, extracting their beneficial properties.

4. After simmering, remove the saucepan from the heat. Strain the elixir through a fine mesh strainer or cheesecloth into a heat-resistant pitcher or teapot, discarding the used herbs.

5. If desired, stir in 1 teaspoon of honey to the warm elixir. Adjust the amount of honey according to your preference for sweetness.

6. Pour the elixir into cups, and if you like, garnish each cup with a slice of lemon for a refreshing touch.

7. Enjoy the elixir warm before bedtime or during moments of stress to experience its calming effects.

Variations

- For a cold version, allow the elixir to cool to room temperature, then refrigerate until chilled. Serve over ice for a refreshing, calming drink.
- Add a cinnamon stick to the saucepan with the passionflower and chamomile for a warming, slightly spicy flavor.
- Incorporate a few fresh mint leaves into the elixir while it simmers for a minty, refreshing twist.

Storage tips

Store any leftover Passionflower and Chamomile Calming Elixir in a sealed glass container in the refrigerator for up to 2 days. Reheat gently on the stove or enjoy cold.

Tips for allergens

For those with allergies to chamomile (which is related to the ragweed family), consider substituting with lavender, which also has calming properties but is less likely to cause allergic reactions. Always ensure that the honey used is pure and free from additives that may trigger allergies.

Hops and Valerian Root Sleep Aid

Beneficial effects

Hops and Valerian Root Sleep Aid leverages the natural sedative properties of both hops and valerian root to promote relaxation and improve sleep quality. Hops, commonly known for their use in brewing beer, contain compounds that have a calming effect on the brain, aiding in reducing insomnia and promoting restful sleep. Valerian root, a herb that has been used for centuries to treat various ailments, is widely recognized for its ability to ease anxiety and improve sleep latency and quality. Together, these herbs create a powerful blend that can help soothe the nervous system, making it easier to fall asleep and stay asleep throughout the night.

Portions
Makes about 20 servings

Preparation time
10 minutes

Cooking time
N/A

Ingredients
- 1/4 cup dried hops flowers
- 1/4 cup dried valerian root
- 1/2 cup boiling water
- Honey or stevia (optional, for sweetness)
- Lemon slice (optional, for flavor)

Instructions
1. Measure 1/4 cup of dried hops flowers and 1/4 cup of dried valerian root. Ensure that both herbs are finely chopped to increase the surface area for extraction.
2. Combine the hops and valerian root in a tea infuser or a small muslin bag. If neither is available, you can directly place the herbs in a cup and strain them out later.
3. Boil 1/2 cup of water using a kettle or a pot on the stove. Once boiling, carefully pour the water over the hops and valerian root in a mug or teapot.
4. Allow the herbs to steep for 10-15 minutes. Covering the mug or teapot with a lid or a small plate will help retain heat and ensure a stronger infusion.
5. After steeping, remove the tea infuser or strain the mixture to separate the liquid from the herbs. Compost or discard the used herbs.
6. If desired, sweeten the sleep aid with honey or stevia according to taste. Adding a slice of lemon can also enhance the flavor and add a refreshing note.
7. Drink the Hops and Valerian Root Sleep Aid about 30 minutes before bedtime to allow the herbs to take effect.

Variations
- For a stronger effect, increase the steeping time to 20 minutes. Be aware that the flavor may become more bitter.
- Add a cinnamon stick or a few cloves to the infusion for a warming, spiced flavor that can also aid in relaxation.
- Combine with chamomile or lavender flowers for additional calming and sleep-promoting benefits.

Storage tips
Store any unused dried hops and valerian root in airtight containers away from direct sunlight and moisture to preserve their potency. The sleep aid is best consumed fresh, but you can prepare a larger batch of the dry blend and store it in a cool, dark place for up to 6 months.

Tips for allergens
Individuals with allergies to plants in the same family as hops or valerian should avoid this sleep aid or consult with a healthcare provider before use. For those sensitive to honey, stevia serves as a suitable sweetener alternative.

CHAPTER 2: HERBS FOR MENTAL FOCUS

Ginkgo Biloba for Cognitive Enhancement

Ginkgo Biloba, a tree native to China, has been used in traditional medicine for thousands of years and is now widely recognized for its potential in enhancing cognitive functions and preventing cognitive decline. The leaves of the Ginkgo Biloba tree contain two types of phytochemicals, flavonoids and terpenoids, which are thought to have strong antioxidant and anti-inflammatory properties. These compounds are believed to protect the nerve cells in the brain from damage and support healthy blood flow, which is crucial for maintaining cognitive health.

For individuals looking to incorporate Ginkgo Biloba into their regimen for cognitive enhancement, the extract from the leaves is commonly used. It is available in various forms, including capsules, tablets, liquid extracts, and teas. The standardized extract, known as EGb 761, has been extensively studied and is recommended for its consistent quality and concentration of active compounds. When selecting a Ginkgo Biloba supplement, look for products that contain 24% flavonoid glycosides and 6% terpene lactones, the proportions typically used in research studies demonstrating cognitive benefits.

The recommended dosage for cognitive enhancement and the prevention of cognitive decline typically ranges from 120 to 240 milligrams per day, divided into two or three doses. Starting with a lower dose and gradually increasing it allows individuals to assess their tolerance and response to the herb. It's important to note that while some people may notice improvements in concentration and memory within a few weeks, it may take up to six months to experience the full benefits. Consistency is key when using Ginkgo Biloba as part of a cognitive health regimen.

In addition to its cognitive benefits, Ginkgo Biloba is also being researched for its potential to improve symptoms of anxiety and depression, further supporting its role in overall brain health. However, individuals taking blood thinners or those with a history of seizures should consult with a healthcare provider before starting Ginkgo Biloba, as it can interact with certain medications and conditions.

To ensure the efficacy and safety of Ginkgo Biloba supplements, it is crucial to store them properly. Keep the supplements in a cool, dry place, away from direct sunlight and moisture, to prevent degradation of the active compounds. Also, ensure that the supplements are kept in their original packaging or an airtight container to protect them from air exposure.

Incorporating Ginkgo Biloba into a holistic approach to cognitive health can also include a balanced diet rich in antioxidants, regular physical exercise, and mental exercises such as puzzles and memory games to stimulate brain function. Together, these practices can support optimal brain health and cognitive function, helping to maintain memory and prevent cognitive decline as one ages.

Rosemary for Mental Alertness

Rosemary, scientifically known as **Rosmarinus officinalis**, is a perennial herb with needle-like leaves and a distinctive, woody aroma. This herb is not only celebrated for its culinary uses but also for its potent stimulant properties that enhance mental alertness and concentration. The active compounds in rosemary, particularly **1,8-cineole**, have been shown to increase blood flow to the brain, thereby improving cognitive performance and memory recall.

To leverage rosemary's benefits for improving concentration, one effective method is through the inhalation of its essential oil. This can be achieved by adding a few drops of **rosemary essential**

oil to a diffuser filled with water. The diffuser should be placed in the area where concentration is needed, such as a study room or office. The aromatic molecules of 1,8-cineole are then dispersed into the air, where they can be inhaled and directly impact the brain's cognitive functions. For optimal results, the diffuser should run for approximately 30 to 60 minutes during periods of work or study.

Another practical application involves creating a **rosemary-infused oil** for topical use. Combine approximately 1 ounce of carrier oil, such as sweet almond or jojoba oil, with 10 to 12 drops of rosemary essential oil in a clean, dry bottle. Shake well to mix. To use, apply a small amount of this blend onto the temples or the back of the neck. The skin absorbs the oil, allowing the active compounds to enter the bloodstream and reach the brain, where they exert their stimulant effects.

For those who prefer a more direct approach, preparing a **rosemary tea** can also be beneficial. Steep 1 teaspoon of dried rosemary leaves in 8 ounces of boiling water for about 5 to 10 minutes. Strain the leaves and enjoy the tea. Drinking rosemary tea can provide a more gradual release of its active compounds, supporting sustained concentration and cognitive performance over time.

When selecting rosemary, whether in its fresh, dried, or oil form, always opt for **organic products** to ensure they are free from pesticides and other harmful chemicals. Organic rosemary is more likely to retain its natural concentration of active compounds, making it more effective for enhancing mental alertness.

Storage of rosemary essential oil and dried leaves should be in **airtight containers** away from direct sunlight and heat to preserve their potency. Essential oils, in particular, should be stored in dark, glass bottles to prevent degradation of the active compounds.

Incorporating rosemary into daily routines can be a simple yet powerful way to boost mental clarity and focus. Whether used aromatically, topically, or as a tea, this herb offers a natural, accessible means to support cognitive functions and enhance productivity.

Gotu Kola for Brain Health

Gotu Kola, scientifically known as Centella asiatica, has been revered for centuries in traditional medicine for its remarkable benefits in enhancing cognitive function and reducing mental fatigue. This herb, native to the wetlands of Asia, is not just another plant but a powerhouse of triterpenoid saponins, mainly asiaticoside, madecassoside, and madasiatic acid, which are credited with its therapeutic effects on the brain. To harness these benefits, it is crucial to understand the optimal ways to incorporate Gotu Kola into one's daily regimen for promoting mental clarity and combating the effects of mental exhaustion.

Firstly, selecting the highest quality of Gotu Kola is paramount. Look for organically grown herbs, as these are less likely to contain pesticide residues that could detract from their health benefits. The leaves of the plant are the most commonly used part, available in various forms such as fresh, dried, powdered, and as extracts. Each form has its specific use and preparation method to maximize its cognitive-enhancing properties.

For those preferring fresh leaves, incorporating them into salads or teas is an excellent way to enjoy their benefits. Ensure the leaves are thoroughly washed under running water to remove any dirt or contaminants. Chopping the leaves finely before adding them to a salad or steeping them in hot water for tea helps in releasing the active compounds. When preparing tea, steeping the leaves for 5 to 10 minutes in boiling water is recommended to extract the maximum amount of saponins.

For dried or powdered Gotu Kola, encapsulation is a convenient option, especially for those with a busy lifestyle. Capsules can provide a precise dosage, making it easier to monitor intake. When purchasing capsules, opt for those that specify the concentration of asiaticoside or total triterpenes, as these are indicators of the product's potency. A daily dosage of 300 to 600 mg of the extract is generally recommended, but it's advisable to start with the lower end of this range to assess tolerance.

Creating a tincture from Gotu Kola offers another method to utilize its brain health benefits. A tincture involves soaking the herb in alcohol or a vinegar solution for several weeks to extract the active compounds. This method allows for a longer shelf life and easy assimilation of the herb's benefits. To prepare a Gotu Kola tincture, fill a jar one-third full with dried Gotu Kola leaves and cover them with a 40% alcohol solution or apple cider vinegar, ensuring the leaves are completely submerged. Seal the jar and store it in a cool, dark place, shaking it daily for 4 to 6 weeks. After this period, strain the liquid through a fine mesh sieve or cheesecloth, squeezing out as much liquid as possible. Store the tincture in amber dropper bottles for easy use. The typical dosage is 20 to 60 drops of tincture in water, taken up to three times daily.

Incorporating Gotu Kola into one's diet or supplement regimen requires understanding and respect for its potent effects on brain health. Whether consumed as a fresh herb, taken in capsule form, or used as a tincture, Gotu Kola stands out as a natural ally in enhancing mental clarity, reducing brain fog, and supporting overall cognitive function. As with any herbal supplement, consulting with a healthcare provider before adding Gotu Kola to your health regimen is essential, especially for those with pre-existing conditions or those taking other medications, to avoid any potential interactions.

Ginkgo and Rosemary Memory Elixir

Beneficial effects

Ginkgo and Rosemary Memory Elixir is designed to enhance cognitive function, improve memory retention, and support overall brain health. Ginkgo Biloba has been widely studied for its ability to increase blood flow to the brain and act as an antioxidant, protecting neurons from oxidative stress. Rosemary, on the other hand, contains compounds such as carnosic acid and rosmarinic acid, which have been shown to have neuroprotective properties and may improve memory performance. Together, these herbs create a potent elixir that can help sharpen focus, improve concentration, and protect the brain from age-related cognitive decline.

Portions

Makes about 2 cups

Preparation time

5 minutes

Cooking time

15 minutes

Ingredients

- 4 cups water

- 2 tablespoons dried Ginkgo Biloba leaves

- 2 tablespoons dried rosemary leaves

- Honey or stevia to taste (optional)

- Lemon slices for garnish (optional)

Instructions

1. Bring 4 cups of water to a boil in a medium saucepan.

2. Once the water is boiling, reduce the heat to low and add 2 tablespoons of dried Ginkgo Biloba leaves and 2 tablespoons of dried rosemary leaves to the saucepan.

3. Cover the saucepan with a lid and let the mixture simmer for about 15 minutes. This allows the water to become infused with the beneficial compounds of the herbs.

4. After simmering, remove the saucepan from the heat. Strain the elixir through a fine mesh strainer or cheesecloth into a heat-resistant pitcher or teapot, discarding the used herbs.

5. If desired, sweeten the elixir with honey or stevia according to taste. Stir well to ensure the sweetener is fully dissolved.

6. Pour the elixir into cups, and if you like, garnish each cup with a slice of lemon for an added touch of flavor and vitamin C.

7. Enjoy the Ginkgo and Rosemary Memory Elixir warm, ideally in the morning or early afternoon to maximize its cognitive-enhancing benefits without interfering with sleep.

Variations

- For a cold version, allow the elixir to cool to room temperature, then refrigerate until chilled. Serve over ice for a refreshing cognitive boost.
- Add a cinnamon stick to the saucepan with the Ginkgo Biloba and rosemary for a warming, slightly spicy flavor that complements the herbal notes.
- Combine with green tea leaves during the simmering process for an added antioxidant boost and a mild caffeine kick.

Storage tips

Store any leftover Ginkgo and Rosemary Memory Elixir in a sealed glass container in the refrigerator for up to 2 days. Reheat gently on the stove or enjoy cold for a revitalizing drink.

Tips for allergens

Individuals with sensitivities to Ginkgo Biloba or rosemary should perform a patch test by applying a small amount of the elixir to the skin before consuming. If allergic reactions occur, discontinue use immediately. For those sensitive to honey, stevia serves as a suitable sweetener alternative that does not trigger allergies.

Scientific references

- "Ginkgo Biloba for Cognitive Enhancement in Healthy Individuals: A Systematic Review," published in the Journal of Alzheimer's Disease, highlights the cognitive benefits of Ginkgo Biloba.
- "Carnosic acid and rosmarinic acid in rosemary (Rosmarinus officinalis L.) as potential neuroprotective agents: A review," published in the International Journal of Molecular Sciences, discusses the neuroprotective properties of compounds found in rosemary.

Bacopa and Lemon Balm Concentration Tea

Beneficial effects

Bacopa and Lemon Balm Concentration Tea is designed to enhance cognitive function, improve memory, and reduce stress. Bacopa monnieri, traditionally used in Ayurvedic medicine, has been shown to support brain health, including enhancing memory and cognitive abilities. Lemon balm, on the other hand, is known for its calming effects, which can help alleviate stress and anxiety, factors that often hinder concentration. Together, these herbs create a synergistic blend that not only aids in improving focus and mental clarity but also promotes a relaxed state of mind, making it easier to concentrate on tasks at hand.

Portions

2 servings

Preparation time

5 minutes

Cooking time

15 minutes

Ingredients
- 2 cups water
- 1 tablespoon dried Bacopa monnieri leaves
- 1 tablespoon dried Lemon balm leaves
- Honey or stevia to taste (optional)
- Lemon slices for garnish (optional)

Instructions
1. Bring 2 cups of water to a boil in a medium-sized saucepan.
2. Once the water is boiling, reduce the heat to a simmer and add 1 tablespoon of dried Bacopa monnieri leaves and 1 tablespoon of dried Lemon balm leaves to the saucepan.
3. Cover the saucepan with a lid and allow the mixture to simmer gently for 10-15 minutes. This slow simmering process helps to extract the active compounds from the herbs, maximizing their cognitive and calming benefits.
4. After simmering, remove the saucepan from the heat. Strain the tea through a fine mesh strainer into two cups, ensuring to press the herbs to extract as much liquid and beneficial properties as possible. Discard the used herbs.
5. If desired, sweeten the tea with honey or stevia according to taste. Stir well to ensure the sweetener is fully dissolved.
6. Garnish each cup with a slice of lemon if using. The lemon not only adds a refreshing flavor but also provides vitamin C, enhancing the health benefits of the tea.
7. Serve the tea warm. Enjoy this Bacopa and Lemon Balm Concentration Tea in the morning or early afternoon to support focus and relaxation throughout the day.

Variations
- For a cold, refreshing version, allow the tea to cool to room temperature, then refrigerate until chilled. Serve over ice for a soothing summer drink.
- Add a cinnamon stick to the saucepan while simmering the herbs for a warming, spicy flavor that complements the herbal notes.
- Mix in a few fresh mint leaves to the tea after straining for an additional refreshing and digestive aid.

Storage tips
Store any leftover tea in a glass container in the refrigerator for up to 2 days. Reheat gently on the stove or enjoy cold for a revitalizing drink.

Tips for allergens
Individuals with sensitivities to any of the herbs used can adjust the recipe by reducing the quantity or substituting with another herb that has similar benefits but is better tolerated. Always perform a patch test or consult with a healthcare provider if unsure about potential allergies.

Scientific references
- "Neurocognitive Effect of Nootropic Drug Brahmi (Bacopa monnieri) in Alzheimer's Disease," published in Annals of Neurosciences, highlights the cognitive-enhancing effects of Bacopa monnieri.
- "Melissa officinalis L. (Lemon balm) extract in the treatment of volunteers suffering from mild-to-moderate anxiety disorders and sleep disturbances," published in Mediterranean Journal of Nutrition and Metabolism, discusses the calming effects of Lemon balm on stress and anxiety.

Gotu Kola and Peppermint Focus Tonic

Beneficial effects

Gotu Kola and Peppermint Focus Tonic is designed to enhance cognitive function, improve concentration, and reduce mental fatigue. Gotu Kola is celebrated for its neuroprotective properties and its ability to improve blood circulation, potentially enhancing brain function and memory. Peppermint, on the other hand, is known to increase alertness and energy. This tonic is an excellent natural remedy for those looking to boost their mental clarity and focus throughout the day.

Portions

Makes about 2 cups

Preparation time

15 minutes

Ingredients

- 2 cups of water
- 1 tablespoon dried Gotu Kola leaves
- 1 tablespoon dried Peppermint leaves
- 1 teaspoon honey (optional, for sweetness)
- A few slices of lemon (optional, for added flavor)

Instructions

1. Bring 2 cups of water to a boil in a medium-sized pot.
2. Once the water is boiling, reduce the heat to a simmer and add 1 tablespoon of dried Gotu Kola leaves and 1 tablespoon of dried Peppermint leaves to the pot.
3. Cover the pot with a lid and allow the mixture to simmer gently for 10 minutes. This process helps to extract the active compounds from the Gotu Kola and Peppermint, infusing the water with their beneficial properties.
4. After simmering, remove the pot from the heat and let it cool slightly for about 5 minutes, allowing the flavors to meld.
5. Strain the tonic through a fine mesh sieve or cheesecloth into a large pitcher or directly into serving cups, discarding the used herbs.
6. If desired, stir in 1 teaspoon of honey to each cup of the tonic to sweeten. Mix well until the honey is completely dissolved.
7. Add a few slices of lemon to each cup for an extra burst of flavor and vitamin C.
8. Serve the tonic warm, or allow it to cool completely and serve over ice for a refreshing drink.

Variations

- For an extra cognitive boost, add a pinch of ground cinnamon to the tonic while it simmers. Cinnamon is known for its anti-inflammatory properties and can enhance the flavor of the drink.
- Incorporate a slice of fresh ginger in the simmering process for added digestive benefits and a spicy kick.
- To make a cold brew version, combine the dried Gotu Kola and Peppermint leaves with cold water in a pitcher and let it steep in the refrigerator overnight. Strain before serving.

Storage tips

Store any leftover Gotu Kola and Peppermint Focus Tonic in a sealed glass container in the refrigerator for up to 2 days. For best flavor, consume within 24 hours.

Tips for allergens

For those with allergies to honey, substitute it with maple syrup or simply enjoy the tonic without any sweeteners. If you're sensitive to caffeine (though Gotu Kola and Peppermint are generally considered low in caffeine compared to traditional teas and coffee), it's best to consume this tonic earlier in the day to avoid any potential impact on sleep.

Scientific references

- "Centella asiatica (L.) Urban: From Traditional Medicine to Modern Medicine with Neuroprotective Potential" published in Evidence-Based Complementary and Alternative Medicine, highlights Gotu Kola's benefits for brain health.

- "Peppermint and Its Functionality: A Review" published in the Journal of Food Science, discusses the invigorating and focus-enhancing effects of peppermint.

CHAPTER 3: NERVOUS SYSTEM TONICS

Oat Straw for Nervous System Health

Oat straw, derived from the green stalks of the oat plant before it fully matures and produces grain, has been a cornerstone in herbal medicine for centuries, primarily for its beneficial impact on the nervous system. Rich in vitamins, minerals, and antioxidants, oat straw offers a gentle yet powerful means to support nervous system health and resilience. Its composition includes B vitamins, magnesium, silica, and calcium, all of which are crucial for nourishing the nervous system, enhancing mood, and supporting overall brain function.

To harness the full potential of oat straw for nervous system nourishment, it's essential to understand the optimal preparation and consumption methods. Oat straw can be consumed in various forms, including teas, tinctures, and capsules, each offering a unique pathway to assimilate its benefits into the body.

For those seeking to incorporate oat straw into their daily routine, starting with a simple tea is often the most accessible approach. To prepare oat straw tea, one would need about one to two teaspoons of dried oat straw per cup of boiling water. The oat straw should be steeped in boiling water for about 10 to 15 minutes to allow the soluble fibers and nutrients to infuse into the water. This tea can be consumed up to three times daily and is known for its soothing effect on the nervous system, potentially aiding in stress reduction and promoting a sense of calm.

For a more concentrated dose, oat straw tincture may be preferred. Creating a tincture involves soaking dried oat straw in a mixture of alcohol and water for several weeks, which extracts a wider range of soluble compounds than tea. The ratio of oat straw to liquid is critical; a common approach is to fill a jar one-third to one-half with dried oat straw, then cover it with a 40-60% alcohol solution. After allowing the mixture to sit in a cool, dark place for about 4 to 6 weeks, shaking it periodically, the liquid is strained and stored in a dark glass bottle. Dosage typically ranges from 1/4 to 1/2 teaspoon, taken up to three times daily.

Capsules offer a convenient alternative for those with a busy lifestyle or those who may not favor the taste of oat straw tea or tincture. When selecting oat straw capsules, it's important to choose products that specify the amount of oat straw extract, ensuring a consistent and effective dosage. The recommended dose can vary, but generally, one to two capsules taken with water up to three times a day is a good starting point.

Regardless of the form chosen, consistency is key in experiencing the full benefits of oat straw. Regular, daily consumption supports the body's natural stress response systems, contributes to healthier sleep patterns, and can improve cognitive function over time. It's also important to source oat straw from reputable suppliers to ensure it's free from contaminants and pesticides, which could undermine its health benefits.

While oat straw is generally considered safe for most people, those with celiac disease or gluten sensitivity should proceed with caution due to the potential for cross-contamination with oat grains. As with any supplement, consulting with a healthcare provider before adding oat straw to one's regimen is advisable, especially for those with pre-existing health conditions or those taking medications.

Incorporating oat straw into one's wellness routine represents a return to ancient, natural methods of supporting the nervous system and enhancing overall well-being. Through mindful selection and consistent use, individuals can tap into the gentle, restorative power of oat straw, fostering resilience against the stresses of modern life.

Ashwagandha for Stress Resilience

Ashwagandha, scientifically known as **Withania somnifera**, is a powerful herb in the world of natural medicine, revered for its adaptogenic properties. Adaptogens are a unique class of healing plants that help balance, restore, and protect the body, making ashwagandha a cornerstone herb for those seeking to mitigate stress and foster resilience against nervous tension. Its roots and leaves contain a wealth of bioactive compounds, including withanolides, alkaloids, and saponins, which contribute to its efficacy in calming overactive nerves and supporting adrenal health.

To incorporate ashwagandha into your wellness routine for stress resilience, consider the following detailed guidance on preparation, dosage, and consumption:

Preparation Methods:

1. **Ashwagandha Tea:** To prepare a soothing cup of ashwagandha tea, measure out 1 teaspoon of dried ashwagandha root powder into a tea infuser. Place the infuser in a cup of hot water and let it steep for 10 to 15 minutes. This method allows for a gentle extraction of the herb's active compounds. For flavor, consider adding honey or cinnamon.

2. **Ashwagandha Tincture:** For a more potent preparation, an ashwagandha tincture can be made by soaking the dried root in alcohol. Fill a jar one-third full with dried ashwagandha root, then cover completely with a 40% alcohol solution. Seal the jar and store it in a cool, dark place, shaking it daily for about 4 to 6 weeks. Strain the liquid through a fine mesh sieve or cheesecloth into a clean bottle. Tinctures offer a concentrated, easily consumable form of ashwagandha.

3. **Capsules:** Ashwagandha capsules provide a convenient and precise dosage option. When purchasing capsules, look for products that specify the withanolide content, as this indicates the potency of the product.

Dosage Recommendations:

- **Tea:** One cup of ashwagandha tea, made from 1 teaspoon of root powder, can be consumed up to twice daily.

- **Tincture:** 20 to 30 drops of ashwagandha tincture can be taken in water or juice, up to three times per day.

- **Capsules:** Follow the manufacturer's instructions, typically ranging from 300 to 500 mg of ashwagandha extract per day.

Consumption Tips:

- Start with a lower dose to assess your body's response, gradually increasing to the recommended dose.

- Consistent daily consumption is key to experiencing the full adaptogenic effects on stress resilience and nervous system support.

- Ashwagandha can be taken at any time of day, but taking it with meals may aid in digestion and absorption.

Safety and Considerations:

- Ashwagandha is generally well-tolerated, but it's advisable to consult with a healthcare provider before beginning any new supplement, especially for those with thyroid conditions, autoimmune diseases, or those taking medications.

- Pregnant or breastfeeding women should avoid ashwagandha due to insufficient safety data.

- Source ashwagandha from reputable suppliers to ensure quality and purity of the product.

By integrating ashwagandha into your daily regimen, you can leverage its adaptogenic properties to fortify your body's stress resilience, calm overactive nerves, and support overall nervous system health. Remember, the key to herbal supplementation is consistency and quality, ensuring you receive the full therapeutic benefits of this ancient herb.

Passionflower for Relaxation

Passionflower, scientifically known as Passiflora incarnata, is a perennial climbing vine renowned for its beautiful flowers and medicinal properties, particularly in supporting the nervous system without inducing sedation. This herb functions as a gentle yet effective nervine, a type of plant that specifically supports the nervous system. It's especially beneficial for individuals experiencing anxiety, stress, or difficulties with sleep, offering a natural way to foster a state of calm and relaxation over time.

The active compounds in passionflower, including flavonoids like vitexin and isovitexin, along with alkaloids such as harman, work synergistically to modulate the body's stress response. These compounds interact with the gamma-aminobutyric acid (GABA) receptors in the brain, a neurotransmitter responsible for reducing neuronal excitability throughout the nervous system. By enhancing GABA's effectiveness, passionflower helps to calm the mind, reduce anxiety, and promote better sleep without the grogginess or dependency risks associated with pharmaceutical sedatives.

To incorporate passionflower into a daily regimen for long-term relaxation and nervous system support, consider the following methods:

1. **Passionflower Tea:** Prepare a soothing tea by steeping 1 teaspoon of dried passionflower in a cup of boiling water for 10 to 15 minutes. This method allows for a gentle extraction of the herb's active compounds. Drinking a cup of passionflower tea one hour before bedtime can aid in easing the transition into sleep.

2. **Passionflower Tincture:** A more concentrated form, tinctures offer a convenient and efficient way to consume passionflower. To use, add 20 to 30 drops of passionflower tincture to water or juice, three times a day. This method is particularly useful for managing daytime anxiety and stress, as it provides a quick and easy way to adjust dosages as needed.

3. **Passionflower Capsules:** For those who prefer a more straightforward approach, capsules containing dried passionflower extract are available. The typical dosage is one to two capsules taken with water, up to three times a day. Capsules are an excellent option for maintaining consistent dosages and for ease of use while traveling or at work.

When selecting passionflower products, it's crucial to source from reputable suppliers to ensure the purity and potency of the herb. Organic or wildcrafted options are preferable, as they minimize exposure to pesticides and other contaminants that could detract from the herb's therapeutic value.

While passionflower is generally considered safe for most people, it's important to note that it may interact with certain medications, such as sedatives and blood thinners. Therefore, consulting with a healthcare provider before adding passionflower to your wellness routine is advisable, especially for those with pre-existing health conditions or those taking prescription medications.

Incorporating passionflower into one's daily routine represents a holistic approach to managing stress and anxiety, promoting relaxation, and supporting overall nervous system health. Its ability to soothe without sedation makes it an invaluable tool for those seeking natural ways to maintain balance and well-being in today's fast-paced world.

Lemon Balm and Passionflower Nerve Tonic

Beneficial effects

Lemon Balm and Passionflower Nerve Tonic is crafted to soothe the nervous system, reduce anxiety, and promote a sense of calm. Lemon balm, with its mild sedative properties, helps to ease stress and improve sleep quality. Passionflower is known for its ability to alleviate symptoms of anxiety and insomnia, making it an excellent herb for those dealing with nervous tension. Together, these herbs create a powerful tonic that can help relax the body and mind, making it easier to unwind and find peace in moments of stress.

Portions
2 servings

Preparation time
10 minutes

Ingredients
- 2 cups of water
- 1 tablespoon dried lemon balm leaves
- 1 tablespoon dried passionflower
- Honey or stevia to taste (optional)
- Lemon slices for garnish (optional)

Instructions
1. Pour 2 cups of water into a medium saucepan and bring to a boil over high heat.
2. Once boiling, reduce the heat to low and add 1 tablespoon of dried lemon balm leaves and 1 tablespoon of dried passionflower to the water.
3. Cover the saucepan with a lid and simmer the mixture on low heat for 5 minutes to allow the herbs to infuse their properties into the water.
4. After simmering, remove the saucepan from the heat and let the tonic steep, covered, for an additional 5 minutes to enhance the extraction of beneficial compounds.
5. Strain the tonic through a fine mesh sieve into two cups, pressing on the herbs to ensure maximum flavor and benefit. Discard the used herbs.
6. If desired, sweeten the tonic with honey or stevia according to your taste preference.
7. Garnish each cup with a slice of lemon for a refreshing twist and added vitamin C.
8. Serve the tonic warm, encouraging slow sipping to fully enjoy its calming effects.

Variations
- For a cooling summer drink, allow the tonic to cool to room temperature, then refrigerate until chilled. Serve over ice with a sprig of fresh mint for a refreshing twist.
- Add a cinnamon stick during the simmering process for a warm, comforting flavor that complements the calming properties of the tonic.
- Mix in a teaspoon of fresh grated ginger with the herbs for an extra soothing effect and a spicy kick.

Storage tips
This tonic is best enjoyed fresh, but if needed, it can be stored in the refrigerator in a sealed glass container for up to 24 hours. Reheat gently on the stove or enjoy chilled.

Tips for allergens
For those with sensitivities to honey, stevia provides a sweetening alternative that is unlikely to cause allergic reactions. If you have allergies to lemon balm or passionflower, consider substituting with chamomile, which also has calming properties but may be more tolerable for those with sensitivities.

Skullcap and Oat Straw Calming Elixir

Beneficial effects

Skullcap and Oat Straw Calming Elixir is a natural remedy designed to soothe the nervous system, reduce anxiety, and promote a sense of calm. Skullcap is known for its sedative properties, making it beneficial for those experiencing stress and sleeplessness. Oat straw, on the other hand, is rich in vitamins and minerals that support nerve health and provide a gentle calming effect. This elixir is perfect for anyone looking to relax after a stressful day or to support overall mental well-being.

Portions

2 servings

Preparation time

10 minutes

Cooking time

5 minutes

Ingredients

- 2 cups water
- 1 tablespoon dried skullcap
- 1 tablespoon dried oat straw
- 1 teaspoon honey (optional)
- 2 slices of lemon (optional, for garnish)

Instructions

1. Bring 2 cups of water to a boil in a medium saucepan.
2. Once boiling, reduce the heat to a simmer and add 1 tablespoon of dried skullcap and 1 tablespoon of dried oat straw to the water.
3. Cover the saucepan and allow the mixture to simmer gently for 5 minutes. This process helps to extract the beneficial compounds from the skullcap and oat straw, infusing the water with their calming properties.
4. After simmering, remove the saucepan from the heat and let it steep, covered, for an additional 5 minutes to enhance the strength of the elixir.
5. Strain the elixir through a fine mesh sieve into two cups, discarding the herbs. This step ensures a smooth drink free from plant material.
6. If desired, sweeten each serving with 1 teaspoon of honey, stirring well until the honey is fully dissolved. Honey adds a natural sweetness that can make the elixir more enjoyable.
7. Garnish each cup with a slice of lemon for a refreshing twist and added vitamin C.

Variations

- For a cooler beverage, allow the elixir to come to room temperature, then refrigerate for 1-2 hours. Serve over ice for a refreshing, calming drink.
- Add a cinnamon stick to the simmering water for a warming, spicy flavor that complements the calming properties of the skullcap and oat straw.
- Incorporate a few fresh mint leaves into the elixir after removing it from heat for a minty, refreshing flavor.

Storage tips

This elixir is best enjoyed fresh, but any leftovers can be stored in a sealed glass container in the refrigerator for up to 24 hours. Gently reheat on the stove or enjoy cold for a soothing treat.

Tips for allergens

For those with allergies to honey, stevia or maple syrup can be used as a sweetener alternative. Always ensure that the skullcap and oat straw are sourced from reputable suppliers to avoid contamination with allergens.

Blue Vervain and Hops Relaxation Tonic

Beneficial effects

Blue Vervain and Hops Relaxation Tonic is crafted to soothe the nervous system, reduce anxiety, and promote a peaceful state of mind. Blue Vervain is known for its nerve-strengthening properties and ability to ease tension and stress, making it an excellent herb for those dealing with anxiety or restlessness. Hops, commonly associated with brewing, also possess sedative qualities that can enhance sleep quality and relaxation. Together, these herbs create a tonic that can help calm the mind, ease into relaxation, and prepare the body for a restful night's sleep.

Portions

2 servings

Preparation time

10 minutes

Cooking time

5 minutes

Ingredients

- 2 cups of water
- 1 tablespoon dried Blue Vervain leaves
- 1 tablespoon dried Hops flowers
- 1 teaspoon honey (optional, for sweetness)
- 1 teaspoon lemon juice (optional, for flavor)

Instructions

1. Begin by bringing 2 cups of water to a boil in a medium-sized saucepan.
2. Once the water reaches a rolling boil, reduce the heat to low and add 1 tablespoon of dried Blue Vervain leaves and 1 tablespoon of dried Hops flowers to the saucepan.
3. Cover the saucepan with a lid to prevent the volatile oils from escaping and let the mixture simmer gently for about 5 minutes. This process allows the water to become infused with the therapeutic properties of the herbs.
4. After simmering, remove the saucepan from the heat and allow the tonic to cool slightly for a more comfortable drinking temperature.
5. Strain the tonic through a fine mesh sieve or cheesecloth into a large glass or pitcher, pressing on the herbs to extract as much liquid as possible. Discard the used herbs.
6. If desired, stir in 1 teaspoon of honey to sweeten the tonic. Mix well until the honey is completely dissolved.
7. Add 1 teaspoon of lemon juice to the tonic for an added refreshing flavor and a boost of vitamin C.
8. Serve the tonic warm in individual cups. Enjoy this relaxation tonic in the evening or before bedtime to maximize its calming effects.

Variations

- For a cold version of the tonic, allow it to cool completely, then refrigerate for 1-2 hours. Serve over ice for a refreshing, calming beverage.

- Add a cinnamon stick to the saucepan while simmering the herbs for a warming, comforting flavor profile.
- Incorporate a slice of fresh ginger in the simmering process for added digestive benefits and a spicy kick.

Storage tips

This tonic is best enjoyed fresh but can be stored in the refrigerator in a sealed glass container for up to 24 hours. Reheat gently on the stove or enjoy cold.

Tips for allergens

Individuals with allergies to any of the herbs used can substitute with chamomile or lavender, which also have calming properties but may be better tolerated. For those sensitive to honey, maple syrup serves as a suitable vegan sweetener alternative that does not compromise the tonic's soothing effects.

Scientific references

- "Nervine Herbs for Treating Anxiety," published in the American Journal of Plant Sciences, discusses the benefits of Blue Vervain and Hops on the nervous system, highlighting their sedative and anxiolytic properties.
- "A Review on the Role of Hops in Sleep Disorders," found in the Journal of Sleep Medicine, examines the sedative effects of Hops and its potential to improve sleep quality and duration.

BOOK 18: HERBAL FIRST AID ESSENTIALS

CHAPTER 1: QUICK-ACTION REMEDIES

Arnica for Bruising and Swelling

Arnica, scientifically known as **Arnica montana**, is a perennial herb native to Europe and Siberia but also cultivated in North America. It is renowned for its potent anti-inflammatory properties, making it an invaluable component of natural first aid for treating **bruises, swelling, and trauma-related injuries**. When applied topically, Arnica works by stimulating the body's healing process, encouraging the dispersal of fluids that accumulate as a result of injury and leading to bruising and swelling.

For effective use in treating sports injuries or trauma-induced conditions, it is crucial to utilize Arnica in the form of a **gel, cream, ointment, or salve**. These preparations should contain a concentration of Arnica extract that is safe for skin application. It is important to note that Arnica should never be applied to open wounds or broken skin, as it can cause irritation and may lead to adverse reactions.

To prepare a simple Arnica topical remedy at home, you can follow these steps:

1. **Purchase Arnica Montana** in either dried herb form for infusing oils or as a pre-made tincture.

2. If using dried Arnica, **infuse the herb into a carrier oil** such as olive oil or sweet almond oil. Use approximately 1 part dried Arnica to 5 parts carrier oil. Gently heat the mixture in a double boiler for up to 3 hours, ensuring the oil does not overheat or boil.

3. After heating, **strain the oil** using a fine mesh strainer or cheesecloth to remove all plant material, ensuring a smooth final product.

4. To the strained oil, add beeswax to thicken the mixture into a salve. A general guideline is to use about 1 ounce (28 grams) of beeswax per cup (240 ml) of infused oil. Melt the beeswax into the oil over low heat.

5. Once fully blended and melted together, **pour the mixture into clean, dry containers** and allow it to cool and solidify.

6. For those opting to use a pre-made Arnica tincture, **mix the tincture with a gel base** such as aloe vera gel at a ratio that achieves the desired consistency and potency, typically starting with a dilution of 1 part tincture to 3 parts gel.

When using Arnica topically, apply a thin layer of the prepared Arnica product to the affected area up to 4 times daily. It is essential to **observe the skin's reaction** to the remedy, and discontinue use if any irritation or rash develops.

Arnica works best when applied at the **first sign of bruising or swelling**, as it can significantly reduce the recovery time by minimizing the body's inflammatory response. However, it's also beneficial for relieving pain and swelling in cases of arthritis or other chronic conditions when used regularly over time.

In summary, Arnica serves as a powerful herbal remedy for managing bruises, swelling, and pain associated with sports injuries and trauma. By preparing and applying Arnica-based products according to these guidelines, individuals can harness the natural healing properties of this herb to support the body's recovery process.

Yarrow for Cuts and Bleeding

Yarrow, scientifically known as Achillea millefolium, is a perennial herb that has been utilized for centuries due to its remarkable styptic and antimicrobial properties, making it an essential component in the realm of natural first aid, especially for treating cuts and bleeding. This herb's ability to quickly staunch blood flow stems from its high content of alkaloids, tannins, and flavonoids, which collectively contribute to the constriction of blood vessels and promotion of clotting, thereby reducing bleeding efficiently.

To harness yarrow's benefits for cuts and bleeding, one can prepare a simple yet effective poultice or infusion. For a poultice, fresh yarrow leaves and flowers are most beneficial. Begin by thoroughly washing the plant material to remove any dirt or debris. Once cleaned, the yarrow can be crushed or chewed (if you're in a survival situation) to release its juices, which are key to activating its medicinal properties. The macerated plant material is then applied directly to the wound, covering it with a clean cloth or bandage to hold the poultice in place. The natural astringent properties of yarrow help to contract the tissues and seal the wound, reducing the risk of infection.

Alternatively, a yarrow infusion can be prepared for cleaning wounds or making compresses. To create an infusion, steep 1 to 2 teaspoons of dried yarrow leaves and flowers in a cup of boiling water for approximately 10 to 15 minutes. Strain the mixture to remove the plant parts, and once cooled to a safe temperature, the infusion can be used to gently clean the wound with a clean cloth or gauze. This method not only aids in stopping the bleeding but also ensures the wound is disinfected, thanks to yarrow's antimicrobial properties.

When collecting yarrow from the wild, it's crucial to positively identify the plant to avoid confusion with similar-looking toxic plants. Yarrow is distinguished by its feathery, fern-like leaves and clusters of small, white to pinkish flowers. It's commonly found in meadows, roadsides, and open forests across various climates and regions.

For those looking to add yarrow to their home apothecary, sourcing high-quality, dried yarrow from reputable suppliers is key to ensuring the potency and safety of the herb. Whether using yarrow in poultices, infusions, or other preparations, it's important to document any reactions and consult with a healthcare professional, especially for individuals with sensitive skin or allergies to plants in the Asteraceae family.

Plantain for Bug Bites

Plantain, scientifically known as **Plantago major**, is a common perennial weed found in many backyards and gardens, yet its medicinal properties are often overlooked. This herb is highly effective in treating **bug bites and stings** due to its anti-inflammatory and antitoxic qualities. The leaves of the plantain are rich in allantoin, an anti-inflammatory phytochemical that speeds up the healing process by stimulating the growth of new skin cells. Additionally, plantain has astringent properties that help in drawing out toxins from bug bites or stings.

To utilize plantain for bug bites or stings, follow these detailed steps to prepare a simple yet effective remedy:

1. **Identification and Harvesting**: First, correctly identify Plantago major, which has broad, oval leaves with parallel veins running their length and a green, flower-bearing spike. Harvest fresh plantain leaves, preferably from areas not treated with pesticides or herbicides. The younger leaves are more tender and potent for topical use.

2. **Cleaning**: Rinse the harvested leaves gently under cool running water to remove any dirt or debris. Pat them dry with a clean towel or let them air dry for a few minutes.

3. **Preparation of a Poultice**: For immediate application, a fresh poultice can be made. This involves crushing the leaves to release their juices. You can use a mortar and pestle or simply chew the leaves if no tools are available. The goal is to break down the leaf enough to release its medicinal compounds.

4. **Application**: Apply the crushed leaves directly onto the affected area. If the skin is broken, place a thin cloth between the poultice and the skin to prevent any plant matter from entering the wound. Secure the poultice in place with a bandage or medical tape.

5. **Alternative Method - Plantain Infusion**: For a less direct method, you can create a plantain infusion. Chop the cleaned leaves finely and place them in a jar. Cover the leaves with boiling water and let them steep for at least 10-15 minutes. Once cooled, strain the infusion. Soak a clean cloth in the liquid and apply it as a compress to the bite or sting.

6. **Frequency of Application**: Reapply the fresh poultice or the infusion-soaked cloth 2-3 times a day until the inflammation and discomfort subside.

7. **Storage**: Any unused plantain leaves can be dried and stored in an airtight container for future use. For the infusion, refrigerate it and use within 24-48 hours for best results.

It's important to note that while plantain is generally safe for topical use, individuals with sensitive skin or plant allergies should perform a patch test on a small area of skin before applying it to affected areas. Additionally, if symptoms persist or if there is a severe allergic reaction to a bite or sting, seek medical attention promptly.

By following these steps, you can effectively harness the natural healing power of **Plantago major** to treat bug bites and stings, providing relief from pain and itching while reducing inflammation and drawing out toxins.

Arnica and Comfrey Bruise Cream

Beneficial effects

Arnica and Comfrey Bruise Cream harnesses the natural anti-inflammatory and healing properties of arnica and comfrey. Arnica is widely recognized for its ability to reduce swelling and decrease pain, making it ideal for treating bruises, sprains, and sore muscles. Comfrey, known for its allantoin content, promotes cell regeneration and speeds up the healing process of the skin. Together, these herbs create a powerful cream that can help accelerate the recovery of bruises and reduce discomfort.

Portions

Makes about 1 cup

Preparation time

20 minutes

Cooking time

30 minutes

Ingredients

- 1/4 cup dried arnica flowers
- 1/4 cup dried comfrey leaves
- 1/2 cup coconut oil
- 1/4 cup shea butter
- 2 tablespoons beeswax pellets
- 10 drops lavender essential oil (for additional anti-inflammatory and soothing properties)
- Dark glass jar for storage

Instructions

1. Begin by infusing the coconut oil with arnica flowers and comfrey leaves. Combine the dried herbs and coconut oil in a double boiler, and gently heat the mixture over low heat for 2-3 hours, ensuring

the oil does not boil. This slow infusion process allows the oil to extract the healing properties of the herbs.

2. After the infusion is complete, strain the oil through a fine mesh strainer or cheesecloth into a clean bowl, discarding the herb residues. Make sure to press the herbs to extract as much oil as possible.

3. Return the infused oil to the double boiler and add shea butter and beeswax pellets. Heat the mixture until the shea butter and beeswax are completely melted, stirring occasionally for a smooth blend.

4. Remove the mixture from heat and allow it to cool slightly for a few minutes. When the mixture is still liquid but has cooled down, stir in the lavender essential oil. This step is crucial as adding essential oils to a very hot mixture can diminish their therapeutic benefits.

5. Carefully pour the warm cream into a dark glass jar. Using a dark glass jar helps protect the cream from light, preserving its therapeutic properties.

6. Allow the cream to cool and solidify completely before sealing the jar. This may take several hours. Do not cover the jar while the cream is still warm as condensation can form inside the jar.

7. Label the jar with the contents and the date of creation.

Variations

- For a vegan version, substitute beeswax pellets with an equal amount of candelilla wax.
- If coconut oil is too heavy for your skin type, jojoba oil can be used as a lighter alternative that is still effective for infusing the herbs.
- For added pain relief, incorporate 5 drops of peppermint essential oil into the cream during step 4.

Storage tips

Store the Arnica and Comfrey Bruise Cream in a cool, dark place. The cream should remain potent for up to 6 months if stored properly. If the cream changes in smell, texture, or color, it should be discarded.

Tips for allergens

Individuals with sensitivities to any of the ingredients, particularly those with allergies to plants in the Asteraceae family (such as arnica), should perform a patch test on a small area of the skin before widespread use. Substitute lavender essential oil with chamomile essential oil for those sensitive to lavender.

Plantain and Yarrow Wound Poultice

Beneficial effects

The Plantain and Yarrow Wound Poultice is a natural remedy designed to accelerate the healing process of wounds, reduce inflammation, and prevent infection. Plantain, known for its antibacterial and anti-inflammatory properties, aids in wound cleaning and promotes faster healing. Yarrow, celebrated for its ability to stop bleeding and act as a natural astringent, helps in tightening the tissues and sealing wounds. Together, these herbs create a potent poultice that can be applied to cuts, scrapes, and other skin injuries to facilitate healing and reduce the risk of infection.

Portions

Enough for 1-2 applications

Preparation time

10 minutes

Ingredients
- 2 tablespoons fresh plantain leaves, finely chopped
- 2 tablespoons fresh yarrow leaves and flowers, finely chopped
- 1 teaspoon water (if needed)
- 1 clean cloth or gauze

Instructions
1. Start by thoroughly washing the plantain leaves and yarrow leaves and flowers under running water to remove any dirt or debris.
2. On a clean cutting board, finely chop both the plantain leaves and yarrow leaves and flowers to increase the surface area that will come into contact with the skin, enhancing the poultice's effectiveness.
3. In a small bowl, combine the chopped plantain and yarrow. If the mixture seems too dry, add 1 teaspoon of water to help the herbs bind together, creating a paste-like consistency.
4. Spread the herb mixture onto a clean cloth or gauze, ensuring it's evenly distributed across the surface where it will be applied to the skin.
5. Place the poultice herb-side down onto the cleaned wound or affected area, applying gentle pressure to ensure it makes good contact with the skin.
6. Secure the poultice in place with a bandage or medical tape, being careful not to wrap it too tightly, which could impede circulation.
7. Leave the poultice on the wound for up to 1 hour, monitoring for any signs of irritation or discomfort. If any adverse reactions occur, remove the poultice immediately.
8. After removing the poultice, gently clean the area with water. The poultice can be applied once or twice daily as needed until the wound shows signs of improvement.

Variations
- For added antimicrobial properties, mix in 1 teaspoon of finely ground sea salt with the herbs before applying to the cloth.
- To enhance the soothing effects, include 1 tablespoon of aloe vera gel to the mixture.
- For larger wounds, increase the quantities of plantain and yarrow proportionally to ensure the entire area can be covered by the poultice.

Storage tips
Fresh plantain and yarrow leaves should be used immediately after preparation for maximum potency. However, if you need to store the herbs, place them in a sealed container in the refrigerator for up to 24 hours before use. Note that the fresher the herbs, the more effective the poultice will be.

Tips for allergens
Individuals with sensitivities to plantain, yarrow, or other Asteraceae family plants should perform a patch test on a small area of skin before applying the poultice to wounds. If an allergic reaction occurs, discontinue use immediately.

Cayenne and Ginger Pain Relief Balm

Beneficial effects
Cayenne and Ginger Pain Relief Balm combines the powerful anti-inflammatory and analgesic properties of cayenne pepper with the soothing, warming effects of ginger to create a topical remedy that can help alleviate muscle pain, reduce arthritis discomfort, and soothe sore joints. Cayenne pepper contains capsaicin, a compound known to reduce pain sensations when applied to the skin.

Ginger, rich in gingerol, helps improve circulation and relieve pain. Together, they offer a natural, effective way to manage pain and inflammation.

Portions

Makes about 4 ounces

Preparation time

20 minutes

Cooking time

10 minutes

Ingredients

- 1/4 cup coconut oil
- 2 tablespoons grated beeswax
- 1 teaspoon cayenne pepper powder
- 1 teaspoon ginger powder
- 10 drops peppermint essential oil
- 5 drops lavender essential oil
- Small glass jar or tin for storage

Instructions

1. Begin by setting up a double boiler: Fill a pot with a few inches of water and place it on the stove over medium heat. Place a heat-safe glass bowl on top of the pot, ensuring the bottom of the bowl does not touch the water.

2. Add 1/4 cup coconut oil and 2 tablespoons grated beeswax to the glass bowl. Stir continuously until the mixture is completely melted and combined.

3. Once melted, carefully remove the bowl from heat. Stir in 1 teaspoon cayenne pepper powder and 1 teaspoon ginger powder to the melted oil and beeswax mixture. Mix thoroughly to ensure the powders are fully incorporated.

4. Allow the mixture to cool for a few minutes before adding the essential oils. Stir in 10 drops of peppermint essential oil and 5 drops of lavender essential oil. Peppermint provides a cooling effect, while lavender offers additional pain relief and a soothing aroma.

5. Quickly pour the mixture into a small glass jar or tin before it begins to solidify. Use caution, as the mixture will be hot.

6. Let the balm cool and solidify completely at room temperature. This may take several hours. Once solidified, secure the lid on the jar or tin.

7. To use, gently rub a small amount of the balm onto the affected area. The balm will melt slightly with the warmth of your skin, making it easy to apply.

Variations

- For extra pain relief, add 5 drops of eucalyptus essential oil to the mixture for its analgesic properties.
- If you have sensitive skin, reduce the amount of cayenne pepper powder to 1/2 teaspoon to minimize any potential irritation.
- For a softer balm, reduce the amount of beeswax to 1 tablespoon.

Storage tips

Store the Cayenne and Ginger Pain Relief Balm in a cool, dark place to preserve the potency of the essential oils and prevent melting. If the balm becomes too soft in warm temperatures, refrigerate for 10 minutes before use.

Tips for allergens

Individuals with sensitive skin or allergies to any of the ingredients should perform a patch test on a small area of skin before applying the balm widely. Substitute beeswax with candelilla wax for a vegan alternative. If allergic to coconut oil, jojoba oil can be used as a substitute due to its similar skin-soothing properties.

CHAPTER 2: ANTISEPTICS AND ANTI-INFLAMMATORIES

Calendula for Wound Care

Calendula, scientifically known as **Calendula officinalis**, is renowned for its potent antibacterial properties, making it an invaluable herb in the realm of natural wound care. The vibrant orange or yellow petals of the calendula flower harbor a wealth of medicinal compounds, including flavonoids, triterpenoids, and carotenoids, which collectively contribute to its ability to fight infection and promote healing.

To effectively utilize calendula for cleaning wounds, follow these detailed steps to prepare a calendula-infused water or oil, which can be used to cleanse wounds and foster a conducive environment for healing:

1. **Harvesting or Sourcing Calendula**: Opt for organically grown calendula flowers to avoid contaminants. If harvesting from your garden, pick the flowers in the morning after the dew has evaporated for optimal potency.

2. **Drying Calendula Flowers**: Spread the calendula flowers on a clean, dry surface away from direct sunlight. Allow them to air dry until the petals are crisp to the touch. This may take several days, depending on humidity levels.

3. **Preparing Calendula-Infused Water**:
   - Place a handful of dried calendula petals in a heat-resistant jar.
   - Boil water and pour it over the petals, ensuring they are fully submerged.
   - Cover the jar and let the mixture steep for at least 4 hours or overnight for a stronger infusion.
   - Strain the infusion using a fine mesh sieve or cheesecloth to remove all plant material, resulting in a clear, golden liquid.

4. **Preparing Calendula-Infused Oil**:
   - Fill a jar halfway with dried calendula petals.
   - Pour a carrier oil, such as olive oil or sweet almond oil, over the petals until the jar is nearly full, ensuring the petals are completely covered.
   - Seal the jar and place it in a warm, sunny spot for 4-6 weeks, shaking it gently every few days.
   - After the infusion period, strain the oil through a fine mesh sieve or cheesecloth, squeezing out as much oil as possible from the petals.

5. **Using Calendula for Wound Cleaning**:
   - For minor cuts and abrasions, soak a clean cloth or gauze in the calendula-infused water and gently clean the wound area. The infusion can be used at room temperature or slightly warmed.
   - For deeper wounds or those requiring more substantial care, apply calendula-infused oil directly to the wound with a clean dropper or sterile gauze. The oil provides a moisture barrier that promotes healing and prevents the wound from drying out.

6. **Storage**:
   - Store the calendula-infused water in a refrigerator and use within one week to ensure freshness and potency. For extended use, consider adding a small amount of alcohol, such as vodka, as a natural preservative, which can extend the shelf life to up to one month.

- Calendula-infused oil should be stored in a cool, dark place. A dark glass bottle is ideal to protect the oil from light degradation. Properly stored, calendula oil can last for up to one year.

Precautions: While calendula is generally safe for topical use, individuals with allergies to plants in the Asteraceae family should perform a patch test before applying it to wounds. Discontinue use if any adverse reactions, such as itching or rash, occur.

By incorporating calendula into your natural first aid kit, you harness the power of this ancient herb to clean wounds effectively, fight infection, and support the body's innate healing process without the need for synthetic chemicals or antibiotics.

Goldenseal as a Natural Antiseptic

Goldenseal, scientifically known as Hydrastis canadensis, is a perennial herb native to the woodlands of the northeastern United States. Recognized for its broad-spectrum antimicrobial properties, goldenseal has been a cornerstone in herbal medicine, particularly as a natural antiseptic. The root of goldenseal contains several alkaloids, with berberine and hydrastine being the most prominent. These compounds are credited with the herb's potent antimicrobial and anti-inflammatory activities, making it highly effective in fighting infections.

When preparing goldenseal for use as a natural antiseptic, it's crucial to source high-quality, sustainably harvested roots due to concerns over the herb's conservation status. Once obtained, the root can be processed into various forms, including tinctures, powders, and creams, each suited for different antiseptic applications.

To create a goldenseal tincture, which can be used to cleanse wounds or as a topical antimicrobial agent, follow these detailed steps:

1. Chop or grind dried goldenseal root to increase its surface area, enhancing the extraction of its medicinal compounds.

2. Place the ground root in a glass jar, covering it with a high-proof alcohol (at least 40% alcohol by volume, such as vodka or grain alcohol) at a ratio of 1 part goldenseal to 5 parts alcohol. This ratio ensures a potent tincture.

3. Seal the jar tightly and store it in a cool, dark place, shaking it daily for 4 to 6 weeks. This period allows for the alcohol to extract the alkaloids from the root.

4. After the infusion period, strain the tincture through a fine mesh sieve or cheesecloth into a clean, dark glass bottle. Compress the plant material to extract as much liquid as possible.

5. Label the bottle with the date and contents. Stored properly, the tincture will remain potent for up to 5 years.

For treating skin infections or as a wound wash, dilute the tincture with sterile water to minimize any potential skin irritation. A typical dilution might be 1 part tincture to 3 parts water, applied directly to the affected area with a clean cloth or cotton pad.

Goldenseal powder, made by finely grinding the dried root, can be applied directly to cuts and wounds to utilize its antiseptic properties. The powder not only aids in infection prevention but also helps in the healing process due to its anti-inflammatory effects. To apply, simply sprinkle a small amount of goldenseal powder onto the cleaned wound before bandaging. This method is particularly useful for minor cuts and abrasions where infection prevention is a priority.

Alternatively, goldenseal can be incorporated into creams for a more soothing application. To make a simple goldenseal cream:

1. Begin with an unscented, natural base cream available at health stores.

2. Mix in goldenseal extract or powder until the desired concentration is achieved. A general guideline is 1 teaspoon of goldenseal powder or 1 tablespoon of tincture per ounce of base cream.

3. Stir the mixture thoroughly to ensure even distribution of the goldenseal.

4. Transfer the cream into a clean container with a lid, labeling it with the date and contents.

This cream can be applied to skin infections, eczema, or psoriasis patches, providing antimicrobial action as well as soothing relief.

Incorporating goldenseal into your herbal first aid kit enhances your ability to manage infections naturally. Its versatility in form—tincture, powder, or cream—allows for tailored applications depending on the need, making goldenseal a valuable ally in natural health and wellness. However, it's important to use goldenseal responsibly, mindful of its conservation status, and consult with a healthcare professional before using it, especially in children, pregnant or breastfeeding women, or individuals with pre-existing conditions.

Witch Hazel for Swelling and Irritation

Witch hazel, scientifically known as Hamamelis virginiana, is a plant native to North America, renowned for its astringent properties derived from its leaves and bark. These properties make witch hazel an invaluable component in the herbal first aid arsenal, particularly for addressing swelling and irritation. The active compounds in witch hazel, including tannins and flavonoids, contribute to its ability to reduce inflammation and soothe irritated skin.

To harness witch hazel's benefits for swelling and irritation, one can prepare a witch hazel extract or use distilled witch hazel water, which is readily available in most health stores. For making a homemade extract, gather fresh leaves and bark from the witch hazel plant during the late fall, as this is when the concentration of active compounds is at its peak. Chop the plant material finely and place it in a jar, covering it with high-proof alcohol, such as vodka or grain alcohol, to extract the tannins effectively. Seal the jar tightly and store it in a cool, dark place, shaking it daily for about four to six weeks. After this period, strain the mixture through a fine mesh sieve or cheesecloth, squeezing out as much liquid as possible, and transfer the clear extract into dark glass bottles for storage.

For topical application, dilute the witch hazel extract with distilled water to create a more skin-friendly solution. Apply this diluted extract gently to the affected area using a clean cotton ball or pad, allowing it to air dry. This method can be particularly effective for minor skin irritations, insect bites, and post-shave astringent to prevent razor burn. Additionally, witch hazel can be incorporated into homemade soothing gels or creams by blending the extract with aloe vera gel and other skin-calming ingredients like lavender essential oil for enhanced effects.

When using witch hazel for swelling, such as that associated with varicose veins or hemorrhoids, applying a cloth soaked in cold witch hazel extract can provide relief. The cooling effect, combined with the astringent properties, helps to constrict blood vessels and reduce swelling. It's important to note, however, that while witch hazel can offer symptomatic relief, it does not replace medical treatment for underlying conditions.

Safety is paramount when using witch hazel, especially for individuals with sensitive skin. Conducting a patch test on a small area of skin before widespread use is advisable to ensure there is no adverse reaction. While allergic reactions to witch hazel are rare, discontinuing use if irritation or sensitivity occurs is important.

Tea Tree and Lavender Antiseptic Spray

Beneficial effects

Tea Tree and Lavender Antiseptic Spray harnesses the natural antiseptic properties of tea tree oil and the soothing, anti-inflammatory benefits of lavender oil. This combination makes for a powerful disinfectant that can be used to cleanse wounds, soothe skin irritations, and even freshen up spaces with its antimicrobial properties. Tea tree oil is well-documented for its ability to fight bacteria, viruses, and fungi, making it an essential component in natural first aid kits. Lavender oil complements this with its ability to reduce redness, calm itchiness, and promote faster healing of minor cuts and burns.

Portions
Makes approximately 8 ounces

Preparation time
5 minutes

Ingredients
- 1/2 cup distilled water
- 1/4 cup witch hazel
- 30 drops tea tree essential oil
- 20 drops lavender essential oil
- 1 tablespoon aloe vera gel
- 1 teaspoon vitamin E oil (optional, for added skin nourishment)
- 8-ounce spray bottle, preferably dark glass to preserve the oils

Instructions
1. Start by pouring 1/2 cup of distilled water into your spray bottle using a funnel to minimize spills.
2. Add 1/4 cup of witch hazel to the bottle. Witch hazel acts as a carrier and enhances the antiseptic properties of the essential oils.
3. Carefully add 30 drops of tea tree essential oil and 20 drops of lavender essential oil to the mixture. These oils are potent, so ensure accurate measurement for the best therapeutic effect.
4. Incorporate 1 tablespoon of aloe vera gel into the bottle. Aloe vera gel adds a soothing, moisturizing component to the spray, making it gentle on the skin.
5. If using, add 1 teaspoon of vitamin E oil to the mixture. Vitamin E oil can help nourish and protect the skin, especially if the spray is used for minor cuts or abrasions.
6. Secure the lid on the spray bottle and shake vigorously for about 30 seconds to ensure all ingredients are well combined.
7. Label the bottle with the contents and date made for future reference.

Variations
- For an extra cooling effect, especially beneficial for soothing sunburns or skin irritations, add 5 drops of peppermint essential oil to the mixture.
- If you prefer a stronger antiseptic spray for household surfaces, increase the tea tree oil to 40 drops and omit the aloe vera gel.
- For a spray that doubles as a refreshing facial mist, reduce the tea tree oil to 20 drops and add 5 drops of rose water for its hydrating properties.

Storage tips
Store the Tea Tree and Lavender Antiseptic Spray in a cool, dark place away from direct sunlight to maintain the efficacy of the essential oils. The spray is best used within 6 months for optimal freshness and potency.

Tips for allergens
For those with sensitivities to tea tree or lavender oil, testing the spray on a small patch of skin before widespread use is recommended. If irritation occurs, diluting the spray with more distilled

water may reduce sensitivity. Alternatively, substituting chamomile essential oil for lavender can offer similar soothing properties with a lower risk of irritation for some individuals.

Calendula and Turmeric Anti-Inflammatory Cream

Beneficial effects

Calendula and Turmeric Anti-Inflammatory Cream harnesses the healing powers of calendula, known for its ability to soothe and repair the skin, and turmeric, celebrated for its anti-inflammatory and antioxidant properties. This cream is designed to reduce inflammation, promote wound healing, and provide relief for irritated skin conditions such as eczema, psoriasis, and acne. The combination of these potent botanicals offers a natural solution for enhancing skin health and restoring a balanced complexion.

Portions

Makes about 8 ounces

Preparation time

15 minutes

Cooking time

10 minutes

Ingredients

- 1/2 cup calendula-infused oil (preferably in olive or almond oil)
- 1/4 cup coconut oil
- 2 tablespoons shea butter
- 1 tablespoon beeswax pellets
- 1 teaspoon turmeric powder
- 10 drops lavender essential oil
- 5 drops frankincense essential oil
- A double boiler
- A glass jar or metal tin for storage

Instructions

1. Begin by setting up your double boiler. Fill the bottom pot with water, about 2 inches deep, and bring to a simmer over medium heat.

2. In the top of the double boiler, combine the calendula-infused oil, coconut oil, shea butter, and beeswax pellets. Stir continuously until the mixture is fully melted and well combined.

3. Once melted, remove from heat and allow to cool for a minute or two, but not solidify.

4. Carefully stir in the turmeric powder until fully incorporated, ensuring no clumps remain.

5. Add the lavender and frankincense essential oils, stirring gently to distribute evenly throughout the mixture.

6. Pour the warm cream into your chosen glass jar or metal tin. Allow to cool and solidify at room temperature, which may take several hours.

7. Once cooled, seal the container. Label with the product name and date made.

Variations

- For a vegan version, substitute beeswax pellets with the same amount of candelilla wax.
- If calendula-infused oil is not available, you can make your own by steeping dried calendula petals in a carrier oil of your choice for 4-6 weeks in a cool, dark place.

- For extra skin nourishment, add a teaspoon of vitamin E oil to the mixture after removing it from heat.

Storage tips

Store the Calendula and Turmeric Anti-Inflammatory Cream in a cool, dark place to preserve its natural properties. If stored properly, the cream should last for up to 6 months. Always use clean hands or a spatula to scoop out the cream to prevent contamination.

Tips for allergens

For those with sensitivities to coconut oil, jojoba oil can be used as a non-comedogenic alternative. If allergic to lavender or frankincense essential oils, they can be omitted or substituted with chamomile essential oil, which also has soothing properties. Always perform a patch test before applying the cream extensively, especially if you have sensitive skin.

Witch Hazel and Chamomile Soothing Antiseptic Gel

Beneficial effects

Witch Hazel and Chamomile Soothing Antiseptic Gel combines the astringent properties of witch hazel with the calming effects of chamomile to create a gentle yet effective antiseptic gel. Witch hazel, known for its ability to tighten skin and reduce inflammation, works in harmony with chamomile, which has been used for centuries to soothe irritated skin and promote healing. This gel is ideal for minor cuts, scrapes, and burns, providing a protective barrier against infection while supporting the skin's natural healing process.

Portions

Makes about 8 ounces

Preparation time

15 minutes

Cooking time

N/A

Ingredients

- 1/2 cup witch hazel extract
- 1/4 cup aloe vera gel, preferably cold-pressed
- 1/4 cup distilled water
- 2 tablespoons dried chamomile flowers
- 1 teaspoon vegetable glycerin (for added moisture)
- 10 drops lavender essential oil (for additional antiseptic and calming properties)
- Small funnel
- Sterilized 8-ounce bottle or jar for storage

Instructions

1. Begin by steeping 2 tablespoons of dried chamomile flowers in 1/4 cup of boiling distilled water. Cover and let it sit for 10 minutes to create a strong chamomile infusion.

2. After steeping, strain the chamomile infusion through a fine mesh sieve or cheesecloth into a clean bowl, ensuring to press out all the liquid from the flowers. Discard the used chamomile flowers.

3. In the bowl with the chamomile infusion, add 1/2 cup of witch hazel extract. Witch hazel serves as the base of this antiseptic gel, providing its astringent properties.

4. Incorporate 1/4 cup of aloe vera gel into the mixture. Aloe vera gel offers soothing and moisturizing benefits, making the antiseptic gel gentle on the skin.

5. Add 1 teaspoon of vegetable glycerin to the mixture. Glycerin is a humectant that helps retain moisture in the skin, enhancing the soothing effect of the gel.

6. Mix in 10 drops of lavender essential oil. Lavender not only adds a calming scent but also contributes additional antiseptic and anti-inflammatory properties to the gel.

7. Using a small funnel, carefully transfer the mixture into a sterilized 8-ounce bottle or jar. Ensure the container is clean to prevent contamination.

8. Seal the container and shake well to ensure all ingredients are thoroughly mixed.

Variations

- For extra skin healing properties, add 5 drops of tea tree essential oil to the mixture for its powerful antimicrobial benefits.
- If you prefer a thicker gel, you can dissolve 1/2 teaspoon of xanthan gum in the distilled water before adding it to the mixture. This will give the gel a more viscous consistency.
- For those sensitive to lavender, substitute with chamomile essential oil to maintain the calming properties without the risk of irritation.

Storage tips

Store the Witch Hazel and Chamomile Soothing Antiseptic Gel in a cool, dark place to preserve its potency. Ideally, keep it in the refrigerator to maintain freshness and provide a cooling effect upon application. Use within 6 months for best results.

Tips for allergens

For individuals with sensitivities to glycerin, it can be omitted without significantly affecting the gel's antiseptic properties. Always perform a patch test on a small area of your skin before applying the gel widely, especially if you have sensitive skin or are prone to allergies.

CHAPTER 3: HERBAL EMERGENCY KIT ESSENTIALS

Portable Herbal Kit Essentials

Creating a portable herbal kit is an essential step for anyone looking to be prepared for minor health emergencies on the go. This kit should contain a well-thought-out selection of herbs that address a wide range of common ailments, from cuts and scrapes to digestive discomforts. The key is to focus on versatility and efficacy, ensuring that each herb serves multiple purposes while also being lightweight and compact for easy transport.

Firstly, select a durable, water-resistant container to house your herbal supplies. This could be anything from a hard-shell case with individual compartments to a soft, padded pouch, depending on your preference and the amount of space you have. The container should be small enough to fit in a backpack or a large purse but large enough to hold several small bottles or tins of herbs, as well as a few essential tools like tweezers, a small pair of scissors, and a mortar and pestle for preparing herbs on the go.

For the herbal contents, begin with dried herbs due to their long shelf life and ease of transport. Dried chamomile flowers are a must-have for their calming and anti-inflammatory properties, making them useful for everything from soothing anxiety to treating minor skin irritations. Peppermint leaves are another versatile choice, as they can help relieve headaches, ease digestive troubles, and even deter insects when crushed. Lavender buds, with their antiseptic and calming properties, are excellent for wound care, promoting relaxation, and aiding in sleep. Yarrow powder is a powerful styptic that can stop bleeding quickly, making it invaluable for cuts and abrasions. Plantain leaves, available in many natural environments, can be chewed or crushed to create a poultice for bug bites, stings, and skin inflammations.

Each herb should be stored in its own small, clearly labeled container. Glass vials with screw-top lids or small, zip-seal bags are both good options, as they protect the herbs from moisture and light degradation. Include a small, laminated card with brief instructions on how to use each herb, such as dosages and preparation methods, to ensure that you or anyone else who might need to use the kit can do so effectively.

In addition to dried herbs, consider including a few small bottles of essential oils for their concentrated therapeutic properties and ease of use. Tea tree oil is a powerful antimicrobial agent, making it ideal for cleaning wounds and treating fungal infections. Eucalyptus oil can serve as a decongestant for respiratory issues and also works as a natural insect repellent. Lavender oil, as mentioned, is useful for stress relief and minor burns. Each oil should be stored in a dark glass bottle to preserve its potency, with a dropper for precise application.

Finally, include a small booklet or a set of cards with detailed information on each herb and oil, including their uses, benefits, and any safety precautions. This reference material should be compact and waterproof, ensuring that it remains readable in any situation.

By carefully selecting and organizing these items, your portable herbal kit will be an invaluable resource for addressing health concerns naturally and effectively, wherever you may be. Remember, the goal is not to replace professional medical treatment but to offer immediate, natural relief for minor ailments and emergencies.

Combining Herbs for First-Aid Blends

Creating blends for common first-aid scenarios involves a thoughtful combination of herbs that can address multiple health concerns efficiently. This process requires an understanding of each herb's properties, potential interactions, and the best methods for preparation and application. To craft effective multi-purpose herbal blends, one must consider the primary health issues that might arise in emergency situations, such as wounds, burns, insect bites, and digestive disturbances. Here, we delve into the specifics of selecting, combining, and utilizing herbs to create versatile first-aid remedies.

To begin, identify a core set of herbs that have broad-spectrum healing properties. For instance, calendula (Calendula officinalis) is renowned for its wound-healing capabilities, anti-inflammatory properties, and ability to reduce infection risk, making it an indispensable herb for any first-aid blend. Lavender (Lavandula angustifolia), with its antiseptic and analgesic properties, not only soothes cuts and burns but also alleviates stress and anxiety, which can be beneficial in traumatic situations. Aloe vera (Aloe barbadensis miller) gel is another versatile ingredient, known for its cooling, healing effects on burns and its soothing properties for skin irritations.

When combining these herbs, consider the most effective form for emergency use. A salve or balm, for example, can be easily applied to wounds, burns, and insect bites. To create a multi-purpose salve, start with a base of beeswax and a carrier oil, such as coconut oil, known for its skin-healing benefits and antimicrobial properties. Melt approximately two parts beeswax to eight parts carrier oil in a double boiler, ensuring the mixture is thoroughly combined. Next, infuse the warm oil with dried calendula petals, lavender buds, and aloe vera gel, allowing the mixture to steep for several hours on low heat to extract the medicinal properties of the herbs.

Once the infusion is complete, strain the mixture to remove the solid herb parts, returning the liquid to the double boiler. At this stage, you can enhance the blend with essential oils such as tea tree (Melaleuca alternifolia) for its potent antimicrobial action and peppermint (Mentha piperita) for its cooling effect and ability to relieve pain and itching. Add these essential oils sparingly, typically a few drops per ounce of the salve base, as they are highly concentrated.

Pour the final mixture into small, sterilized tins or jars, allowing it to solidify. Label each container with the ingredients and the date of creation. This multi-purpose salve can be applied to a variety of skin issues, from minor cuts and scrapes to burns, providing a protective barrier that promotes healing while offering antimicrobial and soothing benefits.

For digestive disturbances, a simple herbal tea blend can be invaluable. Combine dried peppermint leaves, known for their antispasmodic and gas-relieving properties, with ginger root (Zingiber officinale), which can alleviate nausea and stomach upset. To prepare the tea, mix equal parts of peppermint and ginger, storing the blend in a dry, airtight container. To use, steep one teaspoon of the blend in boiling water for ten minutes, strain, and drink as needed for digestive relief.

In creating these herbal first-aid remedies, it's crucial to source high-quality, organic herbs to ensure the potency and safety of your blends. Additionally, understanding the specific needs and sensitivities of those who may use these remedies is essential for effective and safe application. With these considerations in mind, crafting multi-purpose herbal blends can be a rewarding way to provide natural, effective first-aid solutions for a range of common health concerns.

Herbal Kits: Storage and Maintenance

Ensuring that your herbal first aid kit remains organized and effective over time requires meticulous attention to storage and maintenance practices. The longevity and efficacy of the herbs and preparations within your kit are directly influenced by how they are stored, the conditions they are kept in, and how regularly the contents are checked and refreshed. To maintain an organized and potent herbal first aid kit, follow these detailed guidelines.

Firstly, select a storage location that is cool, dark, and dry to prevent degradation of the herbs. Exposure to heat, light, and moisture can lead to the deterioration of active compounds in herbs, reducing their therapeutic value. A cupboard in a room that maintains a consistent temperature and is away from direct sunlight, radiators, and moisture sources is ideal. Ensure the storage area is out of reach of children and pets to avoid accidental ingestion or tampering.

For the containers housing your herbs and preparations, opt for materials that offer protection from light and air. Amber glass jars and metal tins with tight-fitting lids are excellent choices for storing dried herbs, powders, and salves. These materials prevent light from degrading the contents and provide an airtight seal that keeps out moisture and air, which can introduce mold and bacteria. Label each container clearly with the name of the herb or preparation, the date of packaging or preparation, and the expiration date if applicable. This practice not only helps in identifying the contents quickly but also in tracking their shelf life.

Regularly inspect the contents of your herbal first aid kit, ideally every six months, to ensure that everything remains in good condition. Check for any signs of spoilage such as mold, unusual odors, or changes in color and texture. Herbs that have lost their vibrant color, aroma, or flavor are likely to have also lost their medicinal properties and should be replaced. This bi-annual review is also an opportune time to replenish supplies that have been used and to update the kit based on any new health needs or preferences.

For liquid preparations such as tinctures, oils, and syrups, verify that the containers are still sealed tightly and that there are no leaks. Any change in the smell, color, or consistency of liquid preparations could indicate spoilage, and they should be discarded. Store these liquids in dark glass bottles to extend their shelf life and maintain their potency.

In addition to physical maintenance, keep an inventory list as part of your kit. This list should detail the contents, quantities, and expiration dates of all items. Having an inventory aids in the quick assessment of your kit's status and simplifies the process of restocking or updating its contents. Store this list inside your kit, and ensure it is kept current with each inspection and update.

Finally, consider the organization of the kit itself. Group items together based on their use – for example, wound care, digestive aids, and skin treatments – and compartmentalize them within the kit for easy access. Utilize small bags or boxes within larger containers to keep items sorted and prevent them from shifting. This level of organization not only makes it easier to find what you need in an emergency but also helps in monitoring which supplies are running low or nearing their expiration.

By implementing these detailed storage and maintenance practices, you can ensure that your herbal first aid kit remains a reliable resource for natural health care. Regular attention to the condition and organization of your kit guarantees that when the need arises, your herbal remedies will be potent and ready to use.

BOOK 19: GROWING MEDICINAL HERBS

CHAPTER 1: STARTING A MEDICINAL HERB GARDEN

Beginner-Friendly Herbs Selection

When embarking on the rewarding journey of creating a medicinal herb garden, selecting the right plants is crucial, especially for beginners. Focusing on easy-to-grow herbs such as basil, mint, and calendula can ensure a successful start, providing both a bountiful harvest and a foundational learning experience in herbal gardening. These plants have been chosen for their resilience, minimal care requirements, and versatile uses, making them ideal candidates for novice gardeners.

Basil, a beloved culinary herb, thrives in warm, sunny conditions. It requires well-drained soil with a neutral to slightly acidic pH, typically between 6.0 and 7.0. For optimal growth, basil should be planted in an area that receives at least six hours of direct sunlight daily. Watering should be consistent, aiming to keep the soil evenly moist but not waterlogged, as basil is sensitive to overwatering. To encourage a bushier plant and prevent early flowering, pinch off the tip of the central stem after it has developed several sets of leaves. This practice stimulates the growth of lateral branches, increasing leaf production.

Mint, known for its invigorating aroma and flavor, is an incredibly hardy herb that can grow in a variety of conditions, although it prefers moist, well-drained soil and partial to full sunlight. One of the most important considerations when planting mint is its tendency to spread aggressively; therefore, it is advisable to plant it in containers or confined spaces to prevent it from overtaking the garden. Regular harvesting and pinching back the tips of the stems encourage denser growth and prevent the plant from becoming leggy. Mint is relatively pest-resistant and requires little care beyond regular watering and occasional feeding with a balanced fertilizer.

Calendula, with its cheerful, vibrant flowers, is not only aesthetically pleasing but also possesses medicinal properties. It prefers a sunny location but can tolerate partial shade, making it a versatile choice for different garden spots. Calendula grows best in moderately fertile, well-drained soil. While it is drought-tolerant once established, regular watering will promote continuous blooming. Deadheading, or the removal of spent flowers, encourages the plant to produce more blooms. Calendula can be directly sown into the garden after the last frost or started indoors in seed trays before transplanting. It is relatively pest-free, although aphids can sometimes be a problem; these can be managed with a strong spray of water or insecticidal soap.

Incorporating these beginner-friendly herbs into your garden not only sets the foundation for a thriving herbal sanctuary but also offers a gateway to exploring the vast world of medicinal plants. Each herb, with its unique requirements and benefits, provides an opportunity to learn about plant care, harvesting techniques, and the various ways herbs can be used for culinary, medicinal, and aromatic purposes. As your garden grows and your confidence as a herbalist expands, you may find yourself inspired to experiment with more challenging herbs, further enriching your connection to the natural world.

Understanding Soil and Climate Needs

Soil preparation is the bedrock of successful medicinal herb gardening, necessitating a clear understanding and application of specific techniques to create an optimal growing environment. The first step involves assessing the soil's texture, which ranges from sandy to clay-heavy compositions. Ideal soil for most medicinal herbs is loamy, offering a balanced mixture of sand, silt, and clay, along with organic matter to ensure good drainage and nutrient retention. To achieve this, incorporate compost or aged manure into the soil at a depth of 6 to 8 inches. This not only improves soil structure but also enhances microbial life essential for plant health.

The pH level of the soil, a measure of its acidity or alkalinity, significantly affects herb growth by influencing nutrient availability. Most medicinal herbs thrive in a slightly acidic to neutral pH range, between 6.0 and 7.5. Conduct a soil test using a home testing kit or by consulting with a local extension service to determine your soil's pH. If adjustments are needed, apply lime to raise the pH or sulfur to lower it, following the product's guidelines for the amount based on your soil test results.

Sunlight requirements vary among medicinal herbs, but the majority demand full sun, defined as at least six hours of direct sunlight daily. Observe potential garden locations throughout the day to identify areas that meet this criterion. South-facing sites typically receive ample sunlight. However, for herbs that prefer partial shade, such as lemon balm or mint, choose a site that enjoys morning sunlight and afternoon shade. This can be naturally achieved by planting under the dappled light of a tree or on the east side of a structure.

Choosing the right location also involves considering wind exposure and proximity to water sources. Areas that are too exposed can lead to soil drying out quickly and may harm delicate herbs. Implement windbreaks such as fences, shrubs, or tall herbs to protect more sensitive plants. Accessibility to a water source simplifies the irrigation process, essential during dry spells to maintain soil moisture levels conducive to herb growth.

To further tailor the growing environment, raised beds or containers can be utilized for herbs requiring specific soil types or drainage conditions not available in the garden. Raised beds offer improved soil drainage and aeration, beneficial for root development and overall plant health. Containers allow for complete control over the soil environment and can be moved to optimize sunlight exposure.

Incorporating mulch around the plants not only conserves soil moisture but also suppresses weed growth and moderates soil temperature. Organic mulches, such as straw or wood chips, additionally contribute to soil fertility as they decompose.

By meticulously preparing the soil, adjusting its pH, ensuring adequate sunlight, and selecting an appropriate location, gardeners can create a nurturing environment that supports the vigorous growth of medicinal herbs. This foundational work lays the groundwork for a garden that will flourish, providing a bountiful supply of herbs for health and wellness.

Container Gardening for Limited Space

Container gardening is an ideal solution for individuals with limited outdoor space, enabling the cultivation of medicinal herbs in small areas such as balconies, patios, or even windowsills. This method not only maximizes limited space but also offers the flexibility to control the growing environment more effectively than in-ground planting. To embark on container gardening, one must consider the selection of containers, soil composition, watering needs, and the specific requirements of each herb.

Selecting Containers: Choose pots made from materials like clay, ceramic, or recycled plastic, ensuring they have adequate drainage holes at the bottom. The size of the container should accommodate the root system of the herb; generally, a pot with a diameter of 6 to 12 inches is suitable for most herbs. Larger containers can hold multiple herbs, but be mindful to group plants with similar watering and sunlight needs together.

Soil Composition: Use a high-quality potting mix designed for container gardening, which typically includes a blend of peat moss, vermiculite, and perlite. This mix ensures good drainage and aeration, critical factors in preventing root rot and promoting healthy growth. Avoid using garden soil, as it can compact in pots and may contain pests or diseases.

Watering Needs: Herbs in containers require more frequent watering than those in the ground, as soil in pots dries out faster. Check the soil moisture daily by inserting a finger an inch into the soil; if it feels dry, it's time to water. Water the plant until excess water drains out of the bottom, indicating the soil is thoroughly moistened. However, be cautious not to overwater, as standing water can lead to root diseases.

Sunlight Requirements: Most medicinal herbs need at least six hours of direct sunlight daily. Place containers in a south-facing location to maximize light exposure. If sufficient natural light is not available, especially in indoor settings, consider using grow lights. LED grow lights or fluorescent bulbs can provide the necessary spectrum of light for photosynthesis and healthy growth. Position the lights approximately two to four inches above the plants and keep them on for 14 to 16 hours a day to mimic natural sunlight conditions.

Herb Selection: Start with easy-to-grow herbs like basil, mint, and calendula, which adapt well to container life. Basil thrives in warm conditions and requires regular harvesting to prevent flowering, encouraging fuller growth. Mint is vigorous and can easily fill a container; its invigorating aroma makes it a popular choice for indoor gardening. Calendula, with its bright flowers, prefers cooler temperatures and can add a splash of color to your space.

Feeding: Container-grown herbs benefit from regular feeding with a balanced, water-soluble fertilizer, diluted to half the recommended strength. Feed herbs every four to six weeks during the growing season to replenish nutrients that are washed out with frequent watering.

Pest Management: Keep an eye out for common pests such as aphids and spider mites. In most cases, a strong spray of water can dislodge pests. For persistent issues, use insecticidal soap or neem oil, applying according to the product instructions. Always inspect new plants for pests before introducing them to your container garden to prevent infestation.

By following these detailed steps, even those with the smallest of spaces can enjoy the benefits of a medicinal herb garden. Container gardening not only brings the joy of growing your own herbs but also ensures a fresh supply of medicinal plants for health and wellness, right at your fingertips.

CHAPTER 2: HERB GARDEN PLANTING AND CARE

Seed Planting vs. Transplanting

When deciding between seed planting and transplanting for growing medicinal herbs, each method comes with its own set of advantages and challenges. Understanding these can help gardeners choose the approach that best suits their needs, resources, and the specific requirements of the herbs they wish to cultivate.

Seed planting involves sowing seeds directly into the soil or starting them indoors in seed trays or pots. This method is often more cost-effective, as seeds are generally cheaper than seedlings. It also offers a wider variety of herb choices, since many specialty or rare herbs are only available in seed form. Starting from seed allows gardeners to control the growing environment from the very beginning, ensuring that plants are healthy, organic, and free from chemical treatments. However, growing herbs from seeds requires more time and patience. Germination rates can vary widely among different herb types, and some seeds may take a long time to sprout. Additionally, seeds need careful attention to moisture, temperature, and light conditions to germinate successfully. For beginners, this can be a bit daunting, as it requires learning about the specific needs of each herb and possibly investing in equipment like grow lights or heating mats for optimal germination.

Transplanting, on the other hand, involves purchasing young plants or seedlings from a nursery or garden center and planting them directly into the garden or into larger pots. This method offers immediate gratification, as plants are already established and can make a visual impact in the garden sooner. It also reduces the uncertainty of germination and the initial waiting period for seeds to sprout, making it a more straightforward option for beginners or those looking for quicker results. Transplanting can be especially beneficial for slow-growing herbs or those with longer germination times, as it gives them a head start. However, the cost of purchasing seedlings can add up quickly, especially for large gardens or rare herb varieties. There's also a risk of introducing diseases or pests from the nursery to your garden. Additionally, the selection of herbs available as seedlings may be limited compared to seeds, potentially restricting the variety of herbs one can grow.

When planting seeds, it's crucial to use a high-quality, well-draining soil mix and to plant the seeds at the correct depth, which is typically twice the diameter of the seed. For indoor starts, ensure seed trays or pots have adequate drainage and are placed in a location that receives sufficient warmth and light or use a grow light setup to simulate ideal conditions. Regularly mist the soil to keep it moist but not waterlogged, as too much water can cause seeds to rot.

For transplanting, carefully remove the seedling from its container, trying not to disturb the roots too much. Prepare a hole in your garden or pot that is slightly larger than the root ball of the seedling. Gently place the seedling in the hole and fill in around it with soil, pressing down lightly to eliminate air pockets. Water the seedling immediately after transplanting to help settle the soil and provide moisture for the roots. It's important to harden off indoor-grown or greenhouse seedlings before planting them outdoors by gradually exposing them to outdoor conditions over a period of several days. This helps prevent transplant shock, which can occur if plants are moved from a controlled environment to the variable conditions of the outdoors too quickly.

Both seed planting and transplanting have their place in the medicinal herb garden, and the choice between them often comes down to the gardener's preferences, experience level, and the specific herbs being grown. Some gardeners may even find a combination of both methods works best, starting some herbs from seed and purchasing others as seedlings for the best of both worlds.

Seasonal Herb Care and Pest Management

Protecting your medicinal herb garden from pests and diseases through organic solutions requires a proactive and integrated approach. Seasonal care is pivotal, as different seasons bring different challenges. By understanding the life cycles of common pests and the conditions that favor disease outbreaks, you can implement strategies that keep your garden healthy year-round.

Spring: As new growth emerges, so do pests. Aphids, for example, are attracted to the tender new leaves of herbs. An effective organic solution is to spray infested plants with a mixture of water and a few drops of mild liquid soap, which suffocates the aphids. For fungal diseases that thrive in the cool, wet conditions of spring, improve air circulation around your plants by spacing them properly and pruning any overcrowded areas. This reduces humidity around the foliage, making the environment less hospitable for fungi.

Summer: The warm weather can bring about spider mites and whiteflies. These pests prefer dry and dusty conditions, so maintaining adequate moisture through regular watering can deter them. Introducing beneficial insects, such as ladybugs and lacewings, can naturally control these pests by predation. To manage powdery mildew, a common summer fungal issue, mix a tablespoon of baking soda with a gallon of water and a teaspoon of horticultural oil, and spray it on the affected leaves. The baking soda creates an alkaline surface that is inhospitable to the mildew.

Fall: As plants begin to die back, remove any diseased or infested plant material from the garden to prevent pests and pathogens from overwintering in the soil. This is also a good time to apply a layer of compost around your herbs, which can enhance soil health and suppress soil-borne diseases. Slugs and snails, which are active in cooler temperatures, can be managed by setting up traps or barriers, such as copper strips around the base of plants.

Winter: Preparation for winter involves ensuring that your soil is healthy and well-draining to prevent root rot in perennial herbs. Mulching with straw or leaf mold can protect the root zone from freezing temperatures and sudden thaws, which can stress plants and make them more susceptible to disease in the spring. It's also a good time to plan crop rotation for the coming year, which can prevent the buildup of soil-borne pests and diseases.

Throughout the year, practicing good hygiene in your garden is crucial. Regularly clean your tools, especially after working with diseased plants, to prevent the spread of pathogens. Watering in the morning allows foliage to dry before evening, reducing the risk of fungal diseases. Encouraging a diverse ecosystem by planting a variety of herbs and companion plants can create a more resilient garden environment where pests and diseases are less likely to take hold.

By integrating these organic pest and disease management strategies into your seasonal garden care routine, you can maintain a healthy, productive herb garden that thrives throughout the year.

Pruning and Harvesting for Growth

Pruning and harvesting your medicinal herbs are crucial practices that not only influence the current yield but also affect future growth and productivity. To ensure your garden remains vibrant and bountiful, understanding the timing, techniques, and tools for pruning and harvesting is essential.

Pruning involves selectively removing parts of the plant to improve its health, promote growth, and increase the yield of usable parts. Start by identifying dead or dying foliage, which can be removed at any time to prevent disease and pest infestation. For most herbs, pruning is best done in the early spring as plants emerge from dormancy or just after they bloom, to encourage a second flowering. Use clean, sharp pruning shears to make precise cuts just above a leaf node or pair of leaves. This encourages the plant to branch out from that point, leading to a fuller, more productive plant. Regularly removing spent flowers, a practice known as deadheading, can also stimulate further blooming and prevent the plant from going to seed too early in the season.

Harvesting your herbs at the right time maximizes their medicinal properties and flavor. The best time of day for harvesting is in the morning after the dew has evaporated but before the sun becomes too intense. This is when the plants' essential oils are most concentrated. For leaves, the prime time for harvesting is just before the plant flowers, as this is when the concentration of active compounds is highest. Cut leaves or stems with sharp scissors or shears, taking care not to remove more than one-third of the plant at a time to avoid stressing it. For roots, the best harvesting time is in the fall for perennials or late in the season for annuals, once the foliage has begun to die back. Use a garden fork to gently lift the roots from the soil, shaking off excess dirt and trimming away any dead or damaged parts.

Continuous Growth is encouraged by adopting a cycle of pruning and harvesting that aligns with the plant's natural growth phases. After harvesting, provide your plants with a light feeding of balanced, organic fertilizer and ensure they have adequate water to recover and regrow. In climates with a long growing season, you may be able to harvest multiple times by allowing the plant to regrow and then repeating the pruning and harvesting process.

For specific herbs, consider the following tips:

- **Basil**: Pinch off the tips regularly to encourage bushy growth and prevent it from flowering for as long as possible.

- **Mint**: Harvest by cutting the stems just above a set of leaves, which will prompt the plant to branch out.

- **Lavender**: Prune immediately after the first bloom to encourage a second bloom and to maintain shape.

- **Chamomile**: Pick the flowers when they are fully open, just before they begin to wilt, for the best flavor and medicinal properties.

By incorporating these practices into your gardening routine, you can ensure not only a plentiful harvest this season but also a strong, healthy garden ready to produce again in the future. Remember, the key to successful pruning and harvesting is understanding the needs and growth patterns of each herb in your garden.

CHAPTER 3: PRESERVING AND STORING YOUR HARVEST

Drying Herbs for Storage

Drying herbs is a crucial step in preserving their flavor, aroma, and medicinal properties for long-term storage. The process involves removing moisture from the herbs, which helps prevent the growth of mold and bacteria. There are several methods to achieve this, including air-drying, oven-drying, and dehydrating. Each method has its own set of steps, suitable for different types of herbs and the resources available to the harvester.

Air-drying is the most traditional method and is best suited for herbs with low moisture content in their leaves, such as rosemary, thyme, and oregano. Begin by harvesting herbs in the morning after the dew has evaporated but before the sun becomes too intense, as this helps preserve the oils responsible for flavor and aroma. Tie the stems together with twine and hang the bundles upside down in a warm, dry, well-ventilated area out of direct sunlight. A dark, airy attic or a closet are ideal locations. The drying process can take anywhere from one to three weeks, depending on the humidity levels and the type of herb. To test if the herbs are sufficiently dry, check if the leaves crumble easily between your fingers. Once dried, strip the leaves from the stems and store them in airtight containers, labeling each with the herb name and date of drying.

Oven-drying is faster than air-drying and is suitable for herbs with higher moisture content, such as basil, mint, and lemon balm. Preheat your oven to its lowest setting, usually between 150°F to 200°F (65°C to 93°C). While the oven heats, prepare the herbs by washing them gently and patting them dry with a towel. Spread the herbs out on a baking sheet lined with parchment paper, ensuring they are not overlapping. Place the baking sheet in the oven, leaving the door slightly ajar to allow moisture to escape. Check the herbs every 30 minutes, turning them occasionally to ensure even drying. Depending on the herb and the oven's temperature, drying can take between 1 to 4 hours. Herbs are sufficiently dried when they are crispy and crumble easily.

Dehydrating is the most efficient method for drying herbs, especially in humid climates where air-drying may not be feasible. Use a food dehydrator set between 95°F to 115°F (35°C to 46°C). After washing and patting the herbs dry, place them in a single layer on the dehydrator trays. The drying time can vary from 1 to 4 hours, depending on the herb and the dehydrator model. Check the herbs periodically, and once they crumble easily, they are ready for storage. Dehydrators are particularly useful for large batches and can maintain a consistent temperature, ensuring even drying.

Regardless of the method chosen, the key to successful long-term storage is ensuring the herbs are completely dry before sealing them in containers. Any residual moisture can lead to mold growth. Glass jars with tight-fitting lids, vacuum-sealed bags, or metal tins with airtight seals are all suitable storage containers. Store the dried herbs in a cool, dark place to preserve their quality. Properly dried and stored herbs can maintain their potency for up to a year, providing a ready supply of flavors and medicinal properties for your culinary and wellness needs.

Herbal Powders and Infusions

Transforming dried herbs into **powders** and crafting **concentrated infusions** are invaluable skills for anyone interested in harnessing the full potential of their homegrown or foraged botanicals. These processes not only extend the shelf life of your herbs but also enhance their versatility in natural remedies, culinary applications, and personal care products.

Grinding Dried Herbs into Powders

1. **Selection of Dried Herbs**: Ensure that the herbs are completely dry. Any residual moisture can lead to mold growth in the powder. Herbs should crumble easily between your fingers, indicating they are ready for grinding.

2. **Choosing the Right Grinder**: A coffee grinder dedicated to herb processing is ideal due to its fine grinding capability. Ensure the grinder is clean and dry before use to prevent cross-contamination of flavors or medicinal properties.

3. **Grinding in Batches**: To achieve a uniform consistency, grind small quantities at a time. Overloading the grinder can result in unevenly ground particles and may overheat some of the herb powder, potentially degrading its quality.

4. **Sifting the Powder**: After grinding, use a fine-mesh sieve to sift the powder. This step ensures a consistent texture and removes any larger, unground pieces that can be returned to the grinder for further processing.

5. **Storage**: Store the herb powder in airtight containers, away from direct sunlight and moisture. Label each container with the herb name and the date of grinding. Glass jars with tight-fitting lids or metal tins are preferred to preserve the powder's potency.

Creating Concentrated Herbal Infusions

1. **Selecting Herbs and Solvents**: Choose high-quality, dried herbs and a suitable solvent (water, alcohol, glycerin, or oil) based on the intended use of the infusion. Alcohol is commonly used for tinctures due to its efficiency in extracting a wide range of plant constituents and its preservative properties.

2. **Ratio of Herbs to Solvent**: A general guideline for tinctures is a 1:5 ratio of dried herbs to solvent by weight/volume (e.g., 20g of dried herbs to 100ml of alcohol). Adjust the ratio based on the herb's potency and the desired strength of the infusion.

3. **Maceration**: Place the herbs in a clean, dry jar and cover them with the solvent. Seal the jar tightly and label it with the contents and date. Store the jar in a cool, dark place, shaking it daily to encourage extraction.

4. **Straining the Infusion**: After 4-6 weeks, strain the infusion through a cheesecloth or fine-mesh sieve into another clean, dry jar. Press or squeeze the herb material to extract as much liquid as possible.

5. **Bottling and Storage**: Transfer the strained infusion into dark glass bottles to protect it from light, which can degrade its quality. Label each bottle with the herb name, type of solvent, and date of preparation. Store in a cool, dark place. Alcohol-based tinctures can last for several years when stored properly.

By mastering these techniques, you can efficiently convert your herbal harvest into potent powders and infusions, ready to be incorporated into a myriad of natural health and wellness applications.

Freezing and Storing Fresh Herbs

Freezing fresh herbs offers an excellent method for preserving their flavor, aroma, and nutritional value, making them readily available for immediate use. This process involves a few critical steps to ensure the herbs retain their best qualities. First, select fresh herbs that are free from blemishes or signs of wilting. Herbs harvested in the morning, after the dew has evaporated but before the sun is at its peak, tend to have the highest concentration of essential oils, which are key to their flavor and therapeutic properties.

Before freezing, herbs should be thoroughly washed under cold running water to remove any soil or residue. Shake off excess water or use a salad spinner to help dry them quickly. For herbs with larger leaves, such as basil or mint, it's beneficial to pat them dry with a clean kitchen towel or paper towels to remove as much moisture as possible. Excess water can lead to ice crystal formation, which can damage the cell structure of the herbs and result in a loss of flavor.

The next step involves preparing the herbs for freezing. There are two primary methods for freezing herbs: whole and chopped. Freezing herbs whole is the simplest method. Lay the cleaned and dried herbs on a baking sheet in a single layer, ensuring they are not touching. Freeze them for a few hours until they are solid. Once frozen, transfer the herbs to airtight containers or zip-top freezer bags, removing as much air as possible before sealing. Label the containers or bags with the herb name and the date of freezing. This method is particularly suitable for herbs like dill, chives, and rosemary, which can be easily stripped from their stems when frozen and crumbled directly into dishes.

For the chopped method, finely chop the cleaned and dried herbs and pack them into ice cube trays. Cover the herbs with water or olive oil, depending on your future culinary uses. Olive oil is ideal for herbs that you plan to use in sautéing or roasting, as it prevents the herbs from browning and adds an extra layer of flavor. Once the herb cubes are frozen solid, pop them out of the trays and transfer them to airtight containers or zip-top freezer bags, again removing as much air as possible. Label each container or bag with the herb type and freezing date. This method works well for basil, cilantro, parsley, and other soft herbs.

When using frozen herbs, there's no need to thaw them before adding to your cooking. Frozen herbs work best in cooked dishes rather than raw applications, as freezing can alter their texture. Add them directly to soups, stews, sauces, or sauté pans. The heat will thaw the herbs, releasing their flavors into the dish.

By following these detailed steps for freezing and storing fresh herbs, you can extend the life of your herbal harvest, ensuring you have a supply of your favorite flavors on hand year-round for immediate use in your culinary creations.

BOOK 20: SUSTAINABLE HERBAL PRACTICES

CHAPTER 1: ETHICAL WILDCRAFTING AND FORAGING

When engaging in **ethical wildcrafting and foraging**, it's crucial to have a comprehensive understanding of the **ecosystem** you are entering. This involves recognizing not only the plants but also the wildlife that depends on them, ensuring that your harvesting practices do not disrupt local fauna. For instance, if a particular herb serves as a primary food source for an endangered species, it should be left untouched. Always conduct research or consult with local conservationists or botanists to understand the broader ecological impact of removing certain plants from their habitat.

Harvesting Techniques play a significant role in sustainable foraging. When collecting leaves, use sharp scissors or shears to make clean cuts on the plant, taking only the outer leaves to allow the plant to continue growing robustly. For roots, be sure to replant a portion of the root system or seeds to ensure the plant population can regenerate. This technique is particularly important for perennial plants that take several years to mature.

The **time of day** and **season** significantly affect the potency and sustainability of harvested herbs. Early morning is often the best time for harvesting, as plants are full of vital energies and have not yet been stressed by the heat of the day. Moreover, understanding the growth cycle of plants ensures that you harvest at a time when the plant can best recover or when it has the highest concentration of active compounds. For example, many flowers are best harvested just before they fully open, while roots are often most potent in the autumn when the plant's energy is stored below ground.

Responsible foraging also includes the proper **identification** of plants to ensure that you are not harvesting poisonous or protected species. Invest in a good field guide specific to your region and consider taking part in local foraging workshops or walks led by experienced herbalists or botanists. Digital applications that allow you to take photos and identify plants can be helpful, but they should not replace comprehensive knowledge and confirmation from more reliable sources.

By adhering to these practices, foragers can ensure that their activities contribute to the health and sustainability of the ecosystems from which they draw their resources.

CHAPTER 2: COMPOSTING AND RECYCLING IN HERBALISM

Composting is a cornerstone of sustainable herbal practices, transforming organic waste into a nutrient-rich soil amendment that benefits both your garden and the environment. By composting leftover plant materials, you not only reduce waste but also create a valuable resource for growing medicinal herbs. Here's how to start and maintain an effective compost system tailored for herbalists.

Selecting a Compost Bin: Choose a compost bin that fits your space and needs. Options range from open piles to enclosed bins and tumblers. Enclosed systems are ideal for small spaces and can reduce pests and odors. For larger gardens, an open pile might be more practical, allowing for easier turning and aeration.

What to Compost: You can compost most plant-based materials, including herb trimmings, spent plants, and non-diseased plant parts. Avoid composting diseased plants or those treated with pesticides to prevent contaminating your compost. You can also add kitchen scraps like vegetable peels, coffee grounds, and eggshells, but avoid meats, dairy, and oils, which can attract pests.

Creating the Right Mix: A healthy compost pile needs a balance of green (nitrogen-rich) and brown (carbon-rich) materials. Green materials include fresh plant trimmings and kitchen scraps, while brown materials consist of dried leaves, straw, and paper. Aim for a ratio of roughly 2:1, brown to green, to ensure proper decomposition without odors.

Layering Your Compost: Start with a layer of coarse brown material, like straw or twigs, to enhance drainage and aeration. Add layers of green material, followed by brown material. Sprinkle water over each layer to keep the pile moist but not waterlogged. A properly moistened compost pile should feel like a wrung-out sponge.

Turning the Compost: Regularly turning your compost pile increases oxygen flow, speeding up the decomposition process. Use a garden fork to turn the pile every few weeks, moving material from the center to the outside. This aeration is crucial for preventing anaerobic conditions that can slow decomposition and cause odors.

Monitoring Your Compost: Keep an eye on your compost pile's moisture level and temperature. The pile should heat up as the materials break down, a sign that the composting process is working. If the pile is too dry, add water; if it's too wet, add more brown material to absorb excess moisture.

Using Your Compost: Compost is ready to use when it's dark, crumbly, and smells like earth. This process can take anywhere from a few months to a year, depending on factors like temperature, moisture, and material types. Use your finished compost to enrich garden beds, potting mixes, or as a top dressing for plants.

Recycling in Herbal Practices: Beyond composting, sustainable herbal practices include recycling and repurposing materials. Glass jars and bottles can be reused for storing dried herbs, tinctures, and oils. Paper and cardboard can be shredded and added to the compost pile or used as mulch in the garden to suppress weeds and retain soil moisture.

Creating a Zero-Waste Apothecary: Strive for a zero-waste approach by finding creative uses for all parts of the plant. Use leftover herb stems to create infused vinegars or stocks. Repurpose spent herbal material from infusions or decoctions as compost to return nutrients to the soil, completing the cycle of growth and sustainability.

By integrating these composting and recycling practices into your herbal apothecary, you contribute to a sustainable cycle that not only benefits your garden but also the planet. This approach aligns with the principles of permaculture and ecological stewardship, ensuring that the ancient art of herbalism continues to thrive in harmony with the natural world.

Building Nutrient-Rich Compost

To build a nutrient-rich compost for your garden, start by selecting a **compost bin** or designating a **compost area** in your yard. Ideally, this should be a spot that's easily accessible yet out of direct sunlight to maintain moisture without the compost drying out too quickly. A **compost bin** can be purchased or made from materials like wood pallets, wire mesh, or even a simple tarp to cover a pile on the ground.

Begin your compost pile by layering **brown** and **green materials**. **Brown materials**, rich in carbon, include dried leaves, straw, wood chips, and shredded newspaper. **Green materials**, rich in nitrogen, encompass kitchen scraps like fruit and vegetable peels, coffee grounds, and eggshells, as well as green lawn clippings and plant trimmings. Avoid adding meat, dairy, or oily foods to prevent odors and deter pests.

The ideal ratio for a balanced compost is approximately 3:1, three parts brown to one part green. This balance helps to accelerate the decomposition process while minimizing odors. After adding each layer of green material, cover it with a layer of brown material to keep flies away and reduce the smell.

To ensure efficient decomposition, **maintain moisture** in your compost pile. The compost should be as wet as a wrung-out sponge. If it's too dry, add water or green materials. If it's too wet, add more brown materials to absorb excess moisture.

Aeration is another critical factor in composting. Turn your compost pile every two to four weeks with a shovel or pitchfork to introduce oxygen, which is essential for breaking down organic matter. This process also helps to distribute heat and moisture evenly throughout the pile, speeding up the decomposition process.

Monitor the temperature of your compost pile with a compost thermometer. A healthy compost pile will heat up to about 130-160°F in the center. This heat is crucial for killing weed seeds and pathogens. If the pile doesn't heat up, it may need more green materials, water, or aeration.

As the bottom material in the pile turns into compost, it will look and smell like rich, dark soil. This process typically takes anywhere from three to six months, depending on the balance of materials, the size of the pile, and environmental conditions. Once the compost no longer gives off heat and has a crumbly texture, it's ready to use.

To use your compost, spread it around plants, mix it into garden beds, or use it as a potting mix. Compost enriches the soil, provides nutrients to plants, and helps retain moisture in the garden. By recycling kitchen and garden waste into compost, you not only reduce waste sent to landfills but also create a valuable resource for your garden, promoting healthier plant growth and sustainability.

Recycling Herbal Byproducts

Recycling herbal byproducts is a sustainable practice that transforms waste from your herbal preparations into valuable resources. When you've finished making teas, tinctures, or oils, you're often left with stems, leaves, and roots that can be repurposed in several ways. Here's how to make the most of these materials:

1. Creating Herbal Mulches: Dry the leftover plant material thoroughly until it's brittle. Once dried, chop or shred the material into smaller pieces. This can be spread around the base of plants as a mulch. Herbal mulch not only suppresses weeds but can also add nutrients back into the soil as it decomposes. For instance, nitrogen-rich herb leftovers like nettle or comfrey are excellent for this purpose.

2. Making Herbal Composts: Add your dried herbal byproducts to your compost pile. Ensure you maintain the correct balance between green (nitrogen-rich) and brown (carbon-rich) materials in your compost. Since most herbal byproducts are green materials, balance them with brown materials like dried leaves, straw, or shredded paper. This will help in creating a rich, nutritious compost that can be used to enrich your garden soil.

3. Crafting Herbal Paper: For a creative reuse, leftover herbal materials can be turned into homemade paper. Begin by blending the dried plant material with water to create a pulp. Mix this pulp with recycled paper pulp, spread it thinly over a screen, and let it dry. The result is a beautifully textured paper that can be used for writing or as decorative art.

4. Preparing Herbal Smudge Sticks: Certain dried herbal byproducts, especially from aromatic plants like sage, lavender, and rosemary, can be bundled and tied into smudge sticks. Dry the bundles thoroughly until the leaves are crisp. These smudge sticks can be burned for cleansing and purifying the air in your home.

5. Enriching Liquid Fertilizers: Place the leftover fresh or dried herbal material in a bucket, and cover it with water. Allow this mixture to steep for several weeks, stirring occasionally. Strain the liquid, and use it as a nutrient-rich fertilizer for your plants. This liquid fertilizer is particularly beneficial for plants in need of a quick nutrient boost.

6. Crafting Herbal Sachets: Dried herbal byproducts can be sewn into small sachets. These sachets can be tucked into drawers, closets, or even cars to provide a natural fragrance. They're also useful for repelling moths and other insects from stored clothing.

7. Producing Herbal Fire Starters: Combine dried herbal byproducts with other flammable materials like dried pine cones or wood shavings. Dip the mixture in melted wax, let it harden, and you have an aromatic fire starter for grills, fireplaces, or campfires.

8. Herbal Dyeing: Some herbs can be used to create natural dyes for fabric, yarn, or paper. Simmer the plant material in water to extract the color, strain, and then use the dye bath. Mordants such as alum or iron can be added to fix the dye. This method is perfect for achieving unique, earthy tones.

Each of these methods not only reduces waste but also provides a way to further integrate the benefits of herbs into your daily life. By repurposing herbal byproducts, you're contributing to a cycle of sustainability that respects and utilizes the full value of the plants you work with.

Herbal Mulches and Fertilizers

When incorporating **herbal mulches** into your garden, it's crucial to understand their dual role in both weed suppression and soil enrichment. Begin by selecting dried herbal byproducts, such as the stems and leaves from your previous herbal projects. These materials should be thoroughly dried to prevent mold growth when applied as mulch. Chop or shred the dried herbs to increase their surface area, which aids in quicker decomposition and nutrient release.

Apply a layer of this herbal mulch around your plants, approximately 2 to 3 inches thick. This layer will not only suppress weeds by blocking sunlight but also retain soil moisture, reducing the need for frequent watering. As these herbal materials break down, they will release nutrients back into the soil, acting as a slow-release fertilizer. This process enriches the soil with organic matter, improving its structure and fertility over time.

For **herbal fertilizers**, the approach is slightly different. These liquid fertilizers are created by steeping leftover herbal materials in water, essentially creating a nutrient-rich "tea." To make this, fill a large container with fresh or dried herbal remnants. Cover these with water, preferably rainwater, as it's soft and free from chlorine and other chemicals found in tap water. Let this mixture steep for 3 to 4 weeks, stirring occasionally to help release the nutrients into the water.

After steeping, strain the liquid to remove all plant material. This liquid herbal fertilizer can be diluted with water at a ratio of 1:10 (fertilizer to water) and used to water your plants. It's especially beneficial during the growing season when plants require additional nutrients. This homemade fertilizer provides a wide range of micronutrients and growth stimulants naturally found in the herbs.

When selecting herbs for both mulches and fertilizers, consider their specific benefits. For instance, **comfrey** is high in potassium, making it excellent for fruiting plants. **Nettles** are rich in nitrogen, which promotes leafy growth. Understanding the nutrient profile of your herbal byproducts can help you tailor your mulch and fertilizer applications to meet the specific needs of your plants.

Additionally, consider the timing of your applications. Apply herbal mulches in the early spring to suppress weeds and retain moisture during the growing season. Herbal fertilizers are most effective when used during the peak growth periods of spring and early summer, providing plants with the necessary nutrients for growth and development.

By utilizing these sustainable practices, you not only reduce waste but also enhance the health and productivity of your garden. This approach to gardening fosters a deeper connection with the natural cycle of growth and decay, embodying the principles of permaculture and sustainable living.

CHAPTER 3: CREATING A SUSTAINABLE APOTHECARY

Choosing **Eco-Friendly Packaging** is a crucial step in establishing a sustainable apothecary. Opt for **glass jars** for storing dried herbs, tinctures, and salves. Glass is inert, meaning it won't react with the contents, and it's infinitely recyclable, reducing your carbon footprint. For labels, select **recycled paper** and use soy-based inks which are more environmentally friendly than petroleum-based options. When shipping products, utilize **biodegradable packing peanuts** or **recycled paper** as cushioning instead of synthetic bubble wrap. This ensures that your packaging is not only safe for the environment but also aligns with the ethos of natural health and wellness.

Integrating Sustainability into Everyday Herbalism involves more than just the products you create; it's about embodying the principles of sustainability in every aspect of your practice. Start by sourcing **organic herbs** from local growers or cultivating your own to minimize transportation emissions and support local ecosystems. Implement **water-saving techniques** in your garden, such as drip irrigation or rainwater harvesting, to reduce your water usage. For energy needs, consider installing **solar panels** to power your apothecary space or using a **solar dehydrator** for drying herbs. These actions significantly lower your operation's environmental impact.

When crafting herbal remedies, aim to use the **whole plant** to minimize waste. For example, if you're making rosemary oil and have leftover stems, these can be repurposed into herbal brushes for culinary use or ground into mulch for your garden. This approach not only respects the plant but also maximizes your resources.

Engage with your community by offering **workshops** on sustainable herbal practices or creating **online content** that educates about the importance of eco-conscious living. This not only builds your brand but also fosters a community of like-minded individuals who value sustainability.

Finally, continuously **evaluate and adapt** your practices. Sustainability is an evolving field, and new innovations and information can help you further reduce your environmental impact. Stay informed about sustainable practices within the herbalism community and beyond, and be willing to make changes to your operations to reflect best practices in sustainability.

Eco-Friendly Packaging Choices

When selecting glass jars for your apothecary, prioritize those made from recycled glass to further minimize environmental impact. Look for suppliers that offer jars with this specification, as recycled glass uses less energy in production compared to new glass. Ensure the jars come with airtight seals to preserve the potency of your herbal remedies, whether they are dried herbs, tinctures, or salves. The size of the jar should be chosen based on the volume of the product to minimize air exposure, which can degrade the herbal properties over time. For labeling these jars, opt for labels made from recycled paper. Seek out suppliers who use soy-based or vegetable-based inks for printing, as these are less harmful to the environment than traditional petroleum-based inks. These inks provide a high-quality finish and are suitable for both professional and home printers, allowing for customization of labels with minimal environmental impact.

For packaging that needs to be shipped, consider using biodegradable packing peanuts made from materials like cornstarch rather than styrofoam. These biodegradable peanuts dissolve in water and leave no toxic waste, offering a protective cushion for your products without harming the planet. Alternatively, shredded recycled paper or cardboard can be used as a sustainable packing material, providing ample protection for glass jars during transit. This not only recycles waste paper but also ensures that the packaging material can be composted or recycled by the end-user.

When it comes to the outer packaging, choose boxes made from recycled cardboard and avoid using plastic tape. Look for paper tape that is reinforced with natural fibers and uses a natural rubber adhesive. This type of tape is strong enough to secure packages but is fully biodegradable and compostable. Additionally, consider including a note inside the package encouraging customers to reuse or recycle the packaging materials, fostering a culture of sustainability among your customer base.

Implementing these eco-friendly packaging solutions requires initial research to find the right suppliers and materials that align with your sustainability goals. However, the effort pays off by significantly reducing your apothecary's environmental footprint and appealing to customers who value sustainable practices. By making these choices, you not only contribute to the health of the planet but also build a brand that stands for environmental responsibility and care. Remember, every small step towards sustainability makes a difference, and your apothecary can lead by example, inspiring others in the community to adopt eco-friendly practices.

Sustainable Herbal Practices

Incorporating **sustainability into everyday herbalism** requires a conscientious approach to both the sourcing of herbs and the methods used in their preparation and use. One effective strategy is to establish a **personal or community herb garden**. When selecting a site for an herb garden, choose a location that receives at least six hours of direct sunlight daily, ensuring herbs receive adequate light for optimal growth. Utilize **native soil** amended with organic compost to provide a nutrient-rich foundation for your herbs. This not only reduces the need for chemical fertilizers but also promotes healthy, resilient plant growth.

For those without access to garden space, **window boxes** or **container gardening** offers a viable alternative. Select containers made from sustainable materials such as terracotta or recycled plastic. Ensure each container has adequate drainage holes to prevent waterlogging, which can lead to root rot. Use a high-quality, organic potting mix to fill your containers, and position them in areas that receive sufficient sunlight.

Water conservation is another critical aspect of sustainable herbalism. Implement a **drip irrigation system** or use a **watering can** to target the base of plants, minimizing water wastage. Collecting **rainwater** in barrels provides an eco-friendly water source for your garden, reducing reliance on municipal water systems.

When harvesting herbs, practice **sustainable harvesting techniques** to ensure the longevity of your plants. Always leave enough foliage to allow the plant to continue growing. For perennial herbs, such as rosemary and thyme, cutting no more than one-third of the plant at a time is a good rule of thumb. For annuals, like basil and cilantro, frequent harvesting encourages fuller, bushier plants.

After harvesting, drying herbs is a common preservation method. Construct a **solar dehydrator** using recycled materials to dry herbs without electricity. This can be as simple as a wooden frame covered with a clear plastic sheet, allowing sunlight to dry herbs naturally. Alternatively, herbs can be air-dried by hanging bunches in a warm, dry area of your home.

Recycling and repurposing play a significant role in a sustainable apothecary. Glass jars from kitchen use can be cleaned and reused for storing dried herbs or herbal preparations. When labeling, opt for **recycled paper labels** and secure them with a natural adhesive, such as a homemade paste made from flour and water.

In the realm of **herbal waste**, consider composting spent herbs and plant material to create a rich, organic compost for your garden. This not only reduces waste but also returns valuable nutrients to the soil, promoting a cycle of growth and sustainability.

Engaging in **community seed swaps** or **herb exchanges** can further enhance sustainability. This practice not only diversifies your garden but also strengthens community bonds and promotes a shared commitment to environmental stewardship.

By adopting these practices, herbalists can significantly reduce their environmental footprint, contributing to a healthier planet. These actions, when integrated into daily routines, underscore a commitment to sustainability that extends beyond the individual, influencing broader community and environmental health.

BOOK 21: ADVANCED HERBAL EXTRACTION TECHNIQUES

CHAPTER 1: ESSENTIAL OIL DISTILLATION AT HOME

Essential Oil Extraction Tools

To embark on the journey of essential oil extraction at home, one must first familiarize themselves with the necessary tools and equipment, understanding their functions and how they come together to facilitate the distillation process. The cornerstone of home distillation is the distillation kit, which primarily consists of a boiling flask, condenser, receiving flask, and heating source. Each component plays a pivotal role in the transformation of raw herbal materials into pure, potent essential oils.

The boiling flask is where the plant material, combined with water, is heated. For home setups, a 2-liter round-bottom flask is commonly used due to its efficiency in evenly distributing heat and minimizing the risk of hot spots, which could degrade the plant material. It's crucial to select a flask made from borosilicate glass to withstand the high temperatures without cracking.

Next, the condenser, often a Graham or Liebig condenser, is attached to the boiling flask. This apparatus is essential for cooling the vapor produced from the heated plant mixture. A Graham condenser, with its coiled design, maximizes cooling efficiency in a compact form, making it ideal for small-scale operations. The condenser must be connected to a cold water source, with water entering at the bottom and exiting at the top, to ensure the vapor is efficiently condensed into a liquid form.

The receiving flask, also made from borosilicate glass for its thermal resistance, collects the condensed liquid. A 1-liter flask is typically sufficient, but the size may be adjusted based on the expected yield of essential oil. It's connected to the lower end of the condenser, ready to capture the distilled essential oil and hydrosol as they emerge from the cooling unit.

A reliable heating source is vital for maintaining a consistent temperature throughout the distillation process. An electric heating mantle is preferred for its ability to provide uniform heat and its built-in temperature control. This is particularly important when distilling essential oils, as precise temperature management can significantly impact the quality of the oil extracted.

In addition to the primary distillation equipment, several accessories are necessary to streamline the process and ensure safety. Glass tubing, silicone tubing, and clamps are required to securely connect the components of the distillation kit. A thermometer is crucial for monitoring the temperature within the boiling flask, while a water pump may be needed to circulate cooling water through the condenser.

When assembling your home distillation setup, it's imperative to prioritize safety. Ensure all connections are secure to prevent leaks of steam or hot water. Always use heat-resistant gloves when handling the equipment, especially during operation, as surfaces can become extremely hot. Ventilation is another critical factor; conducting the distillation in a well-ventilated area or under a fume hood can prevent the accumulation of vapor in the air, reducing the risk of inhalation or flammable situations.

By meticulously selecting and assembling the appropriate tools and equipment for essential oil extraction, enthusiasts can efficiently and safely distill their own oils at home. This process not only offers a deeper understanding of herbal properties and essential oil production but also provides the satisfaction of creating pure, personalized remedies from the comfort of one's own space.

Essential Oil Distillation Process

With the distillation kit assembled and safety measures in place, the next step is to embark on the essential oil distillation process, focusing on extracting oils from herbs such as lavender, rosemary, and eucalyptus. Each herb requires a specific approach due to its unique oil content and properties. Here, we break down the process into detailed steps, ensuring clarity and effectiveness in extracting high-quality essential oils.

Firstly, prepare the plant material by harvesting at the optimal time, which for most herbs is when their oil content is highest, usually in the morning after the dew has evaporated but before the sun is at its peak. For lavender and rosemary, this means selecting healthy, undamaged leaves and flowers. Eucalyptus leaves, preferably young and supple, are also ideal. Chop the plant material into smaller pieces to increase the surface area for more efficient oil extraction. Approximately 500 grams of plant material is a good starting point for a 2-liter distillation flask.

Fill the boiling flask with the chopped plant material, then add distilled water until the plant matter is fully submerged. The water acts as a carrier for the essential oil vapors as they are released from the plant material. For a 2-liter flask, using about 1.5 liters of water is typically sufficient. It's crucial to leave some space in the flask to allow for efficient boiling and vapor production.

Attach the filled flask to the heating mantle and connect the condenser, ensuring the cold water supply is functioning correctly. The water should flow into the condenser at the lower connection point, rise up through the system, and exit through the upper connection, removing heat from the vapor as it passes through.

Turn on the heating mantle and gradually increase the temperature to bring the water to a gentle boil. Monitor the temperature closely with a thermometer inserted in the flask. The ideal boiling range for extracting essential oils is between 212°F (100°C) and 245°F (118°C), depending on the plant material. Lavender and rosemary typically require lower temperatures, while eucalyptus may need slightly higher temperatures due to its robust leaves.

As the water heats, the steam will carry the essential oil vapors up into the condenser, where they cool and condense back into a liquid. This liquid, a mixture of water and essential oil, will drip into the receiving flask. The process of distillation can take several hours, depending on the amount of plant material and the desired yield of essential oil.

Once distillation is complete, carefully remove the receiving flask and allow the liquid to settle. Essential oils will naturally separate from the water due to their lighter density. Using a pipette or a separating funnel, gently collect the essential oil layer from the top. Store the collected oil in dark glass bottles to protect it from light, which can degrade its quality. Label the bottles with the name of the essential oil and the date of extraction.

The remaining water, known as hydrosol, also contains valuable therapeutic properties and can be used in skincare, aromatherapy, or as a room spray. Store the hydrosol in clean, sterilized bottles, ensuring they are also labeled and dated.

This step-by-step guide to essential oil distillation at home empowers individuals to harness the natural benefits of herbs like lavender, rosemary, and eucalyptus. By following these detailed instructions, enthusiasts can produce their own essential oils and hydrosols, capturing the essence of these plants for use in natural remedies, skincare, and holistic wellness practices.

Essential Oil Safety and Storage

Handling and storing essential oils require careful consideration due to their potent and volatile nature. These concentrated plant extracts can degrade or become hazardous if not managed properly. To ensure the longevity and efficacy of essential oils, follow these detailed guidelines for safety and storage.

Safety Precautions for Handling Essential Oils:

1. **Wear Protective Gear:** Always use gloves when handling essential oils to prevent skin irritation or sensitization. Consider wearing eye protection, especially when transferring oils or working with large quantities, to guard against accidental splashes.

2. **Work in a Well-Ventilated Area:** Essential oils can be potent and overwhelming in enclosed spaces. Ensure adequate ventilation to disperse fumes and reduce inhalation exposure.

3. **Avoid Direct Contact with Skin:** Unless diluted, essential oils should not come into direct contact with the skin. Use a carrier oil, such as coconut or jojoba oil, to dilute essential oils before topical application.

4. **Keep Away from Flames:** Essential oils are flammable. Keep them away from open flames, sparks, and heat sources, including candles and stovetops.

Storage Recommendations for Essential Oils:

1. **Use Dark Glass Bottles:** Store essential oils in dark (amber or cobalt blue) glass bottles to protect them from light, which can accelerate degradation. Dark glass helps maintain the integrity of the oil by blocking harmful UV rays.

2. **Maintain Cool Temperatures:** Heat can alter the chemical composition of essential oils. Store them in a cool, dark place away from direct sunlight. Consider using a refrigerator for long-term storage of citrus oils, which are more prone to oxidation. However, ensure the oils are brought to room temperature before use to avoid condensation inside the bottle.

3. **Tightly Seal Containers:** Essential oils can evaporate and lose their efficacy if not properly sealed. Ensure the cap is tightly closed after each use. For added protection, consider using a bottle with an orifice reducer, which controls the flow of oil and minimizes exposure to air.

4. **Label Clearly:** Each bottle should be clearly labeled with the name of the essential oil and the date of bottling. This practice helps track the age of the oil and prevents cross-contamination.

5. **Organize by Shelf Life:** Some essential oils, like citrus oils, have a shorter shelf life (1-2 years) compared to others, such as sandalwood or patchouli, which can last longer (4-8 years). Organizing oils by their expiration date ensures that older oils are used first.

6. **Keep Out of Reach of Children and Pets:** Essential oils can be toxic if ingested or applied inappropriately. Store them in a secure location, out of reach of children and pets, to prevent accidental ingestion or contact.

By adhering to these safety and storage guidelines, you can preserve the quality and therapeutic properties of essential oils, ensuring they remain effective for natural health and wellness applications. Proper handling and storage not only extend the life of these precious oils but also safeguard the well-being of those who use them, aligning with the principles of responsible and sustainable herbal practice.

CHAPTER 2: ALCOHOL-FREE TINCTURES AND EXTRACTS

Glycerites: Alcohol-Free Herbal Extracts

Glycerites, or glycerin-based extracts, offer a versatile and alcohol-free alternative for those seeking to harness the therapeutic properties of herbs without using alcohol as a solvent. Glycerin, a clear, odorless liquid also known as vegetable glycerine, is derived from plant oils and is recognized for its ability to extract and preserve the medicinal compounds of herbs. Its sweet flavor makes glycerites particularly appealing for children's remedies, or for anyone with sensitivities or objections to alcohol. Here, we detail the process of creating glycerites, ensuring clarity and effectiveness in extracting high-quality herbal extracts.

To begin, select high-quality dried or fresh herbs for your glycerite. While both can be used, fresh herbs should be wilted for a day to reduce their moisture content, as excess water can dilute the glycerin and potentially lead to spoilage. For dried herbs, ensure they are not too old or stale, as this can affect the potency of your extract.

Measure your herbs and glycerin. The ratio of glycerin to herb can vary depending on the herb's density and the desired strength of your extract. A common starting point is a 1:4 ratio of herbs to glycerin by weight for dried herbs and a 1:3 ratio for fresh, wilted herbs. This means for every one part of herb, you use four parts of glycerin for dried herbs or three parts for fresh.

Place your herbs in a clean, dry jar. Pour the glycerin over the herbs, ensuring they are completely covered. If using fresh herbs, make sure to press them down to release any trapped air bubbles and to fully saturate them with glycerin.

Seal the jar tightly with a lid. Label the jar with the name of the herb, the date, and the type of extract (glycerite). This helps in tracking and identifying your extracts, especially if you are making multiple batches.

Store the jar in a warm, dark place. A cupboard or shelf away from direct sunlight is ideal. The warmth helps to facilitate the extraction process. Shake the jar once or twice a day to mix the herbs and glycerin, ensuring a thorough extraction.

The maceration period for glycerites can range from 4 to 6 weeks. During this time, the glycerin will draw out the soluble constituents of the herbs. After the desired maceration time, strain the mixture through a fine mesh strainer or cheesecloth to separate the liquid extract from the herb material. For a clearer glycerite, strain a second time or allow the extract to settle and then decant the clear liquid into another container.

Transfer the strained glycerite into dark glass bottles for storage. Amber or cobalt blue bottles are preferred to protect the extract from light, which can degrade its quality over time. Ensure the bottles are labeled with the herb name, type of extract (glycerite), and date of production.

Store the glycerite in a cool, dark place. While glycerites have a longer shelf life than alcohol tinctures due to glycerin's preservative properties, they should ideally be used within 1-2 years for maximum potency.

Glycerites can be used internally for their medicinal properties or added to foods and beverages for flavor and health benefits. They can also be incorporated into topical applications such as creams, lotions, or salves for skin care.

By following these detailed steps, individuals can create their own glycerin-based herbal extracts at home, offering a sweet, alcohol-free alternative to traditional tinctures. This method allows for the safe and effective use of herbal remedies, catering to a wide range of preferences and needs.

Vinegar Infusions for Health

Vinegar infusions, particularly those made with apple cider vinegar, harness the natural acidity and preservative qualities of vinegar to extract and preserve the medicinal components of herbs. Apple cider vinegar, rich in acetic acid, has been valued for its health benefits, including digestive support and antimicrobial properties. When combined with various herbs, these infusions create potent remedies that can be easily incorporated into daily wellness routines. To create a medicinal vinegar infusion, follow these detailed steps to ensure a potent and effective product.

Select high-quality, organic apple cider vinegar as your base. The vinegar should be raw, unfiltered, and contain the "mother" – a cobweb-like amino acid-based substance found at the bottom of the bottle – to ensure it contains the most enzymes and nutrients. The acidity of apple cider vinegar is ideal for extracting the active constituents from herbs, making it an excellent medium for creating medicinal infusions.

Choose your herbs based on the desired health benefits. For digestive aid, herbs like fennel, ginger, and peppermint are excellent choices. For a detoxifying effect, consider dandelion root, burdock, and milk thistle. Ensure the herbs are dried and finely chopped or crushed to maximize the surface area exposed to the vinegar, which facilitates a more efficient extraction of medicinal properties.

For every cup of vinegar, use approximately ¼ cup of dried herbs. This ratio can be adjusted based on personal preference for strength, but this is a good starting point for general medicinal infusions. If using fresh herbs, the ratio shifts to 1 cup of loosely packed herbs per cup of vinegar due to the higher water content in fresh plant material.

Combine the herbs and vinegar in a clean, dry glass jar. Fill the jar with enough vinegar to completely submerge the herbs, leaving about an inch of space at the top. Stir the mixture thoroughly to ensure all the herbs are wetted by the vinegar. If necessary, add more vinegar to cover the herbs completely.

Seal the jar with a plastic lid or place a piece of parchment paper under a metal lid to prevent corrosion from the vinegar. Label the jar with the contents and date. Store the jar in a cool, dark place, shaking it daily to agitate the herbs and promote extraction.

Allow the infusion to macerate for 4 to 6 weeks. The length of time will depend on the herbs used and the desired potency. Taste the infusion periodically to gauge its strength. Once the infusion has reached the desired potency, strain the herbs from the vinegar using a fine mesh strainer or cheesecloth. For a clearer infusion, strain a second time or allow the infusion to settle and decant the clear liquid into another container.

Transfer the strained medicinal vinegar into clean, dark glass bottles to protect it from light, which can degrade its quality. Ensure the bottles are labeled with the herb name, type of extract (vinegar infusion), and date of production.

Store the finished vinegar infusion in a cool, dark place. While vinegar is a natural preservative, ensuring proper storage will maintain the potency and effectiveness of the infusion. Medicinal vinegar infusions can be used internally, taking a tablespoon diluted in water before meals for digestive support, or externally, applying to the skin as a toner for its astringent properties.

Honey-Based Herbal Syrups

Honey-based herbal syrups serve as a delightful and effective way to incorporate the healing properties of herbs into your daily routine, especially for respiratory and immune support. Honey, a natural preservative and sweetener, also brings its own therapeutic benefits, including soothing sore throats, acting as a cough suppressant, and offering antioxidant properties. To create a potent and beneficial honey-based herbal syrup, follow these detailed steps:

Select Your Herbs: Choose herbs known for their respiratory and immune-boosting properties. For respiratory support, herbs like **eucalyptus, thyme,** and **mullein** are excellent for clearing congestion and soothing irritated airways. For immune support, consider **elderberry, echinacea,** or **astragalus**. These herbs can be used singly or in combination to enhance the syrup's effectiveness.

Prepare the Herbal Decoction: Begin by measuring **1 cup of dried herbs** or **2 cups of fresh, finely chopped herbs**. Place the herbs in a medium saucepan and cover with **4 cups of cold water**. Slowly bring the mixture to a boil, then reduce the heat and simmer gently until the volume is reduced by half, which typically takes about 30 to 40 minutes. This process extracts the medicinal properties from the herbs, creating a concentrated decoction.

Strain and Measure the Decoction: Once reduced, remove the saucepan from heat and let it cool slightly. Strain the decoction through a fine mesh strainer or cheesecloth to remove the herb particles, pressing or squeezing to extract as much liquid as possible. Measure the remaining liquid; you should have approximately **2 cups**. If you have less, add enough water to reach this volume.

Combine with Honey: Pour the strained decoction back into the saucepan. Add an equal volume of honey to the herbal liquid, which should be around **2 cups of honey** for a 1:1 ratio. Gently heat the mixture over low heat, stirring constantly, until the honey is fully dissolved into the herbal decoction. Avoid boiling the mixture to preserve the beneficial enzymes and properties of the honey.

Add Optional Enhancers: For additional flavor and health benefits, consider adding **1 tablespoon of lemon juice** or **ginger root** during the last few minutes of simmering. Lemon juice adds a refreshing flavor and vitamin C, while ginger offers additional anti-inflammatory and immune-boosting properties.

Cool and Bottle: Remove the saucepan from heat and allow the syrup to cool to room temperature. Once cooled, transfer the syrup into sterilized dark glass bottles using a funnel. Dark glass helps protect the syrup from light, which can degrade its potency over time.

Label and Store: Label each bottle with the name of the syrup, ingredients, and date made. Store the bottles in the refrigerator to maintain freshness. Properly stored, the syrup should last for **4-6 months**.

Dosage: For adults, take **1 tablespoon of syrup** up to three times a day for immune support or respiratory relief. For children over one year of age, the dosage is **1 teaspoon** up to three times a day. Always consult with a healthcare provider before giving herbal remedies to children or if you have specific health concerns.

Creating honey-based herbal syrups is a simple and rewarding process, allowing you to harness the natural healing powers of herbs in a delicious and accessible form. Whether used for soothing a cough, bolstering the immune system, or simply as a natural sweetener in tea, these syrups offer a versatile addition to your home apothecary.

CHAPTER 3: ADVANCED PRESERVATION METHODS

Solar Infusion for Herbal Oils is a method that harnesses the power of the sun to gently heat carrier oils infused with herbs, facilitating the extraction of the herbs' beneficial properties. This method is ideal for creating potent herbal oils for use in massage, skincare, or as a base for further herbal preparations. To begin, select a high-quality carrier oil such as **cold-pressed virgin olive oil**, **coconut oil**, or **sweet almond oil** due to their stable nature and ability to effectively extract and preserve the essence and therapeutic properties of herbs. Choose fresh or dried herbs that align with your desired outcome, such as **lavender** for relaxation, **calendula** for skin healing, or **rosemary** for its invigorating properties.

1. **Preparation of Herbs and Oil**: Begin by filling a clean, dry glass jar about halfway with your chosen herbs. If using fresh herbs, ensure they are dry to the touch to reduce the risk of water contamination, which can lead to spoilage. Pour the carrier oil over the herbs until they are completely submerged, leaving about an inch of oil above the herbs to account for expansion.

2. **Infusing the Oil**: Seal the jar tightly with a lid to prevent moisture from entering. Place the jar in a location where it will receive direct sunlight, such as a windowsill or a sunny spot in your garden. The gentle warmth from the sun will heat the oil, allowing the herbs to release their therapeutic properties into the oil over time.

3. **Duration of Infusion**: The duration of the infusion can vary depending on the herbs used and the desired potency, but a general guideline is to allow the oil to infuse for 2-4 weeks. Gently shake the jar every few days to mix the herbs and oil, ensuring a thorough infusion.

4. **Straining the Infused Oil**: Once the infusion period is complete, strain the oil through a fine mesh strainer or cheesecloth to remove the herb particles. For a clearer oil, strain multiple times or use a coffee filter for the final strain.

5. **Storage**: Transfer the strained oil into clean, dry bottles, preferably made of dark glass to protect the oil from light, which can degrade its quality. Label the bottles with the type of oil, the herbs used, and the date of infusion. Store the bottles in a cool, dark place to preserve the oil's therapeutic properties. Properly stored, solar-infused herbal oils can last up to a year or more, depending on the carrier oil's shelf life.

6. **Safety and Usage Tips**: Always perform a patch test before using the oil extensively on the skin, especially if you have sensitive skin or are prone to allergies. If infusing oils with herbs known for their strong properties, such as **hot peppers** or **strongly scented herbs**, consider the end use and potential skin sensitivity.

Solar infusion is a simple, energy-efficient method that allows for the creation of personalized herbal oils without the need for direct heat or electricity. By following these steps and guidelines, you can harness the natural power of the sun to create a variety of herbal oils tailored to your specific health and wellness needs.

Solar Infusion for Herbal Oils

To ensure the **solar infusion process** is successful, attention to detail is crucial at every step. After preparing your herbs and oil, and placing them in direct sunlight, monitoring the infusion's progress is essential. Here are further instructions to maximize the effectiveness of your solar-infused herbal oils:

1. **Monitoring Sun Exposure**: The jar should receive direct sunlight for most of the day. If possible, position the jar in a location that tracks the sun's movement from east to west. This maximizes the infusion process by ensuring consistent warmth. If you live in an area with limited

sunlight, consider using a reflective surface, such as aluminum foil or a mirror, to direct more light onto the jar.

2. **Temperature Considerations**: While sunlight is necessary for the infusion, too much heat can degrade the oil and the herbs' beneficial properties. If temperatures exceed 95°F (35°C), it's advisable to move the jar to a spot that receives partial shade during the hottest part of the day. A simple thermometer placed near the jar can help you monitor the temperature.

3. **Shaking the Jar**: Beyond the initial few shakes during the first days, it's beneficial to gently rotate the jar once a day to ensure all parts of the herbs are exposed to the oil. This action helps release the herbs' essential oils and compounds into the carrier oil more effectively.

4. **Checking for Condensation**: Periodically inspect the inside of the jar's lid for condensation, which can indicate moisture inside the jar. Moisture can lead to mold growth and spoilage. If condensation is present, open the jar and carefully wipe the inside of the lid and the jar's opening with a clean, dry cloth. Ensure the herbs are still fully submerged; add more oil if necessary.

5. **Straining the Infused Oil**: Use a fine mesh strainer lined with cheesecloth or a nut milk bag for straining. For an extra-clear oil, a second straining through a coffee filter placed inside the strainer can remove the finest particles. Ensure all equipment used for straining is thoroughly clean and dry to prevent contamination.

6. **Bottling**: Choose bottles made of dark amber or cobalt blue glass to filter out damaging UV light, extending the shelf life of the infused oil. Using a small funnel can help transfer the oil into bottles without spillage. Ensure the bottles are labeled with the type of carrier oil, the herb(s) used, and the date of infusion to keep track of freshness.

7. **Storage**: Store the bottled oil in a cool, dark place such as a cabinet or pantry. Avoid storing the oil near heat sources like stoves or in direct sunlight. Properly stored, the oil should maintain its potency for at least 6 months to a year. Over time, check the oil for any changes in smell, color, or texture, which can indicate spoilage.

By adhering to these detailed steps and considerations, you can craft high-quality solar-infused herbal oils. These oils can serve as the foundation for a variety of natural health and wellness products, from skincare to massage oils, each imbued with the healing properties of the chosen herbs.

Encapsulation of Herbal Powders

Encapsulation of herbal powders is a method that allows for the convenient intake of herbs in a concentrated form. This process involves filling empty capsules with powdered herbs, which can be done manually or with the aid of a capsule filling machine. To begin, you will need high-quality herbal powders, which can be obtained by grinding dried herbs using a coffee grinder or purchasing pre-ground powders from a reputable source. Ensure the herbs are completely dry to prevent any mold growth within the capsules.

First, select the appropriate size of capsules for your needs. Capsules come in various sizes, typically ranging from "000" (largest) to "5" (smallest). For most herbal supplements, sizes "00" or "0" are commonly used, as they offer a good balance between ease of swallowing and capacity for herbal powder. It's important to use capsules made from vegetarian or gelatin bases, depending on personal or dietary preferences.

For manual encapsulation, a capsule filling tray can significantly streamline the process. This tray allows you to fill multiple capsules simultaneously and is designed to hold the capsule halves securely. Begin by separating the capsule halves and placing the larger bottom halves into the base of the filling tray. If you are using a grinder to prepare your herbal powders, aim for a fine consistency to ensure even filling and optimal absorption when ingested.

Using a spoon, sprinkle the herbal powder over the base of the capsule tray, ensuring an even distribution. A straight edge, such as a plastic card or spatula, can be used to spread the powder and fill the capsules. Gently tap the base of the tray to settle the powder, adding more until each capsule is filled to the desired level. Once filled, place the smaller top halves of the capsules onto the filled bases. The capsule machine will typically have a mechanism to secure the tops and bottoms together.

For those preferring not to use a capsule filling tray, encapsulation can also be done by hand, although this method is more time-consuming. Simply hold the larger half of the capsule in one hand and use a small spoon or spatula to fill it with powder. Once filled, carefully place the top half of the capsule over the bottom and press together until sealed.

After the capsules are filled and assembled, store them in a cool, dry place, away from direct sunlight. An airtight container or zip-lock bag is ideal for storage to prevent moisture from compromising the quality of the herbal powders. Labeling the container with the herb name, dosage, and date of encapsulation will help keep track of your supplements and ensure they are used within an appropriate timeframe. Properly stored, these capsules can last for several months, providing a convenient and effective way to incorporate herbal supplements into your daily health regimen.

The encapsulation of herbal powders offers a tailor-made approach to herbal supplementation, allowing for the combination of different herbs to suit individual health needs. By following these detailed steps, individuals can create personalized herbal supplements that are easy to consume, transport, and store, making it simpler to maintain a natural health regimen tailored to their specific wellness goals.

Freezing Tinctures and Infusions

Freezing tinctures and infusions can be an effective method to extend their shelf life while preserving their potency. However, it's crucial to approach this preservation method with care to ensure the herbal preparations remain effective after thawing. Here are detailed steps and considerations for successfully freezing and thawing your herbal tinctures and infusions:

1. **Select Appropriate Containers**: Use only glass containers designed to withstand freezing temperatures. Regular glass may crack or shatter with temperature changes. Containers made of borosilicate glass are recommended due to their thermal resistance. Ensure containers are clean and dry before use.

2. **Leave Space for Expansion**: When filling containers with tinctures or infusions, leave at least a half-inch of space at the top. Liquids expand when frozen, and this space allows for expansion without causing the container to break.

3. **Label Clearly**: Use waterproof labels to indicate the contents, concentration, and date of freezing. This practice helps in identifying and tracking the usability period of the frozen product.

4. **Freeze at Stable Temperatures**: Place your tinctures and infusions in the back of the freezer where the temperature is most constant. Fluctuations in temperature can cause the contents to thaw and refreeze, potentially degrading their quality.

5. **Thawing Process**: To thaw, transfer the container from the freezer to the refrigerator and allow it to thaw slowly. Avoid using direct heat or leaving it out at room temperature, as rapid temperature changes can affect the preparation's efficacy.

6. **Check for Separation or Changes**: Once thawed, inspect the tincture or infusion for any separation or changes in color, smell, or texture. Gently shake the container to recombine ingredients if separation has occurred. If there are noticeable changes in the appearance or smell, it's best to discard the preparation as these can indicate spoilage or degradation.

7. **Use Thawed Preparations Promptly**: Once thawed, use the tinctures and infusions within a week to ensure you're benefiting from their full potency. Keep them refrigerated until use.

BOOK 22: HERBS FOR RARE AND CHRONIC CONDITIONS

CHAPTER 1: HERBAL MANAGEMENT OF AUTOIMMUNE DISEASES

Turmeric for Reducing Inflammation

Turmeric, a vibrant yellow spice commonly used in culinary practices, particularly in South Asian cuisine, holds a significant place in herbal medicine for its potent anti-inflammatory and antioxidant properties. The active compound in turmeric, curcumin, is credited with these effects. In the context of autoimmune diseases, where the body's immune system mistakenly attacks its own tissues, causing inflammation and pain, turmeric can play a crucial role in managing and mitigating these symptoms. Autoimmune conditions, such as rheumatoid arthritis, lupus, and psoriasis, can benefit from the incorporation of turmeric into one's daily regimen, not only for symptom management but also for the potential to improve overall health and wellness.

To harness the benefits of turmeric for reducing inflammation associated with autoimmune diseases, it's essential to understand the optimal ways to incorporate it into the diet and lifestyle. Curcumin's bioavailability, or the body's ability to absorb and utilize the compound, is relatively low on its own. However, combining turmeric with certain other substances can significantly enhance its absorption and efficacy.

One of the most effective ways to increase curcumin's bioavailability is by pairing turmeric with black pepper. Black pepper contains piperine, a natural substance that enhances the absorption of curcumin by up to 2000%. A practical approach to this is adding a pinch of black pepper to turmeric-infused dishes or beverages. For instance, when preparing a turmeric latte, also known as golden milk, incorporate a small amount of ground black pepper into the mix. The recipe could include 1 teaspoon of turmeric powder, a pinch of black pepper, 1 cup of almond or coconut milk, a dash of cinnamon, and honey to taste, heated gently over the stove until warm.

Another method to increase the absorption of turmeric is to consume it with healthy fats. Curcumin is fat-soluble, meaning it dissolves in fat, which can then be absorbed into the bloodstream more efficiently. Integrating turmeric into meals that contain healthy fats, such as avocados, nuts, seeds, or olive oil, can facilitate better absorption. For example, adding turmeric to a smoothie that includes avocado or almond butter can enhance its bioavailability.

For those considering turmeric supplements, especially individuals with autoimmune diseases seeking a more concentrated intake, it's crucial to select high-quality products that contain piperine or are formulated to improve curcumin's bioavailability. It's advisable to consult with a healthcare provider before starting any new supplement regimen, particularly for individuals with autoimmune conditions, to ensure it aligns with their overall treatment plan and to avoid any potential interactions with medications.

Incorporating turmeric into the daily diet can be as simple as adding the spice to vegetable dishes, soups, and stews, or preparing a turmeric tea by steeping 1 teaspoon of turmeric powder in hot water for about 10 minutes, then adding lemon and honey to taste. For topical applications, particularly for localized inflammation and joint pain, creating a paste of turmeric powder with water or coconut oil and applying it to the affected area can provide relief. However, it's important to note that turmeric can stain the skin and fabrics, so precautions should be taken when using it topically.

Ashwagandha for Adrenal Support

Ashwagandha, scientifically known as Withania somnifera, stands out as a pivotal herb in the realm of herbal management for autoimmune diseases, particularly due to its profound adaptogenic properties. This ancient herb, deeply rooted in Ayurvedic medicine, has been revered for centuries for its ability to fortify the body's resilience against stress and chronic fatigue, conditions often associated with autoimmune disorders. The adaptogenic nature of Ashwagandha lies in its capacity to modulate the body's stress response systems, thereby offering a stabilizing effect on the hypothalamic-pituitary-adrenal (HPA) axis, which plays a crucial role in stress regulation and adrenal function.

To harness the adrenal support benefits of Ashwagandha, it is essential to understand the optimal methods of preparation and dosage. The most effective form of Ashwagandha for addressing adrenal fatigue and stress is the standardized root extract, which ensures a consistent concentration of its active compounds, withanolides. These compounds are credited with the herb's stress-reducing effects. For those experiencing chronic stress or adrenal fatigue, a daily dosage ranging from 300 to 500 mg of Ashwagandha root extract, ideally divided into two doses taken with meals, is recommended. This regimen can help in significantly reducing cortisol levels, a stress hormone, thereby alleviating symptoms of stress and enhancing energy levels.

Incorporating Ashwagandha into one's daily routine requires attention to quality and sourcing. Opt for organic, non-GMO Ashwagandha supplements that provide transparent information about the concentration of withanolides. This ensures you are receiving a potent and clean product that maximizes the herb's adaptogenic benefits. Additionally, while Ashwagandha is generally well-tolerated, it's prudent to start with a lower dose to assess individual tolerance before gradually increasing to the recommended dosage. It's also advisable to consult with a healthcare provider before adding Ashwagandha to your regimen, especially for those with autoimmune conditions, to ensure it complements your overall treatment plan without any contraindications.

Beyond supplementation, incorporating lifestyle practices that support adrenal health and reduce stress, such as mindfulness meditation, gentle yoga, and adequate sleep, can enhance the benefits of Ashwagandha. These practices, in conjunction with Ashwagandha supplementation, create a holistic approach to managing stress and adrenal fatigue, offering a pathway to improved well-being for individuals navigating the challenges of autoimmune diseases.

Astragalus for Immune Modulation

Astragalus, scientifically known as **Astragalus membranaceus**, is a cornerstone herb in the management of autoimmune diseases due to its remarkable ability to modulate the immune system. This herb, deeply ingrained in Traditional Chinese Medicine, has been utilized for centuries to bolster the body's defense mechanisms and promote overall vitality. Its role in balancing overactive immune responses makes it particularly beneficial for individuals with autoimmune conditions, where the immune system mistakenly attacks the body's own cells.

The active components in Astragalus, including **polysaccharides, saponins, and flavonoids**, contribute to its immune-modulating effects. These compounds enhance the body's immune response, making it more efficient at fighting off pathogens while simultaneously preventing the immune system from becoming overactive and causing harm to the body. To effectively incorporate Astragalus into a regimen for autoimmune disease management, it is crucial to understand the optimal preparation methods and dosages.

For immune modulation, the root of Astragalus is most commonly used. It can be prepared in several forms, including **teas, tinctures, and capsules**. A standard approach is to use dried Astragalus root to prepare a decoction. To do this, one would typically simmer 15 to 30 grams of the root in water for 30 to 60 minutes. This process extracts the water-soluble active ingredients, resulting in a potent brew that can be consumed daily. For those seeking convenience, Astragalus is also available in capsule form, with dosages ranging from **250 to 500 mg taken twice daily**.

When sourcing Astragalus, look for **organic** or **wildcrafted** options to ensure the herb is free from pesticides and contaminants. The quality of the herb significantly impacts its efficacy, so choosing a reputable supplier is paramount. Additionally, it's important to note that while Astragalus is generally considered safe, it should be used with caution in individuals with autoimmune diseases due to its immune-stimulating properties. Starting with a lower dose and gradually increasing allows for monitoring of any adverse reactions.

Incorporating Astragalus into one's daily routine should be viewed as part of a holistic approach to managing autoimmune diseases. This includes a balanced diet, regular exercise, and stress management techniques. Combining these lifestyle factors with Astragalus supplementation can help create a more balanced immune response, reducing the frequency and severity of autoimmune flare-ups.

For those interested in exploring the benefits of Astragalus further, consulting with a healthcare professional, especially one experienced in herbal medicine, is advisable. This ensures that Astragalus is an appropriate choice for your specific health condition and that it complements any existing treatments.

Turmeric and Black Pepper Anti-Inflammatory Tonic

Beneficial effects

Turmeric and Black Pepper Anti-Inflammatory Tonic is designed to leverage the powerful anti-inflammatory and antioxidant properties of turmeric, enhanced by the bioavailability-boosting effects of black pepper. Curcumin, the active compound in turmeric, has been extensively studied for its potential to reduce inflammation and support joint and muscle health. However, curcumin's absorption is significantly enhanced when combined with piperine, a compound found in black pepper. This tonic aims to provide a natural way to alleviate inflammation, support immune health, and promote overall well-being.

Portions

2 servings

Preparation time

5 minutes

Cooking time

N/A

Ingredients

- 2 cups of filtered water
- 1 tablespoon of turmeric powder
- 1/2 teaspoon of ground black pepper
- 1 tablespoon of honey, or to taste
- Juice of 1/2 lemon
- A pinch of cinnamon (optional for flavor)

Instructions

1. Start by pouring 2 cups of filtered water into a large glass jar or pitcher.

2. Add 1 tablespoon of turmeric powder to the water, ensuring it's evenly dispersed throughout the liquid.

3. Incorporate 1/2 teaspoon of ground black pepper into the mixture. The piperine in black pepper enhances the absorption of curcumin by the body, making the turmeric more effective.

4. Stir in 1 tablespoon of honey, adjusting the amount according to your sweetness preference. Honey not only sweetens the tonic but also brings its own anti-inflammatory and antimicrobial properties.

5. Squeeze the juice of 1/2 lemon into the jar, adding a refreshing and vitamin C-rich component to the tonic. Lemon juice also helps to balance the earthy flavor of turmeric.

6. If desired, add a pinch of cinnamon for an additional layer of flavor and its own anti-inflammatory benefits.

7. Secure the lid on the jar or pitcher and shake vigorously for about 30 seconds to ensure all the ingredients are well combined and the turmeric is fully dissolved.

8. Let the mixture sit for a few minutes to allow the flavors to meld together. Serve the tonic over ice or at room temperature, stirring well before pouring into glasses.

Variations

- For a warm tonic, gently heat the water before adding the turmeric and other ingredients. This is especially comforting during colder months.
- Add a slice of fresh ginger for an extra anti-inflammatory kick and a spicy flavor profile.
- Substitute honey with maple syrup for a vegan-friendly sweetener option that complements the flavors of the tonic.

Storage tips

This tonic is best enjoyed fresh but can be stored in the refrigerator for up to 24 hours. If sediment settles at the bottom, simply stir or shake well before serving.

Tips for allergens

For those with allergies to honey, maple syrup or stevia are suitable alternatives that do not compromise the anti-inflammatory benefits of the tonic. If you have a sensitivity to black pepper, reducing the quantity to a minimal amount may lessen the likelihood of irritation while still enhancing curcumin absorption.

Scientific references

- "Curcumin: A Review of Its' Effects on Human Health," published in Foods, highlights the wide-ranging health benefits of curcumin, including its anti-inflammatory properties.
- "Influence of Piperine on the Pharmacokinetics of Curcumin in Animals and Human Volunteers," published in Planta Medica, demonstrates how piperine enhances the bioavailability of curcumin, making it more effective.

Licorice Root and Ginger Immune Support Tea

Beneficial effects

Licorice Root and Ginger Immune Support Tea is crafted to bolster the immune system, offering a natural way to fight off colds, flu, and other respiratory infections. Licorice root has antiviral and antimicrobial properties that enhance the body's ability to defend against harmful pathogens, while ginger adds potent anti-inflammatory and antioxidant benefits, aiding in symptom relief and recovery. Together, these ingredients create a warming, soothing tea that not only supports immune function but also provides a comforting, healing experience during times of illness.

Portions

2 servings

Preparation time

5 minutes
Cooking time
15 minutes
Ingredients
- 2 cups water
- 1 tablespoon dried licorice root
- 1 tablespoon fresh ginger, thinly sliced
- Honey to taste (optional)
- Lemon slices for garnish (optional)

Instructions

1. Pour 2 cups of water into a medium saucepan and bring to a boil over high heat.

2. Once the water is boiling, add 1 tablespoon of dried licorice root and 1 tablespoon of thinly sliced fresh ginger to the saucepan.

3. Reduce the heat to low, cover the saucepan with a lid, and allow the mixture to simmer gently for 15 minutes. This slow simmering process helps to extract the active compounds from the licorice root and ginger, infusing the water with their immune-supporting properties.

4. After simmering, remove the saucepan from the heat. Carefully strain the tea through a fine mesh sieve into two mugs or cups, discarding the licorice root and ginger pieces.

5. If desired, sweeten each serving with honey to taste. Stir well until the honey is fully dissolved.

6. Garnish each cup with a slice of lemon for an added boost of vitamin C and a refreshing flavor contrast to the spicy-sweet taste of the tea.

7. Serve the tea warm, encouraging slow sipping to fully enjoy its therapeutic benefits.

Variations

- For an added immune boost, include a cinnamon stick in the saucepan while simmering the licorice root and ginger.
- If you prefer a caffeine kick, add a bag of green tea to each cup when pouring the strained tea and let it steep for 3 minutes before removing.
- To enhance the soothing effect on the throat, mix in a teaspoon of apple cider vinegar to each serving.

Storage tips

This tea is best enjoyed fresh but can be stored in a thermos or insulated bottle to retain warmth for up to 2 hours, making it convenient for sipping throughout the day as needed.

Tips for allergens

Individuals with hypertension should be cautious when consuming licorice root, as it can affect blood pressure levels. A substitute for licorice root for those concerned can be echinacea, which also supports immune health without affecting blood pressure.

Boswellia and Ashwagandha Joint Relief Elixir

Beneficial effects

The Boswellia and Ashwagandha Joint Relief Elixir combines the anti-inflammatory properties of Boswellia, also known as Indian Frankincense, with the stress-reducing and rejuvenating effects of Ashwagandha. This elixir is specifically formulated to support joint health, reduce pain and inflammation associated with conditions like arthritis, and enhance the body's resilience to stress, which can exacerbate joint discomfort. Boswellia has been shown in studies to inhibit pro-inflammatory markers in the body, while Ashwagandha is known for its adaptogenic qualities, helping to balance the body's response to stress and potentially reducing inflammation.

Portions
Makes about 2 cups

Preparation time
15 minutes

Ingredients
- 2 cups filtered water
- 1 tablespoon dried Boswellia serrata resin
- 1 tablespoon dried Ashwagandha root
- 1 teaspoon ground turmeric
- 1/2 teaspoon black pepper (to enhance turmeric absorption)
- Honey or stevia to taste (optional)

Instructions
1. Pour 2 cups of filtered water into a medium saucepan and bring to a gentle boil over medium heat.
2. Add 1 tablespoon of dried Boswellia serrata resin and 1 tablespoon of dried Ashwagandha root to the boiling water.
3. Reduce the heat to low and simmer the mixture for 10 minutes, allowing the water to become infused with the herbs.
4. Stir in 1 teaspoon of ground turmeric and 1/2 teaspoon of black pepper into the simmering water. The black pepper increases the bioavailability of curcumin, the active compound in turmeric, enhancing its anti-inflammatory effects.
5. After simmering for an additional 5 minutes, remove the saucepan from the heat and allow the elixir to cool slightly.
6. Strain the elixir through a fine mesh strainer or cheesecloth into a heat-resistant pitcher or jar, discarding the solid residues.
7. If desired, sweeten the elixir with honey or stevia according to taste. Stir well to ensure the sweetener is fully dissolved.
8. Serve the elixir warm, or allow it to cool completely and refrigerate for a refreshing cold drink.

Variations
- For an added immune boost, include a slice of fresh ginger during the simmering process. Ginger's anti-inflammatory properties complement those of turmeric and Boswellia.
- To make a more potent elixir, double the amount of Boswellia and Ashwagandha, steeping for a longer period of up to 20 minutes.
- For those who prefer a creamier texture, blend the strained elixir with a tablespoon of coconut oil before serving. The healthy fats in coconut oil can also aid in the absorption of the herbs' active compounds.

Storage tips
Store any leftover Boswellia and Ashwagandha Joint Relief Elixir in a glass container in the refrigerator for up to 3 days. Gently reheat on the stove or enjoy cold. Shake well before using if separation occurs.

Tips for allergens

For individuals with sensitivities to honey or stevia, the elixir can be enjoyed unsweetened or with an alternative sweetener of choice. Ensure to source high-quality, organic Boswellia and Ashwagandha to avoid potential contaminants and allergens.

Scientific references

- "The effectiveness of Boswellia serrata in treating osteoarthritis: A review of clinical trials," published in the Journal of Alternative and Complementary Medicine, highlights the anti-inflammatory and pain-reducing effects of Boswellia.

- "An overview on Ashwagandha: A Rasayana (Rejuvenator) of Ayurveda," published in the African Journal of Traditional, Complementary, and Alternative Medicines, discusses the adaptogenic and anti-inflammatory properties of Ashwagandha.

CHAPTER 2: HERBAL REMEDIES FOR CHRONIC PAIN

Willow Bark for Pain Relief

Willow bark, known scientifically as **Salix alba**, has been recognized for centuries for its pain-relieving properties. Its effectiveness in easing discomfort stems from the presence of a compound called **salicin**, which in the body converts to salicylic acid, a precursor of aspirin. This natural remedy offers a gentler alternative to synthetic aspirin, making it suitable for those seeking relief from headaches, lower back pain, osteoarthritis, and other inflammatory conditions without the harsh side effects often associated with over-the-counter pain medications.

To utilize willow bark effectively for pain relief, it's important to understand the proper preparation and dosage. The bark can be harvested from young or mature willow trees; however, young branches tend to have higher concentrations of salicin. After collecting the bark, it should be dried thoroughly in a well-ventilated, shaded area to prevent mold and decay. Once dried, the bark can be stored in airtight containers away from direct sunlight to preserve its potency.

For making a **willow bark tea**, a common method of consumption, follow these steps:

1. Measure approximately 2 teaspoons of dried, chopped willow bark for each cup of water.

2. Bring water to a boil in a stainless steel or glass pot.

3. Add the willow bark to the boiling water and simmer for about 10-15 minutes. This slow simmering process allows for the extraction of salicin into the water.

4. Remove from heat and let the tea steep for an additional 30 minutes to enhance the strength of the infusion.

5. Strain the tea to remove the bark pieces. The resulting liquid can be consumed once cooled. For taste, consider adding honey or lemon, as willow bark has a naturally bitter flavor.

The recommended dosage for willow bark tea varies, but starting with one cup per day and observing the body's response is advisable. Adjustments can be made based on personal tolerance and the severity of pain. It is important to note that while willow bark is a natural product, it can still interact with certain medications and conditions. Individuals who are allergic to aspirin, taking blood-thinning medications, or who have kidney issues should avoid willow bark. Additionally, it is not recommended for children or pregnant women due to the lack of research on its effects in these groups.

For those preferring a more convenient form, willow bark is also available in capsule or tincture form. When choosing these options, look for products that specify the salicin content, ensuring a standardized dose. A general guideline for capsules is to take 240-320 mg of salicin daily for relief from chronic conditions, but it's crucial to follow the manufacturer's instructions or consult with a healthcare provider.

Devil's Claw for Joint Pain Relief

Devil's Claw, scientifically known as Harpagophytum procumbens, is a potent herb native to the deserts of South Africa. Renowned for its anti-inflammatory and analgesic properties, it has been a cornerstone in traditional medicine for addressing joint and muscle pain. The primary active component, harpagoside, is credited with the herb's ability to reduce inflammation and alleviate pain, making it particularly beneficial for individuals suffering from arthritis, rheumatism, and other musculoskeletal conditions.

To harness the therapeutic benefits of Devil's Claw for joint and muscle pain, it is crucial to understand the appropriate preparation methods and dosages. The root of Devil's Claw is the part most commonly used for medicinal purposes. It can be prepared in various forms, including tinctures, capsules, and teas, each offering a different method of delivery with its own set of considerations for effective use.

For those opting to prepare a Devil's Claw tea, the process involves:

1. Taking 1-2 teaspoons of dried Devil's Claw root and adding it to approximately 2 cups of water.

2. Bringing the water to a boil, then reducing the heat to allow the mixture to simmer gently for 8-10 minutes. This slow simmering process aids in extracting the harpagoside from the root into the water.

3. After simmering, remove the pot from the heat and allow the tea to steep for another 10-15 minutes, enhancing the strength of the infusion.

4. Strain the tea to remove the root pieces, and the liquid is ready for consumption. Given the bitter taste of Devil's Claw, adding a natural sweetener like honey or mixing it with another herbal tea to improve palatability may be beneficial.

For those who prefer a more straightforward approach, Devil's Claw is available in capsule form. The recommended dosage for capsules generally ranges from 400 to 600 mg taken three times daily with meals. This form is particularly convenient for maintaining consistent dosages and for those who might find the taste of the tea unpalatable.

Another effective preparation method is a tincture, which involves:

1. Soaking the dried root in a mixture of alcohol and water for several weeks, shaking the container periodically to ensure thorough extraction.

2. After the soaking period, the liquid is strained and bottled, preserving the extract.

3. The typical dosage for a Devil's Claw tincture is 1-2 ml taken three times daily. Tinctures offer a concentrated form of the herb, allowing for easier dosage adjustments and rapid absorption.

When incorporating Devil's Claw into a regimen for joint and muscle pain relief, it's important to consider the quality of the herb. Opting for organically grown Devil's Claw ensures the product is free from pesticides and other contaminants that could undermine its therapeutic value. Additionally, while Devil's Claw is generally well-tolerated, it's advisable to start with a lower dose to assess individual tolerance and gradually increase as needed.

It's also crucial to be aware of potential interactions and contraindications. Devil's Claw may interact with certain medications, such as blood thinners and antacids, and is not recommended for individuals with stomach ulcers or gallstones due to its stimulating effect on stomach acid production. As with any herbal remedy, consulting with a healthcare provider before starting Devil's Claw, especially for those with existing health conditions or who are taking other medications, ensures safe and effective use.

Incorporating lifestyle modifications that support joint and muscle health, such as regular gentle exercise, maintaining a healthy weight, and adopting an anti-inflammatory diet, can amplify the benefits of Devil's Claw. Combining these practices with the herb's use offers a comprehensive approach to managing pain and inflammation, contributing to improved mobility and quality of life for individuals dealing with chronic musculoskeletal conditions.

Boswellia for Pain Relief

Boswellia, also known as frankincense, is derived from the resin of the Boswellia tree, which is native to India, North Africa, and the Middle East. This resin has been used for thousands of years in traditional medicine to treat various chronic inflammatory conditions, including arthritis. The active components in Boswellia resin, boswellic acids, have been shown to inhibit pro-inflammatory enzymes in the body, thereby reducing inflammation and pain.

To utilize Boswellia for arthritis and chronic inflammation effectively, it's essential to select a high-quality source of the resin or a standardized extract containing a high percentage of boswellic acids. The market offers Boswellia in various forms, including raw resin, powder, capsules, and tinctures. Each form requires specific preparation methods to ensure optimal absorption and effectiveness.

For those opting to use the raw resin, it can be ground into a fine powder using a mortar and pestle or a spice grinder. This powder can then be mixed with a carrier oil, such as cold-pressed virgin olive oil or coconut oil, to create a topical ointment. The recommended ratio is about one part Boswellia powder to five parts carrier oil. This mixture should be gently heated in a double boiler for 20-30 minutes, allowing the boswellic acids to infuse into the oil. Once cooled, the ointment can be applied directly to the affected joints to alleviate pain and inflammation. It's advisable to perform a patch test on a small skin area before widespread application to ensure no allergic reactions occur.

For oral consumption, Boswellia capsules or tablets are the most convenient option. These should be taken according to the manufacturer's dosage recommendations, typically ranging from 300 to 500 mg of Boswellia extract taken two to three times daily with meals. It's crucial to choose products that specify their boswellic acid content, as this ensures potency and effectiveness.

Another effective method is the use of Boswellia tinctures, which offer a liquid form of the herb for those who may have difficulty swallowing capsules. The typical dosage for tinctures is 1 ml (about 20 drops) taken three times a day, mixed into water or juice. The alcohol in the tincture serves as a solvent, extracting the active compounds from the resin, and also aids in preserving the extract.

When incorporating Boswellia into a treatment plan for arthritis and chronic inflammation, it's important to give the herb time to exhibit its effects. While some individuals may notice improvements within a few days, it may take several weeks for the full benefits to manifest. Consistency is key, as the anti-inflammatory effects build up over time.

Additionally, combining Boswellia with other natural anti-inflammatory compounds, such as turmeric (which contains curcumin), can enhance its pain-relieving properties. A holistic approach, including a balanced diet rich in anti-inflammatory foods, regular gentle exercise, and stress management techniques, can further support joint health and reduce symptoms of chronic inflammation.

It's also important to consult with a healthcare provider before adding Boswellia to your regimen, especially if you are taking prescription medications or have existing health conditions. This ensures that Boswellia supplements do not interact with medications or exacerbate health issues.

White Willow Bark Pain Relief Tea

Beneficial effects

White Willow Bark Pain Relief Tea utilizes the natural pain-relieving properties of white willow bark, known as nature's aspirin, to reduce inflammation and alleviate pain. This herbal remedy has been used for centuries to treat headaches, muscle pain, menstrual cramps, and rheumatic conditions. The active compound in white willow bark, salicin, is converted by the body into salicylic acid, which is the precursor to aspirin. Unlike synthetic aspirin, white willow bark offers a gentler approach to pain relief without the common gastrointestinal side effects associated with over-the-counter NSAIDs.

Portions
2 servings

Preparation time
5 minutes

Cooking time

15 minutes

Ingredients

- 2 cups of water
- 2 teaspoons of dried white willow bark
- 1 teaspoon of dried peppermint leaves (for flavor and additional pain-relieving properties)
- Honey or stevia to taste (optional, for sweetness)

Instructions

1. Pour 2 cups of water into a medium-sized saucepan and bring to a boil over high heat.
2. Once the water reaches a rolling boil, add 2 teaspoons of dried white willow bark to the saucepan.
3. Reduce the heat to low, allowing the mixture to simmer gently. Cover the saucepan with a lid to prevent the volatile oils from escaping.
4. Simmer the mixture for 10 minutes to allow the active compounds in the white willow bark to be released into the water.
5. After 10 minutes, add 1 teaspoon of dried peppermint leaves to the saucepan. Peppermint not only enhances the flavor of the tea but also contributes additional pain-relieving and anti-inflammatory benefits.
6. Continue to simmer the mixture for an additional 5 minutes with the peppermint leaves.
7. Remove the saucepan from the heat and allow the tea to cool slightly for a comfortable drinking temperature.
8. Strain the tea through a fine mesh sieve or cheesecloth into two mugs or cups, pressing on the herbs to extract as much liquid as possible. Discard the used herbs.
9. If desired, sweeten the tea with honey or stevia according to taste. Stir well until the sweetener is fully dissolved.
10. Serve the tea warm, encouraging slow sipping to fully enjoy its therapeutic benefits.

Variations

- For a stronger anti-inflammatory effect, add a slice of fresh ginger to the saucepan along with the white willow bark. Ginger's potent anti-inflammatory properties can enhance the pain-relieving effects of the tea.
- To create a more complex flavor profile, include a cinnamon stick during the simmering process. Cinnamon adds a warming, slightly spicy note that complements the herbal flavors.
- For those sensitive to the taste of white willow bark, blending the strained tea with a bag of your favorite herbal or green tea can mask the bitterness and make the remedy more palatable.

Storage tips

This tea is best enjoyed fresh but can be stored in a thermos or insulated bottle to retain warmth for up to 2 hours, making it convenient for sipping throughout the day as needed.

Tips for allergens

Individuals with allergies to aspirin or other salicylates should avoid white willow bark, as it may cause similar reactions. A suitable alternative for pain relief without the use of salicylates is turmeric tea, which also offers significant anti-inflammatory benefits.

Turmeric and Ginger Anti-Inflammatory Smoothie

Beneficial effects
The Turmeric and Ginger Anti-Inflammatory Smoothie combines the powerful anti-inflammatory properties of turmeric and ginger, both known for their ability to reduce inflammation and aid in digestion. Turmeric contains curcumin, a compound that has been shown to decrease inflammation markers in the body, while ginger can help alleviate muscle pain and soreness. This smoothie is an excellent choice for those looking to naturally manage inflammation, improve immune function, and support overall health.

Portions
2 servings

Preparation time
10 minutes

Ingredients
- 1 cup unsweetened almond milk
- 1 ripe banana, sliced
- 1/2 cup frozen pineapple chunks
- 1 tablespoon freshly grated turmeric root (or 1 teaspoon turmeric powder)
- 1 tablespoon freshly grated ginger root
- A pinch of black pepper (to enhance turmeric absorption)
- 1 tablespoon chia seeds
- 1 teaspoon honey (optional, for sweetness)
- Ice cubes (optional, for a colder smoothie)

Instructions
1. In a blender, combine 1 cup of unsweetened almond milk with the sliced banana and 1/2 cup of frozen pineapple chunks. Blend on high speed until smooth.
2. Add 1 tablespoon of freshly grated turmeric root (or 1 teaspoon of turmeric powder) and 1 tablespoon of freshly grated ginger root to the blender. The fresh roots provide a potent flavor and maximum health benefits, but powdered versions can be used for convenience.
3. Incorporate a pinch of black pepper into the mixture. Black pepper contains piperine, which significantly enhances the absorption of curcumin from turmeric, making it more effective.
4. Add 1 tablespoon of chia seeds to the blender. Chia seeds are rich in omega-3 fatty acids and fiber, contributing to the anti-inflammatory and digestive benefits of the smoothie.
5. If a sweeter taste is desired, include 1 teaspoon of honey. Blend all the ingredients until the mixture is smooth and creamy.
6. For a colder smoothie, add a few ice cubes to the blender and blend until the desired consistency is reached.
7. Pour the smoothie into two glasses and serve immediately for the freshest taste and the most nutritional benefits.

Variations
- For an extra protein boost, add a scoop of your favorite plant-based protein powder. This can make the smoothie a more filling meal replacement or post-workout recovery drink.
- Substitute almond milk with coconut water for a lighter version that adds electrolytes, making it an excellent choice for hydration.

- Add a handful of spinach or kale to incorporate greens into your smoothie without significantly altering the taste, enhancing its nutritional profile.

Storage tips

It's best to consume the Turmeric and Ginger Anti-Inflammatory Smoothie immediately after preparation to ensure maximum freshness and potency of the ingredients. However, if necessary, it can be stored in a sealed container in the refrigerator for up to 24 hours. Give it a good stir or shake before consuming as the ingredients may settle or separate.

Tips for allergens

For those with nut allergies, almond milk can be replaced with oat milk or another non-nut-based milk alternative. Ensure that any added protein powders or supplements are free from allergens that may affect you. If using honey, ensure it is pure and not processed in facilities that handle allergens you are sensitive to.

Scientific references

- "Curcumin: A Review of Its' Effects on Human Health," published in Foods, highlights the wide-ranging health benefits of curcumin, including its anti-inflammatory properties.
- "Ginger consumption is associated with decreased risk of obesity, diabetes, and heart disease: A comprehensive review on its health benefits," published in the Journal of Nutrition and Metabolism, discusses the benefits of ginger on inflammation and overall health.

Devil's Claw Joint Support Tincture

Beneficial effects

Devil's Claw Joint Support Tincture is designed to alleviate joint pain and inflammation, making it an excellent natural remedy for individuals suffering from arthritis, gout, and other conditions affecting joint health. Devil's Claw, scientifically known as Harpagophytum procumbens, contains harpagoside, a compound known for its anti-inflammatory and analgesic properties. This tincture aims to reduce pain, enhance mobility, and improve the quality of life for those dealing with chronic joint discomfort.

Portions

Makes about 1 pint

Preparation time

24 hours for maceration

Cooking time

N/A

Ingredients

- 1/2 cup dried Devil's Claw root
- 2 cups high-proof alcohol (e.g., vodka or brandy, at least 80 proof)
- Dark glass bottle with a tight-fitting lid

Instructions

1. Measure 1/2 cup of dried Devil's Claw root and place it into a clean, dry dark glass bottle.
2. Pour 2 cups of high-proof alcohol over the Devil's Claw root, ensuring the roots are completely submerged. If necessary, add more alcohol until the roots are covered by at least an inch of liquid.
3. Secure the lid tightly on the bottle and shake gently to mix the Devil's Claw with the alcohol.
4. Label the bottle with the date and contents. Store the bottle in a cool, dark place.

5. Allow the mixture to macerate for at least 24 hours, shaking the bottle gently once or twice a day to agitate the roots and ensure a potent extraction.

6. After maceration, strain the tincture through a fine mesh strainer or cheesecloth into another clean, dry dark glass bottle or jar. Press or squeeze the root material to extract as much liquid as possible.

7. Discard the spent Devil's Claw root. Transfer the strained tincture into dark glass dropper bottles for easy use.

8. Label the dropper bottles with the tincture's name and the date of completion.

Variations

- For a non-alcoholic version, glycerin can be used in place of alcohol, though the extraction process may differ slightly, and the resulting tincture may have a shorter shelf life.
- Add ginger root to the maceration process for additional anti-inflammatory benefits and to enhance the tincture's flavor.
- Incorporate turmeric root in the mixture for its curcumin content, known to synergize with harpagoside in Devil's Claw, enhancing anti-inflammatory effects.

Storage tips

Store the Devil's Claw Joint Support Tincture in a cool, dark place, such as a cabinet or pantry. The alcohol acts as a natural preservative, allowing the tincture to maintain its potency for up to 2 years. Ensure the dropper bottles are tightly sealed to prevent evaporation and contamination.

Tips for allergens

Individuals with allergies to Devil's Claw or other plants in the sesame family should avoid this tincture. As always, consult with a healthcare provider before starting any new herbal regimen, especially if you have allergies, are pregnant, nursing, or taking prescription medications.

CHAPTER 3: HERBS FOR RECOVERY AND HEALING

Comfrey for Tissue Regeneration

Comfrey, known scientifically as Symphytum officinale, has been revered through the ages for its remarkable ability to promote tissue regeneration, making it an invaluable herb for those recovering from fractures and deep wounds. The active compound in comfrey responsible for its healing prowess is allantoin, which accelerates cell proliferation, thereby speeding up the healing process. To harness the benefits of comfrey for tissue regeneration, it is essential to understand the proper preparation and application methods to ensure both efficacy and safety.

For topical applications, creating a comfrey poultice is one of the most effective methods to facilitate healing. Begin by harvesting fresh comfrey leaves, preferably from plants that are young and vibrant, as they contain the highest concentration of allantoin. Wash the leaves thoroughly to remove any dirt or debris. Using a mortar and pestle, crush the leaves into a fine paste. If a mortar and pestle are not available, a blender can be used as an alternative, adding a small amount of water to aid in the process. The goal is to extract as much of the juice from the leaves as possible.

Once the comfrey paste is ready, spread it directly over the affected area, if the skin is not broken, or on a clean, thin cloth if the skin is open or if there's concern about direct contact. Apply the poultice to the fracture or wound site, securing it with a bandage or wrap to keep it in place. It's crucial to ensure that the poultice is not applied too tightly, as circulation should not be restricted. The poultice should be left in place for up to four hours before being removed. This process can be repeated two to three times daily, monitoring the skin for any signs of irritation or allergic reaction, as comfrey should not be used for prolonged periods on broken skin due to the presence of pyrrolizidine alkaloids, which can be absorbed through the skin and are toxic to the liver in large quantities or over extended use.

For those who prefer a less hands-on approach, comfrey ointments and creams are available and can be applied according to the product instructions. These commercial preparations typically contain a standardized concentration of allantoin, minimizing the risk associated with pyrrolizidine alkaloids, making them safe for regular use over unbroken skin.

In addition to topical applications, integrating comfrey into a holistic recovery plan can be beneficial. This includes maintaining a balanced diet rich in vitamins and minerals essential for bone health and tissue repair, such as calcium, vitamin D, magnesium, and zinc. Hydration is also crucial, as water plays a key role in transporting nutrients to damaged cells and removing waste products from the body.

While comfrey is a powerful herb for promoting tissue regeneration, it is important to consult with a healthcare professional before beginning any new treatment, especially for those with underlying health conditions or those who are pregnant or breastfeeding. With proper use, comfrey can be a safe and effective component of a natural healing regimen, offering a time-honored solution for accelerating recovery from fractures and deep wounds.

Schisandra for Liver Support

Schisandra, scientifically known as **Schisandra chinensis**, is a potent adaptogenic herb renowned for its comprehensive support of liver function and its therapeutic role in the recovery from chronic conditions. The liver, being a vital organ for detoxification, metabolizes toxins and various metabolic by-products. Schisandra enhances this detoxification process, aids in liver cell regeneration, and protects the liver from toxic damage.

To leverage **Schisandra** for liver support, it's essential to understand its active components and optimal preparation methods. Schisandra berries contain lignans, particularly **schizandrins**, which are responsible for their hepatoprotective properties. These lignans act as antioxidants, combating free radical damage and supporting the liver's natural detoxification pathways.

Preparation of Schisandra for Liver Support involves several steps to ensure the bioavailability of its beneficial compounds. A common method is the preparation of a **Schisandra decoction**, which involves simmering the dried berries in water to extract the active compounds. To prepare this decoction:

1. Measure 1-2 teaspoons of dried **Schisandra berries** per cup of water. For a stronger decoction, adjust the amount of berries accordingly.

2. Place the berries in a saucepan and add the measured water.

3. Slowly bring the mixture to a boil, then reduce the heat to a simmer.

4. Cover and simmer for approximately 20-30 minutes. The liquid should reduce by about a third, concentrating the decoction.

5. Strain the decoction to remove the berries. The remaining liquid contains the extracted compounds.

6. Consume the decoction while warm. For liver support, drinking 1-2 cups daily is recommended, especially before meals to enhance digestion and absorption.

For those seeking a more convenient option, **Schisandra extract** in the form of tinctures or capsules is available. When selecting a Schisandra supplement, opt for products that specify the content of schizandrins or other active lignans, as these are indicative of the product's potency.

Dosage is crucial for achieving therapeutic effects without adverse reactions. While Schisandra is generally considered safe, starting with lower doses and gradually increasing based on tolerance can help minimize potential side effects such as gastrointestinal upset. The standard dose for Schisandra extract varies depending on the concentration, but generally, 100-500 mg per day is a safe range for most adults. Always consult with a healthcare provider before starting any new supplement, especially for individuals with existing liver conditions or those taking medications that may interact with Schisandra.

Incorporating **Schisandra** into a holistic approach to liver health involves not only regular consumption of the herb but also adopting a liver-friendly diet rich in antioxidants and essential nutrients. Foods high in omega-3 fatty acids, fiber, and low in processed sugars support liver function and complement the benefits of Schisandra. Additionally, maintaining adequate hydration, regular physical activity, and avoiding excessive alcohol consumption are key lifestyle factors that support liver health and enhance the detoxifying effects of Schisandra.

By understanding the properties of Schisandra and implementing these detailed preparation and consumption guidelines, individuals can effectively utilize this ancient herb to support liver function and aid in the recovery from chronic conditions, harnessing its full potential for natural health and wellness.

Milk Thistle for Liver Health

Milk thistle, scientifically known as Silybum marianum, stands out for its profound impact on liver health, particularly in cellular repair and recovery from damage. This herb's active ingredient, silymarin, is a complex of flavonolignans that includes silibinin, silidianin, and silicristin, which collectively contribute to its therapeutic properties. Silymarin acts as an antioxidant, anti-inflammatory, and antifibrotic agent, making milk thistle a pivotal component in managing liver diseases and detoxification processes.

To harness milk thistle's benefits for liver health, it's crucial to focus on quality sourcing and proper preparation. Opt for milk thistle supplements that specify the percentage of silymarin, as this indicates the potency and effectiveness of the product. A standardized extract containing 70% to 80% silymarin is ideal for therapeutic use.

For daily supplementation, the recommended dosage of milk thistle extract varies depending on the concentration of silymarin. Generally, 140 milligrams taken two to three times daily is considered effective for liver support. However, it's essential to consult with a healthcare provider to determine the appropriate dosage based on individual health needs and conditions.

Incorporating milk thistle into a holistic liver health regimen involves more than just supplementation. A diet rich in antioxidants, such as fruits, vegetables, whole grains, and lean proteins, supports liver function and enhances the detoxifying effects of milk thistle. Additionally, minimizing exposure to liver toxins, such as alcohol, certain medications, and environmental pollutants, is crucial for reducing liver stress and allowing milk thistle to aid in cellular repair and regeneration effectively.

For those preferring a more direct approach to consuming milk thistle, preparing a tea from the seeds offers a traditional method of intake. To prepare milk thistle tea, crush one teaspoon of milk thistle seeds in a mortar and pestle. Boil one cup of water and pour it over the crushed seeds, allowing it to steep for 15-20 minutes. Strain the tea to remove the seed particles before drinking. Consuming one to two cups of milk thistle tea daily can provide a gentle liver detox and support overall liver health.

It's also possible to integrate milk thistle into the diet by incorporating the ground seeds into smoothies, yogurts, or cereals. This not only ensures the intake of silymarin but also increases dietary fiber, which supports digestive health.

Monitoring the body's response to milk thistle is vital, as individual reactions can vary. While milk thistle is generally well-tolerated, some individuals may experience mild digestive disturbances. Starting with a lower dose and gradually increasing it allows for assessing tolerance and effectiveness, ensuring a positive impact on liver health.

In conclusion, milk thistle's role in promoting liver health and aiding in cellular repair is supported by its antioxidant, anti-inflammatory, and antifibrotic properties. Through careful selection of supplements, appropriate dosing, and integration into a healthy lifestyle, milk thistle can significantly contribute to liver recovery and overall well-being.

Arnica and St. John's Wort Healing Balm

Beneficial effects

Arnica and St. John's Wort Healing Balm combines the anti-inflammatory and pain-relieving properties of Arnica montana with the nerve-restorative benefits of St. John's Wort (Hypericum perforatum). This balm is specifically formulated to soothe bruises, reduce inflammation, and aid in the healing of minor wounds and nerve pain. Arnica has been traditionally used to treat physical trauma, sprains, and muscle soreness, while St. John's Wort is known for its effectiveness in repairing nerve damage and reducing symptoms of neuralgia. Together, they create a potent topical remedy for natural pain relief and skin healing.

Portions

Makes about 4 ounces

Preparation time

30 minutes

Cooking time

10 minutes

Ingredients
- 1/4 cup Arnica montana flowers, dried
- 1/4 cup St. John's Wort flowers, dried
- 1/2 cup olive oil or almond oil
- 2 tablespoons beeswax pellets
- 10 drops lavender essential oil (for additional soothing properties)
- Dark glass jar for storage

Instructions
1. Begin by infusing the olive or almond oil with Arnica montana and St. John's Wort flowers. Combine the dried flowers and oil in a double boiler, gently heating the mixture over low heat for 2-3 hours to allow the herbs to infuse their properties into the oil. Stir occasionally to ensure even heat distribution.
2. After the infusion period, strain the oil through a fine mesh strainer or cheesecloth into a clean bowl, pressing the herbs to extract as much oil as possible. Discard the herb residues.
3. Return the infused oil to the double boiler, and add 2 tablespoons of beeswax pellets. Heat the mixture until the beeswax is completely melted, stirring constantly for a smooth consistency.
4. Remove the mixture from heat and allow it to cool for a few minutes. Before the balm starts to solidify, stir in 10 drops of lavender essential oil for its calming and anti-inflammatory effects.
5. Carefully pour the warm balm into a dark glass jar to protect the active ingredients from light degradation. Allow the balm to cool and solidify completely at room temperature.
6. Once cooled, seal the jar tightly. Label the jar with the product name and date of creation.

Variations
- For a vegan version, replace beeswax pellets with the same amount of candelilla wax or carnauba wax.
- If you prefer a softer balm, adjust the amount of beeswax to 1 tablespoon. This will make the balm easier to apply, especially in colder temperatures.
- For additional pain relief, incorporate 5 drops of peppermint essential oil into the balm during step 4. Peppermint oil can provide a cooling sensation and further aid in soothing sore muscles and joints.

Storage tips
Store the Arnica and St. John's Wort Healing Balm in a cool, dark place. The balm should remain effective for up to 1 year if stored properly. Avoid exposing the balm to direct sunlight or heat, as this can cause the ingredients to degrade more quickly.

Tips for allergens
Individuals with sensitivities to Arnica, St. John's Wort, or lavender should perform a patch test on a small area of skin before widespread use. If irritation occurs, discontinue use immediately. For those allergic to nuts, ensure that almond oil is not used; olive oil is a safe alternative.

Gotu Kola and Ashwagandha Recovery Tonic

Beneficial effects
The Gotu Kola and Ashwagandha Recovery Tonic is a potent blend designed to support the body's natural healing processes, enhance mental clarity, and promote overall wellness. Gotu Kola, known for its neuroprotective and cognitive-enhancing properties, aids in improving memory and reducing anxiety. Ashwagandha, an adaptogen, helps the body manage stress, boosts brain function, and supports adrenal health. Together, these herbs create a tonic that not only aids in physical recovery

but also in mental and emotional well-being, making it an excellent choice for those seeking to rejuvenate their body and mind.

Portions
2 servings

Preparation time
10 minutes

Ingredients
- 2 cups of water
- 1 tablespoon dried Gotu Kola leaves
- 1 tablespoon dried Ashwagandha root
- 1 teaspoon honey (optional, for sweetness)
- 1/2 teaspoon lemon juice (optional, for flavor)

Instructions
1. Bring 2 cups of water to a boil in a medium saucepan.

2. Once boiling, reduce the heat to low and add 1 tablespoon of dried Gotu Kola leaves and 1 tablespoon of dried Ashwagandha root to the saucepan.

3. Cover the saucepan with a lid and simmer the mixture on low heat for 5 minutes to allow the herbs to infuse their properties into the water.

4. After simmering, remove the saucepan from the heat and let it steep, covered, for an additional 5 minutes to enhance the strength of the tonic.

5. Strain the tonic through a fine mesh sieve into a large glass or pitcher, pressing on the herbs to extract as much liquid as possible. Discard the used herbs.

6. If desired, stir in 1 teaspoon of honey to sweeten the tonic. Mix well until the honey is completely dissolved.

7. Add 1/2 teaspoon of lemon juice to the tonic for an added refreshing flavor and a boost of vitamin C.

8. Serve the tonic warm, or allow it to cool completely and refrigerate for a refreshing cold drink.

Variations
- For an added immune boost, include a slice of fresh ginger during the simmering process. Ginger's anti-inflammatory properties complement those of Gotu Kola and Ashwagandha.

- To make a more potent tonic, increase the amount of Gotu Kola and Ashwagandha to 2 tablespoons each, steeping for up to 10 minutes.

- For those who prefer a creamier texture, blend the strained tonic with a tablespoon of coconut milk before serving. The healthy fats in coconut milk can also aid in the absorption of the herbs' active compounds.

Storage tips
Store any leftover Gotu Kola and Ashwagandha Recovery Tonic in a glass container in the refrigerator for up to 48 hours. Gently reheat on the stove or enjoy cold. Shake well before using if separation occurs.

Tips for allergens
For individuals with sensitivities to honey, maple syrup or stevia are suitable alternatives that do not compromise the anti-inflammatory benefits of the tonic. If you have a sensitivity to Ashwagandha or Gotu Kola, it's best to start with a smaller dose to assess tolerance.

Scientific references

- "Neuroprotective effects of Asiatic acid in brain injury and neurodegenerative diseases," published in the Journal of Pharmacological Sciences, highlights Gotu Kola's benefits for brain health.
- "An Overview on Ashwagandha: A Rasayana (Rejuvenator) of Ayurveda," published in the African Journal of Traditional, Complementary, and Alternative Medicines, discusses Ashwagandha's adaptogenic and neuroprotective properties.

Turmeric and Boswellia Joint Healing Elixir

Beneficial effects

The Turmeric and Boswellia Joint Healing Elixir is designed to alleviate joint pain and inflammation, harnessing the potent anti-inflammatory properties of both turmeric and Boswellia. Turmeric, containing the active compound curcumin, has been widely recognized for its ability to reduce inflammation and is often recommended for managing conditions like arthritis. Boswellia, also known as Indian Frankincense, contains acids that have been shown to inhibit the production of pro-inflammatory enzymes. Together, these herbs offer a synergistic approach to reducing joint pain and improving mobility, making this elixir a valuable addition to natural health practices.

Ingredients

- 2 cups of water
- 1 tablespoon turmeric powder
- 1 tablespoon Boswellia serrata powder
- A pinch of ground black pepper (to enhance curcumin absorption)
- Honey or stevia to taste (optional for sweetness)
- Juice of half a lemon (optional, for flavor and vitamin C)

Instructions

1. Pour 2 cups of water into a medium saucepan and bring to a gentle boil over medium heat.
2. Reduce the heat to low and add 1 tablespoon of turmeric powder and 1 tablespoon of Boswellia serrata powder to the simmering water.
3. Stir in a pinch of ground black pepper. The piperine in black pepper is known to significantly enhance the bioavailability of curcumin, making the turmeric more effective.
4. Allow the mixture to simmer on low heat for 10 minutes, stirring occasionally to ensure the powders are well dissolved and the ingredients are fully infused into the water.
5. After simmering, remove the saucepan from the heat and let the elixir cool for a few minutes.
6. Strain the elixir through a fine mesh sieve into a large mug or heat-resistant glass to remove any undissolved particles.
7. If desired, sweeten the elixir with honey or stevia according to taste. Stir well until the sweetener is fully dissolved.
8. Squeeze the juice of half a lemon into the elixir for an added boost of flavor and vitamin C, enhancing the anti-inflammatory and antioxidant properties of the drink.
9. Enjoy the Turmeric and Boswellia Joint Healing Elixir warm, ideally in the morning or evening to support joint health throughout the day.

Variations

- For those who prefer a cold beverage, allow the elixir to cool completely and then refrigerate. Serve over ice for a refreshing anti-inflammatory drink.
- Add a slice of fresh ginger while simmering the elixir for an additional anti-inflammatory boost and a spicy flavor profile.

- Mix in a teaspoon of coconut oil before drinking. The healthy fats can aid in the absorption of turmeric and Boswellia's fat-soluble compounds.

Storage tips

This elixir is best enjoyed fresh but can be stored in the refrigerator for up to 2 days. Store in a glass container with a lid to preserve the flavors and health benefits. Gently reheat on the stove or enjoy cold.

Tips for allergens

For individuals with sensitivities to honey, stevia provides a sweetening alternative that does not compromise the anti-inflammatory benefits of the elixir. If allergic to black pepper, omitting it will reduce the bioavailability of curcumin but still offer anti-inflammatory benefits.

BOOK 23: COMBINING HERBS FOR SYNERGY

When exploring the realm of herbal synergy, it's paramount to understand the concept of **complementary actions**. This principle is foundational in creating blends that not only coexist but enhance each other's therapeutic effects. For instance, when combining herbs with calming properties, such as **lavender** and **chamomile**, with adaptogens like **ashwagandha**, the blend targets stress relief from multiple angles. Lavender and chamomile provide immediate soothing effects, while ashwagandha addresses the underlying stress response system, offering a more comprehensive approach to stress management.

Another critical aspect is the **ratio of herbs** in a blend. The efficacy of a synergistic blend can be significantly influenced by the proportions of each herb. For example, in a tea blend aimed at enhancing sleep, a higher ratio of **valerian root** to **lemon balm** might be used to capitalize on valerian's potent sedative properties, with lemon balm acting to moderate the blend and add a pleasant flavor. Precise measurements, such as one part valerian to two parts lemon balm, ensure that the final product is both effective and enjoyable to consume.

The **method of preparation** also plays a crucial role in maximizing the benefits of a herbal blend. Different herbs release their active compounds under different conditions. A decoction, which involves simmering herbs in water over a period, might be suitable for tougher materials like roots or bark, such as **ginger** or **cinnamon**, to extract their full potency. In contrast, delicate leaves or flowers, such as **rose petals** or **peppermint**, are better suited to an infusion, where boiling water is poured over the herbs and allowed to steep. This method preserves the volatile oils and flavors that would be destroyed by boiling.

Carrier substances can also impact the effectiveness of a herbal blend. When creating a salve for skin irritation, the choice of carrier oil—be it **coconut oil**, known for its moisturizing properties, or **jojoba oil**, which closely mimics the skin's natural sebum—can enhance the therapeutic effects of the added herbs, such as **calendula** for healing or **tea tree oil** for its antimicrobial action. The carrier not only dilutes essential oils to a safe concentration for topical application but can also contribute additional benefits to the blend.

Understanding the **interactions between different herbs** is essential to avoid counterproductive effects. Some herbs can negate or diminish the effects of others when combined. For instance, combining **sedative herbs** with **stimulants** like **green tea** could result in a blend that is neither particularly relaxing nor energizing, effectively canceling out the desired effects of both components. Therefore, knowledge of herb profiles is indispensable in crafting synergistic blends.

In creating herbal blends for **digestive support**, combining **carminatives** like **fennel** or **peppermint**, which relieve gas and bloating, with **bitters** such as **dandelion root**, which stimulate digestive juices, can offer a more holistic approach to digestive health. This combination addresses both the symptoms and the root causes of digestive discomfort, illustrating the power of synergy in herbal medicine.

As we delve deeper into the art and science of combining herbs for synergistic effects, it becomes clear that a thoughtful and informed approach is necessary for crafting effective and harmonious herbal remedies. The next part of this discussion will further explore the intricacies of herbal synergy, including advanced techniques for blending and the role of modern research in validating traditional knowledge.

Advanced techniques for blending herbs take into account not only the individual properties of each herb but also how they interact with each other to create a balanced and effective remedy. For instance, when creating a blend for respiratory support, herbs like **eucalyptus** and **thyme**, which have expectorant properties, can be combined with **marshmallow root**, known for its soothing mucilage. This combination allows for both the breaking up of mucus and the protection of mucous membranes, offering a comprehensive approach to respiratory health.

Modern research plays a pivotal role in validating the traditional knowledge of herbal synergy. Studies on phytochemical interactions provide scientific backing for the efficacy of certain combinations, such as the pairing of **turmeric** with **black pepper**. The piperine in black pepper enhances the bioavailability of curcumin in turmeric, making the blend more potent than either herb alone. This evidence-based approach supports the development of herbal remedies that are both safe and effective.

When considering the creation of a synergistic herbal blend, it's also important to factor in the **form of the herb**. Whole herbs, powders, tinctures, and extracts each offer different benefits and considerations. For example, tinctures may provide a more concentrated form of the herb, allowing for smaller dosages, while whole herbs may offer a broader spectrum of compounds. The choice of form will depend on the desired strength and immediacy of the remedy's effect.

The **timing of administration** is another critical consideration. Some blends are best taken on an empty stomach, where they can be rapidly absorbed, while others may be more effective after meals, particularly if they are intended to aid digestion. Additionally, the circadian rhythm can influence the efficacy of herbal remedies, with certain herbs offering more benefits when taken at specific times of the day.

Finally, the **duration of use** for a herbal blend is a key factor in its overall effectiveness. Some combinations are intended for short-term relief, such as a blend for acute stress, while others may be designed for long-term support, such as a tonic for adrenal health. Understanding the appropriate duration of use is essential to avoid potential tolerance or adverse effects.

In crafting synergistic herbal blends, the practitioner must consider a multitude of factors, from the properties and ratios of the herbs to the method of preparation and timing of administration. This holistic approach ensures that the final remedy is not only effective but also tailored to the individual's needs. By leveraging both traditional wisdom and modern research, herbalists can create powerful remedies that harness the full potential of plant medicine.

CHAPTER 1: THE SCIENCE OF HERBAL SYNERGY

The exploration of **herbal synergy** extends into the realm of **flavor enhancement** and **nutritional benefits** when herbs are incorporated into daily meals. The concept of **food as medicine** underscores the importance of selecting herbs not only for their therapeutic properties but also for their ability to enhance the nutritional profile of dishes. For instance, adding **turmeric** to rice or vegetables not only imparts a vibrant color and a warm, earthy flavor but also introduces **curcumin**, a compound known for its anti-inflammatory and antioxidant properties. To maximize the absorption of curcumin, it's recommended to include a pinch of **black pepper** in the dish, which contains **piperine**, enhancing curcumin's bioavailability by up to 2000%.

When creating a synergistic herbal blend for culinary purposes, consider the **complementary flavors** as well as the health benefits. A blend of **rosemary**, **thyme**, and **lavender** can create a Provencal-inspired mix that not only elevates the taste of roasted meats and vegetables but also offers **antimicrobial** and **relaxing** effects. The key is to balance the robust flavors of rosemary and thyme with the subtle sweetness of lavender, typically using a ratio of 2:2:1 to avoid overpowering the dish.

Incorporating **herbs into beverages** presents another avenue for achieving synergy. A tea blend combining **ginger**, **lemon balm**, and **peppermint** can offer digestive relief while providing a refreshing and soothing drink. Ginger acts as a **carminative**, aiding in the reduction of gas and bloating, while lemon balm and peppermint offer **calming** and **antispasmodic** effects. For a single serving, use about one teaspoon of dried ginger, one teaspoon of dried lemon balm, and half a teaspoon of dried peppermint. Steep in boiling water for 5-10 minutes, adjusting the time based on desired strength.

The **method of incorporating herbs** into meals and beverages significantly impacts their therapeutic value. For instance, delicate herbs like **cilantro** or **parsley**, rich in **vitamin C** and **iron**, should be added towards the end of the cooking process or used fresh to preserve their nutrient content and vibrant flavor. In contrast, hardier herbs such as **oregano** or **sage** can be added earlier in the cooking process, allowing their flavors to meld with the dish while still imparting their **digestive** and **antioxidant** benefits.

Preservation of herbs plays a critical role in maintaining their potency. Drying and storing herbs correctly ensures that their essential oils and active compounds are preserved. For drying, herbs should be placed in a well-ventilated, dark, and dry area, with temperatures ideally between 68-86°F (20-30°C). Once dried, herbs should be stored in airtight containers away from direct sunlight. This method is particularly effective for herbs like **basil** and **mint**, which can lose their aromatic oils if not properly dried and stored.

The practice of **layering flavors** with herbs in cooking not only enhances the taste experience but also allows for the creation of dishes that can positively impact health. A dish seasoned with **garlic** (known for its **cardiovascular benefits**) and **basil** (with **anti-inflammatory** properties) not only offers a depth of flavor but also contributes to heart health and inflammation reduction. Understanding the individual properties of each herb and how they can complement each other is key to creating dishes that are both nutritious and delicious.

In summary, the science of herbal synergy extends far beyond traditional remedies and into the kitchen, where the principles of complementary actions, ratios, and preparation methods can transform everyday meals into therapeutic experiences. By thoughtfully selecting and combining herbs, one can enhance both the flavor profile and nutritional value of dishes, embodying the true essence of food as medicine.

CHAPTER 2: SYNERGISTIC HERBAL BLENDS

When considering the creation of **synergistic herbal blends**, it's crucial to understand the individual properties of each herb and how they can work together to amplify the desired effects. For example, when blending herbs for a **sleep aid**, combining **lavender**, known for its calming and relaxing properties, with **valerian root**, which acts as a powerful natural sedative, can provide a more potent remedy than using either herb alone. The key is to balance the herbs in such a way that they complement and enhance each other's effects without overwhelming the user.

Choosing the Right Herbs: Start by selecting herbs that have a history of being used together or have complementary medicinal properties. For instance, **ginger** and **turmeric** both have anti-inflammatory properties, but when combined, the presence of ginger enhances the absorption of curcumin, the active compound in turmeric, making the blend more effective.

Determining the Correct Ratios: The ratio of herbs in a blend is critical. Too much of one herb can overpower the others, potentially leading to imbalances or side effects. A general guideline is to use equal parts of each herb, but adjustments should be made based on the potency of individual herbs. For example, in a blend designed for **stress relief**, you might use two parts **ashwagandha** to one part **lavender** to ensure the adaptogenic properties of ashwagandha are balanced with the gentle calming effect of lavender.

Method of Preparation: The way you prepare your herbal blend also affects its synergy. For teas, infusions, or decoctions, the preparation method can significantly influence the extraction of medicinal compounds. **Decoctions** are best for hard, woody substances or roots, such as **licorice root**, which requires boiling for a longer period to extract its full benefits. **Infusions** are suitable for delicate parts of the plant, like leaves or flowers, where boiling water is poured over the herbs and steeped. This method is ideal for herbs like **chamomile** or **peppermint**, where overheating can destroy their delicate oils.

Formulation Considerations: When creating a blend, consider the final form it will take. Will it be a tea, tincture, capsule, or topical application? The form influences how the herbs are processed and combined. For **tinctures**, alcohol or glycerin is used to extract the active compounds, which may involve macerating the herbs for several weeks. The solvent used can affect the solubility of certain compounds, thereby influencing the blend's effectiveness.

Adjusting for Taste and Aroma: The sensory properties of a blend, such as taste and aroma, can also play a role in its therapeutic effects. Aroma, in particular, can have a direct impact on the brain's limbic system, influencing emotions and stress levels. Adding **citrus peels** or **cinnamon** can improve the flavor and aroma of a blend, making it more pleasant to consume while still providing health benefits.

Testing and Adjusting: Once your blend is created, it's important to test it for efficacy and palatability. Start with small batches and adjust the ratios or ingredients based on the results. Keep detailed notes on the proportions used and any feedback received to refine the blend over time.

Safety and Interactions: Always consider the potential for allergic reactions or interactions with medications when crafting herbal blends. Research each herb thoroughly and consult with healthcare professionals if necessary, especially for blends intended for internal use or for individuals with existing health conditions.

CHAPTER 3: PERSONALIZING HERBAL REMEDIES

Adjusting Blends for Individual Needs

Adjusting herbal blends to cater to individual needs requires a nuanced understanding of each herb's properties, potential interactions, and the unique health conditions or sensitivities of the person using them. This process begins with a comprehensive evaluation of the individual's health history, current conditions, and any medications or supplements they may be taking to avoid adverse interactions. For instance, someone with a history of liver issues should approach herbs known for their potent effects on the liver, such as milk thistle or dandelion root, with caution and under professional guidance.

When tailoring herbal remedies, it's crucial to consider the method of preparation that best suits the individual's lifestyle and preferences. For example, a tincture might offer a more concentrated and easily absorbed form of the herb for someone who requires a potent, fast-acting remedy. In contrast, teas and infusions can provide a gentler effect for those with sensitivities or for long-term use. The choice between using fresh or dried herbs also plays a role, as fresh herbs generally offer a different potency and spectrum of active compounds compared to their dried counterparts.

Dosage adjustments are another critical aspect of personalizing herbal blends. Factors such as body weight, age, and the presence of chronic conditions can significantly influence the appropriate dosage. Children, pregnant women, and the elderly, in particular, often require modified dosages to ensure safety and efficacy. Starting with the lowest possible dose and gradually increasing it while monitoring for any adverse reactions is a prudent strategy to find the optimal dosage for an individual.

The flavor profile of the blend should also be considered, especially for those who may be sensitive to certain tastes or have dietary restrictions. Adding natural sweeteners, citrus, or mint can improve palatability for those who find certain herbal tastes too strong or bitter. This consideration is especially important for remedies intended for long-term use, as acceptance and compliance are key to their effectiveness.

Furthermore, understanding the energetics of herbs—such as warming, cooling, drying, or moistening properties—allows for the creation of blends that not only address specific symptoms but also harmonize with the individual's constitution. For instance, a person with a naturally warm and dry constitution experiencing inflammation might benefit from cooling and moistening herbs like marshmallow root or cucumber seed, rather than warming and drying herbs like ginger or cayenne, which could exacerbate their underlying imbalance.

Incorporating feedback and observations is an ongoing part of adjusting herbal blends. Regular check-ins to discuss the effects of the remedy, any side effects, and overall progress can provide valuable insights that guide further customization. This iterative process ensures that the herbal blend remains aligned with the individual's evolving health needs and preferences.

Lastly, it's essential to document any changes made to the blend, including the reasons for adjustments, the effects observed, and any feedback provided by the individual. This documentation serves as a valuable reference for future adjustments and can help in understanding the long-term impacts of the herbal remedy on the individual's health.

Blending for Age and Lifestyle

Creating age-appropriate herbal blends requires careful consideration of the physiological differences and specific health needs across different life stages. For **children**, the focus is on gentle, safe herbs with a pleasant taste to ensure compliance. Herbs like **chamomile** and **lemon balm** are ideal for their calming effects and can be administered in small, diluted doses. For instance, a soothing tea blend for children might consist of 1 teaspoon of dried chamomile flowers and 1 teaspoon of dried lemon balm leaves steeped in 8 ounces of boiling water for 5-10 minutes. This mild infusion can be offered to help ease restlessness or digestive discomfort.

For **adults**, the herbal blends can be more robust and targeted towards common concerns such as stress, energy, and overall wellness. Adaptogens like **ashwagandha** and **rhodiola** are suitable for managing stress and enhancing energy levels. A daily tonic for adults could include 1 gram of ashwagandha powder and 500 milligrams of rhodiola extract, mixed into a smoothie or warm beverage. This blend supports resilience to stress and boosts stamina without overstimulating the system.

When formulating blends for **seniors**, it's crucial to consider herbs that support joint health, cognitive function, and circulatory health, while being mindful of potential interactions with medications. **Ginkgo biloba** and **turmeric** are beneficial for cognitive and circulatory support, respectively. A senior-friendly blend might involve incorporating 120 milligrams of ginkgo biloba extract and 500 milligrams of turmeric extract into a daily regimen, possibly in capsule form for ease of use. This combination helps enhance memory and circulation while offering anti-inflammatory benefits.

In all cases, it's essential to adjust the form of the herb to match the individual's ability to digest and absorb it. For children, liquid extracts or teas are often best, as they allow for easy adjustment of dosages and are easier for young bodies to assimilate. Adults may prefer capsules, tinctures, or powders that can be conveniently incorporated into their daily routine. Seniors might benefit from softer forms such as teas, soft capsules, or gels that are easier to swallow and digest.

Moreover, when blending herbs for any age group, it's important to consider the taste and aroma of the final product. Enhancing the flavor with natural sweeteners like **honey** (for those over one year of age) or using aromatic herbs can make the remedies more palatable. For instance, adding a cinnamon stick to a pot of herbal tea can improve its flavor, making it more appealing without compromising the therapeutic benefits.

Lastly, the timing of when herbs are taken can also be tailored to the lifestyle of the individual. For working adults, an energizing blend might be best taken in the morning, while a calming blend would be more beneficial in the evening. For seniors who may have a more flexible schedule, spacing out doses to coincide with meal times can improve absorption and effectiveness.

By considering these factors, herbalists can create personalized blends that respect the unique needs and preferences of children, adults, and seniors, ensuring that each individual receives the maximum benefit from their herbal regimen.

Creating Seasonal Herbal Formulas

Crafting seasonal herbal formulas requires an understanding of how the body's needs change with the seasons. This approach not only aligns with the natural rhythms of the earth but also optimizes health by preemptively addressing seasonal health challenges.

Spring often brings about allergies and a need for detoxification after a winter of heavier foods and less activity. A formula for this time might include **nettles** for their natural antihistamine properties and support of kidney function, **dandelion root** for liver detoxification, and **burdock root** to cleanse the blood. These herbs can be combined in a tea, with a suggested ratio of 1 part dandelion root, 1 part burdock root, and 2 parts nettles. Steep 1 tablespoon of this blend in 8 ounces of boiling water for 10-15 minutes. This tea can be consumed daily throughout the spring to support detoxification and alleviate allergy symptoms.

Summer requires cooling and hydration to combat the heat and increased activity levels. Herbs like **peppermint** and **hibiscus** offer cooling effects, while **cucumber seeds** are excellent for hydration. A refreshing summer drink can be made by infusing water with ¼ cup of dried hibiscus flowers, a handful of fresh peppermint leaves, and 2 tablespoons of dried cucumber seeds in 1 quart of water. Let this mixture infuse overnight in the refrigerator for a cooling, hydrating beverage.

Autumn is a time to support the immune system and prepare the body for the colder months ahead. Herbs such as **elderberry**, **echinacea**, and **astragalus** can boost immune function. A simple syrup can be made by combining 1 part elderberry juice, ½ part echinacea tincture, and ¼ part astragalus tincture. This syrup can be taken in 1 tablespoon doses daily throughout the autumn to enhance immune resilience.

Winter calls for warming and nourishing herbs to combat the cold and damp. **Ginger**, **cinnamon**, and **cardamom** are excellent for warming the body and stimulating circulation. A warming tea blend can consist of 2 parts ginger root, 1 part cinnamon bark, and 1 part cardamom pods. Use 1 tablespoon of this blend per 8 ounces of boiling water, steeping for 10-15 minutes. This tea can be enjoyed daily during the winter months to maintain warmth and vitality.

For each season, it's crucial to source high-quality, organic herbs to ensure the maximum therapeutic benefit. Additionally, the exact proportions and dosages can be adjusted based on individual needs and responses to the herbs. It's also important to consult with a healthcare provider, especially for those with existing health conditions or who are pregnant, to ensure these herbal formulas are appropriate.

When transitioning from one season to the next, gradually incorporating the upcoming season's herbs can help the body adjust more smoothly. This proactive approach to wellness harnesses the power of nature to maintain balance and health throughout the year.

BOOK 24: HERBAL BUSINESS BASICS

CHAPTER 1: STARTING YOUR HERBAL BUSINESS

Developing a brand identity is a crucial step in distinguishing your herbal business in a competitive market. Your brand represents your business's personality, values, and the promises you make to your customers. It encompasses everything from your logo and packaging to your customer service and online presence. A strong brand identity not only attracts customers but also builds loyalty and trust over time.

Logo Design: Your logo is often the first interaction potential customers have with your brand. It should be memorable, simple, and reflective of your herbal business's ethos. Consider hiring a professional graphic designer who can translate your vision into a visually appealing logo. The design should work well across various mediums, from product labels to your website.

Packaging: Packaging plays a significant role in branding, especially in the herbal product market. It's not just about protecting the product; it's an opportunity to make a statement about your brand's commitment to sustainability, quality, and aesthetics. Use eco-friendly materials to align with the natural and health-conscious values of your target audience. Ensure that the packaging design is consistent with your logo and color scheme to enhance brand recognition.

Unique Value Proposition (UVP): Clearly define what sets your herbal products apart from others. Your UVP should address the specific benefits your products offer, such as organic ingredients, locally sourced herbs, or unique formulations for health and wellness. This proposition should be prominently featured in your marketing materials and on your website.

Website and Online Presence: In today's digital age, a professional website is indispensable for any business. Your website should be easy to navigate, aesthetically pleasing, and informative, providing customers with everything they need to know about your products, your story, and how to purchase. Utilize search engine optimization (SEO) strategies to improve your site's visibility online. Additionally, establish a strong presence on social media platforms relevant to your target audience, such as Instagram and Facebook, to engage with customers and promote your products.

Customer Service: Exceptional customer service is a cornerstone of a strong brand identity. Be responsive to customer inquiries, feedback, and complaints. Establish clear policies for shipping, returns, and refunds that are customer-friendly. Personal touches, such as handwritten thank-you notes or samples with orders, can significantly enhance the customer experience and foster brand loyalty.

Community Engagement: Building a community around your brand can be incredibly beneficial. Host workshops, attend local markets, or create online content that educates your audience about the benefits of herbal remedies and sustainable living. Engaging with your community not only raises brand awareness but also establishes your business as a trusted authority in the herbal market.

Consistency: Consistency across all touchpoints of your brand is key to building recognition and trust. Ensure that your visual elements, tone of voice, and messaging are coherent and reflect your brand's values and personality. This consistency should be maintained in your product quality, customer interactions, and marketing efforts.

Finding Your Herbal Market Niche

Identifying your niche within the herbal market is a critical step for setting your business apart and targeting your ideal customer base effectively. The herbal market is vast, encompassing a wide range of products from medicinal tinctures to beauty creams, each catering to different segments of consumers with unique needs and preferences. To carve out a niche, you must first conduct thorough market research to understand the existing demand, identify gaps in the market, and evaluate the competition. This involves analyzing trends in the herbal industry, such as the growing interest in organic and sustainably sourced products, and considering how your products can meet these demands in ways that others do not.

Once you have a grasp of the market landscape, the next step is to define your target audience. Consider factors such as age, lifestyle, health concerns, and values. For instance, if you decide to focus on herbal skincare products, your target audience might include individuals with sensitive skin who prefer natural over chemical ingredients. Understanding your audience's pain points and desires allows you to tailor your product formulations, marketing messages, and branding to resonate with them deeply.

Specializing in a particular category of herbal products, such as teas for digestive health or tinctures for stress relief, enables you to become an expert in that area. This specialization can be based on your personal passions, expertise, or a noticeable lack in the market. For example, if you have a background in aromatherapy, you might focus on creating herbal essential oils that offer both therapeutic and aromatic benefits. It's essential to ensure that your chosen niche aligns with your interests and strengths, as this passion will be evident in your product quality and brand story.

Developing a unique selling proposition (USP) is crucial for distinguishing your products from those of competitors. This could involve innovative product formulations, unique packaging, or a compelling brand story that highlights the origins and benefits of your herbs. For example, if you're focusing on herbal teas, your USP could be a commitment to direct trade with organic herb farmers, ensuring both the highest quality ingredients and support for sustainable farming practices.

Product development should be guided by both your niche and your target audience's needs. This means choosing the right herbs, formulations, and packaging that appeal to your customers. For skincare products, this might involve selecting herbs known for their soothing properties, such as chamomile or lavender, and using eco-friendly packaging that reflects your brand's commitment to sustainability.

Marketing strategies should also be tailored to your niche. This could involve content marketing that educates your audience on the benefits of your herbs, social media campaigns that showcase customer testimonials, or collaborations with influencers who align with your brand values. Engaging with your community through workshops or herbal remedy classes can further establish your expertise and build trust with your audience.

Finally, continuously gathering feedback from your customers and staying informed about industry trends will help you refine your products and marketing strategies over time. This iterative process ensures that your herbal business remains relevant and continues to meet the evolving needs of your target market. By focusing on a specific niche and deeply understanding your customers, you can build a loyal following and achieve long-term success in the herbal market.

Setting Up a Legal Herbal Business

Navigating the legal landscape is a fundamental step in establishing a herbal business, ensuring that operations comply with local, state, and federal regulations. The process begins with obtaining the necessary permits and certifications, which serve as official endorsements of your business's adherence to industry standards and legal requirements. This section delves into the specifics of these legal prerequisites, offering a comprehensive guide to setting up a legal herbal business.

Firstly, registering your business is the initial legal step. This involves selecting a business structure, such as a sole proprietorship, partnership, limited liability company (LLC), or corporation. Each structure offers different benefits and liabilities, particularly concerning taxation, ownership, and legal responsibilities. For instance, an LLC provides personal liability protection and tax flexibility, making it a popular choice among small business owners. The registration process typically requires submitting a business name, obtaining a Federal Employer Identification Number (FEIN) from the IRS for tax purposes, and registering with state and local tax authorities.

Secondly, acquiring the appropriate business licenses and permits is crucial. The specific requirements vary significantly depending on your location and the nature of your herbal business. For example, if you plan to manufacture herbal products, a manufacturing license may be necessary, along with health department permits if your products are intended for consumption. Retail businesses require a sales permit to legally sell products. Researching local regulations through your city or county's business licensing office can provide clarity on the exact permits needed.

Thirdly, certifications play a vital role in establishing credibility and trustworthiness in the herbal market. Certifications such as organic, GMP (Good Manufacturing Practices), and fair trade not only assure customers of your commitment to quality and ethical standards but also may be legally required for certain operations. Obtaining organic certification, for instance, involves adhering to strict guidelines on how your herbs are grown, processed, and handled, overseen by the USDA's National Organic Program. GMP certification, regulated by the FDA, ensures that products are consistently produced and controlled according to quality standards.

Moreover, understanding and complying with labeling and marketing regulations is essential to avoid legal pitfalls. The FDA oversees the labeling of herbal products, requiring accurate ingredient lists, nutritional information, and disclaimers if health claims are made. Misleading or unverified claims about the therapeutic benefits of your products can result in severe penalties. Familiarizing yourself with the FDA's guidelines on dietary supplements and the FTC's regulations on advertising can help navigate these complexities.

Insurance is another critical consideration for legal protection. General liability insurance, product liability insurance, and professional liability insurance can safeguard your business from lawsuits related to product defects, accidents, or negligence. Consulting with an insurance agent who specializes in small businesses or herbal products can tailor coverage to your specific needs.

Lastly, maintaining compliance involves regular reviews and updates to your legal documents and practices as laws and regulations change. Joining professional associations, attending industry conferences, and subscribing to trade publications can keep you informed about legal trends affecting the herbal market.

By meticulously addressing each of these legal requirements, you can lay a solid foundation for your herbal business, ensuring not only compliance but also building a reputation for reliability and integrity in the herbal community.

Developing a Brand Identity

Developing a brand identity for your herbal business involves creating a visual and thematic representation that communicates your values, mission, and what sets you apart from competitors. The cornerstone of this identity is your logo, which should be distinctive, memorable, and reflective of the herbal realm in which your business operates. When designing a logo, consider incorporating elements that are synonymous with nature and healing, such as leaves, plants, or a mortar and pestle. Choose colors that evoke a sense of calm, healing, or vitality, such as greens, blues, or earth tones. The font should be readable yet convey the essence of your brand, whether that's elegant and refined or rustic and earthy.

Packaging plays a crucial role in establishing your brand identity and can significantly influence a customer's purchasing decision. Opt for packaging that not only protects and preserves your products but also aligns with your brand's commitment to sustainability. This could mean using recyclable or biodegradable materials, minimalistic designs to reduce waste, or reusable containers that encourage customers to return for refills. The packaging should clearly display your logo and include essential product information in a legible font. Incorporating your brand's color scheme and thematic elements into the packaging design will enhance brand recognition and cohesion across your product line.

Crafting a unique value proposition (UVP) involves succinctly articulating what makes your herbal products or services special and why customers should choose them over others. Your UVP should highlight the benefits and results that customers can expect from using your products, such as improved wellness, relief from specific ailments, or the enjoyment of all-natural ingredients. It's also important to emphasize any unique aspects of your sourcing, production processes, or company ethos, such as locally sourced herbs, handcrafted preparations, or a commitment to environmental stewardship. This statement should be prominently featured on your website, marketing materials, and packaging to ensure it resonates with your target audience.

In developing your brand identity, consistency is key. Ensure that your logo, packaging, and UVP are consistently applied across all platforms and points of contact with your customers, including your website, social media profiles, product labels, and promotional materials. This consistency helps to build trust and recognition, making it easier for customers to remember and recommend your brand. Additionally, engaging storytelling that shares the origins of your business, the passion behind your products, and the impact you hope to have can further deepen the connection with your audience, making your herbal business not just a choice, but a community they want to be part of.

CHAPTER 2: CREATING AND PACKAGING PRODUCTS

Once your brand identity is firmly in place, the next crucial step is to **focus on the product itself**. This involves selecting the right **herbs** and **materials** for your products. For instance, when creating a herbal tea blend aimed at promoting relaxation, consider herbs like **chamomile, lemon balm, and lavender** for their calming properties. It's essential to source these herbs from reputable suppliers to ensure they are **organic, non-GMO, and free from contaminants**. This not only guarantees the quality and efficacy of your products but also aligns with a brand that values purity and sustainability.

The **creation process** should be meticulously documented, including the **ratios of herbs** used, **steeping times**, and **temperatures** to ensure consistency in your product line. For a herbal tea, a typical ratio might be **1 part lavender, 2 parts chamomile, and 1 part lemon balm**. Steeping times should be around **5-7 minutes** at **205°F** to extract the optimal flavor and therapeutic benefits without bitterness.

Packaging is where your brand's visual identity comes to life. For herbal teas, consider **biodegradable tea bags** and **recyclable cardboard boxes** or **tin containers** that can be reused or recycled. The packaging should clearly state the **ingredients, benefits, brewing instructions**, and any **warnings** for allergies or interactions. For instance, the front of the package might feature your logo and product name, such as "Soothing Herbal Blend," while the back provides a detailed list of ingredients, a brief description of the blend's calming effects, and a QR code linking to more in-depth information on your website.

Finally, **marketing your products** effectively is key to reaching your target audience. Utilize social media platforms to share engaging content about the **benefits of herbal remedies**, **behind-the-scenes looks** at your creation process, and **customer testimonials**. Collaborations with influencers who align with your brand's values can also help introduce your products to a wider audience. Offering samples at local markets or health food stores can provide direct feedback and foster community connections, further establishing your brand's presence in the herbal wellness space.

CHAPTER 3: MARKETING YOUR HERBAL PRODUCTS

Creating an Online Presence

Creating an online presence is a multifaceted process that begins with the establishment of a professional website. This digital storefront is where potential customers can learn about your herbal products, understand your brand's ethos, and make purchases. To set up a website, select a domain name that is both memorable and reflective of your herbal business. Use a platform that offers user-friendly website builders, such as WordPress or Shopify, which come with e-commerce capabilities and customizable templates. Ensure your website's design is clean, navigable, and mobile-friendly, as a significant portion of online shopping is done via smartphones and tablets. Incorporate high-quality images of your products, detailed descriptions, and information about your sourcing and production processes to build trust and transparency with your audience.

Integrating an e-commerce platform into your website is crucial for facilitating online sales. Platforms like Shopify, WooCommerce, and BigCommerce offer tools for inventory management, secure payment processing, and order fulfillment. Choose an e-commerce solution that aligns with your business size, budget, and technical expertise. Make sure it supports various payment methods to accommodate the preferences of a broad customer base, including credit cards, PayPal, and Apple Pay. Setting up an SSL certificate for your website is essential for encrypting data and protecting customer information, which further enhances trust in your brand.

Leveraging social media is another critical component of building an online presence. Identify which platforms your target audience frequents the most, whether it's Instagram, Facebook, Twitter, or Pinterest, and create profiles on those sites. Use social media to share engaging content that resonates with your audience, such as educational posts about the benefits of herbal remedies, behind-the-scenes looks at your production process, and customer testimonials. Utilize high-quality visuals and consistent branding across all platforms to strengthen your brand identity. Engaging with your audience through comments, direct messages, and interactive content like polls and live videos can foster a sense of community and loyalty around your brand.

Selling on e-commerce platforms beyond your website can significantly expand your reach. Consider listing your products on marketplaces like Etsy, Amazon, or eBay, which attract millions of shoppers worldwide. Each platform has its own set of rules and fees, so research thoroughly to determine the best fit for your herbal products. When listing products, use keyword-rich titles and descriptions to improve visibility in search results. High-quality photos and detailed product descriptions are crucial for convincing shoppers to choose your herbal remedies over competitors.

In conclusion, creating an online presence for your herbal business involves a strategic blend of a well-designed website, effective e-commerce integration, active social media engagement, and leveraging additional online marketplaces. By meticulously executing each step, you can establish a robust digital footprint that attracts and retains customers, driving the success of your herbal business in the digital age.

Engaging with Your Audience

Engaging with your audience through blogs, videos, and direct interactions is a dynamic way to build trust and foster a community around your herbal business. This approach not only showcases your expertise but also demonstrates your commitment to providing value beyond just selling products. To effectively engage with your audience, start by identifying the topics that resonate most with them. This could range from the basics of herbal remedies, how-to guides on using your products, to deeper dives into the science behind herbalism. Each blog post should be well-researched, citing credible sources and including practical advice that readers can implement in their daily lives. Use a conversational tone to make complex information accessible and relatable. Incorporate high-quality images of herbs, your products, or step-by-step processes to visually complement your written content.

Creating videos is another powerful tool for engagement. Videos can range from short, informative clips about a specific herb to longer, detailed tutorials on making your own herbal remedies at home. Utilize platforms like YouTube or Instagram TV for hosting these videos. When creating video content, ensure the lighting is bright enough to clearly see the content, and the audio quality is clear without background noise. It's beneficial to script your videos beforehand to ensure you cover all key points succinctly while maintaining a natural, engaging delivery.

Direct interactions with your audience can take many forms, including responding to comments on your blog, social media posts, and videos. This immediate, two-way communication helps to humanize your brand and shows that you value your customers' opinions and feedback. Additionally, hosting live Q&A sessions on social media platforms can provide a real-time opportunity to connect with your audience, answer their questions, and discuss topics of interest in the herbal community.

To further personalize these interactions, consider sending out newsletters that include exclusive content, such as early access to new products, special discounts, or behind-the-scenes looks at your herbal business. Use an email marketing service to manage your subscriber list and analyze the performance of your newsletters, such as open rates and click-through rates, to continually refine your approach based on what content performs best.

Remember, the goal of engaging with your audience is not just to educate and inform but also to listen. Encourage feedback, conduct surveys, and ask your audience what content they would like to see. This not only helps in tailoring your content strategy to better meet their needs but also strengthens the relationship between your brand and its customers, fostering a loyal community of herbal enthusiasts.

BOOK 25: SPIRITUAL AND ENERGETIC HERBAL PRACTICES

CHAPTER 1: HERBS FOR CLEANSING AND GROUNDING

Sage and Palo Santo for Energy Clearing

Sage and Palo Santo have been revered for centuries for their potent energy-clearing properties. These sacred herbs are used in rituals to cleanse spaces, objects, and individuals of negative energy, fostering a harmonious and positive environment.

Sage, particularly white sage (Salvia apiana), is celebrated for its strong aromatic properties that are believed to purify spaces of negative energies. When burned, sage releases a thick, purifying smoke that attaches to negative energies and, as the smoke clears, it takes these energies with it. To perform a sage smudging ritual, you will need a bundle of dried white sage, a fireproof container, and matches or a lighter. Begin by lighting the tip of the sage bundle until it produces a steady stream of smoke. Gently wave the sage in the air to encourage the smoke to spread throughout the room. Move clockwise around the space, paying special attention to corners and behind doors where stagnant energy can accumulate. As you move, visualize the smoke absorbing negativity and chaos, leaving behind tranquility and positive vibes. It's crucial to keep windows open during the smudging process to allow the negative energy to escape.

Palo Santo, or "holy wood" from the Bursera graveolens tree native to South America, is used similarly to sage but carries a sweeter, more uplifting scent. Palo Santo is believed to not only cleanse negative energy but also to bring positive energy and healing to the space. To use Palo Santo for energy clearing, you'll need a stick of Palo Santo wood, a fireproof container, and a means to ignite it. Light one end of the Palo Santo stick, allowing it to burn for about 30 seconds to a minute before blowing it out. The wood will smolder and release smoke. Carry the Palo Santo around the room, allowing the smoke to waft around, especially in areas that need an energetic cleanse. While sage is often used for heavy cleansing, Palo Santo is preferred for its gentler, uplifting qualities, making it suitable for daily use.

For both sage and Palo Santo, it's important to source these materials ethically and sustainably, respecting their sacred origins and the cultures from which they come. Always ensure that your sage and Palo Santo are harvested sustainably and responsibly.

Incorporating sage and Palo Santo into your regular spiritual practice can help maintain a cleansed and balanced energetical space, conducive to healing, meditation, and general well-being. Whether used separately or together, these powerful tools serve as a bridge to the ancient wisdom of energy cleansing, grounding, and renewal.

Lavender and Rosemary for Emotional Balance

Lavender and rosemary, when used in conjunction, offer a powerful duo for enhancing emotional balance and mental clarity, particularly during meditation practices. Lavender, known for its soothing and calming properties, helps to reduce stress and anxiety, creating a serene environment conducive to meditation. To harness these benefits, consider adding a few drops of lavender essential oil to a diffuser before beginning your meditation session. The diffuser should be placed in a stable position, ideally at a central location within the room where you meditate, to ensure even distribution of the scent. For a more direct application, dilute lavender oil with a carrier oil, such as jojoba or almond oil, at a ratio of 1:10 (essential oil:carrier oil), and apply to the temples or wrists. This method allows the calming properties of lavender to work through both olfactory senses and skin absorption.

Rosemary, on the other hand, is celebrated for its ability to enhance memory, concentration, and overall brain performance. These cognitive benefits make rosemary an excellent herb for meditation, as it aids in maintaining focus and intention. Incorporating rosemary into your meditation routine can be as simple as placing a sprig of fresh rosemary beside you or using rosemary essential oil in combination with lavender in your diffuser. If opting for the essential oil method, a ratio of three parts lavender to one part rosemary can create a balanced blend that promotes both relaxation and mental sharpness. Ensure that the essential oils used are of therapeutic grade for maximum efficacy.

For individuals seeking a more tactile experience, creating a sachet filled with dried lavender flowers and rosemary leaves offers a portable and natural option. To prepare a sachet, select a small, breathable fabric bag and fill it with equal parts of dried lavender and rosemary. This sachet can be placed near your meditation space, squeezed gently to release the aromas, or carried with you throughout the day for moments of mindfulness and grounding.

Additionally, incorporating these herbs into a pre-meditation tea can also be beneficial. A simple tea can be made by steeping a teaspoon of dried lavender and a teaspoon of dried rosemary in boiling water for five to ten minutes. Strain the herbs and enjoy the tea before meditation to prepare your body and mind for the practice. Ensure the herbs are culinary grade and have not been treated with pesticides or chemicals to ensure safety for consumption.

The combination of lavender and rosemary not only supports a deeper meditation experience but also fosters an environment of emotional balance and mental clarity. By integrating these herbs into your meditation practice through aromatherapy, topical application, sachets, or herbal teas, you can enhance your ability to relax, focus, and connect with your inner self. Remember to experiment with different methods of incorporating lavender and rosemary to find what best suits your personal preferences and meditation style, allowing these ancient herbs to deepen your practice.

Mugwort for Intuition and Psychic Energy

Mugwort, scientifically known as **Artemisia vulgaris**, has been revered across various cultures for its ability to enhance intuition and psychic energy, particularly in dream work. To harness mugwort's properties for these purposes, it's essential to understand the specific methods of preparation and application.

For enhancing intuition and psychic energy through dream work, creating a **mugwort dream pillow** is a highly effective method. Begin by selecting dried mugwort leaves, ensuring they are free from any pesticides or contaminants. You'll need approximately one to two handfuls of dried mugwort leaves for a standard-sized dream pillow.

Select a small, breathable fabric pouch, preferably made of natural materials like cotton or linen, to fill with the dried mugwort. The size of the pouch should be small enough to fit comfortably within your regular pillowcase but large enough to hold the mugwort leaves. Before filling the pouch, consider adding a few drops of **lavender essential oil** to the mugwort leaves. Lavender's calming properties can complement mugwort's effects, promoting a more relaxed state conducive to intuitive dreams.

Once the pouch is filled, securely close it, either by tying it with a natural string or sewing it shut if it doesn't have a built-in closure. Place the mugwort dream pillow inside your pillowcase, near where your head rests. The aromatic properties of mugwort will be released as you sleep, facilitating a state of heightened awareness and receptivity to intuitive insights and psychic dreams.

For those who prefer a more direct approach, brewing a **mugwort tea** before bedtime can also be beneficial. Use one teaspoon of dried mugwort per cup of boiling water, steeping it for approximately 5-10 minutes. Strain the tea to remove the leaves, and drink it 30 minutes before going to bed. It's important to note that mugwort tea has a bitter taste, so you may want to sweeten it with honey or mix it with other herbal teas to improve its flavor. Additionally, mugwort tea should be consumed in moderation, and it's not recommended for pregnant women or individuals taking certain medications, so consulting with a healthcare provider before use is advised.

Another method to utilize mugwort for enhancing intuition and psychic energy involves creating a **mugwort-infused oil** that can be applied to the forehead or temples before sleep. To prepare the oil, fill a jar with dried mugwort leaves, then cover them completely with a carrier oil such as almond or olive oil. Seal the jar and place it in a sunny window for about 4-6 weeks, shaking it gently every few days. After the infusion period, strain the oil to remove the mugwort leaves. Store the infused oil in a dark glass bottle in a cool, dry place. Before bedtime, apply a small amount of the oil to your temples or forehead to promote psychic awareness and intuitive dreams.

Incorporating mugwort into your spiritual or energetic practices requires mindfulness and respect for the herb's powerful properties. Whether choosing to create a dream pillow, brew a tea, or use an infused oil, mugwort can serve as a valuable ally in exploring the depths of your intuition and enhancing your psychic energy.

CHAPTER 2: RITUALS AND HERBAL PRACTICES

Frankincense and Myrrh have been used for thousands of years in various cultural and spiritual rituals for meditation and healing purposes. These resins, when burned, release aromatic smoke that is believed to elevate prayers to the divine, cleanse spaces of negative energies, and aid in meditative practices. To utilize Frankincense and Myrrh effectively in your rituals and practices, follow these detailed steps:

Selecting Frankincense and Myrrh: Choose high-quality, ethically sourced Frankincense (Boswellia sacra) and Myrrh (Commiphora myrrha) resins. These can be found at specialty spiritual shops or online. The resins should be in their natural, unprocessed form, often appearing as small, irregularly shaped tears or chunks.

Preparation for Burning: You will need a heat-resistant vessel, traditionally a charcoal burner or censer, and natural charcoal discs designed for burning resins. Ensure your space is well-ventilated, as the smoke can be quite potent.

Igniting Charcoal: Using tongs, hold a charcoal disc and light it with a match or lighter. You'll know it's ready when you see sparks traversing the disc, and it starts to glow red. Place the charcoal in your burner and wait a few minutes for it to become evenly ignited, indicated by a layer of gray ash forming on its surface.

Applying Resins to Charcoal: With a small spoon or your fingers, carefully place a few pieces of Frankincense and Myrrh onto the hot charcoal. The heat will melt the resins, releasing their aromatic smoke. Start with a small amount, as you can always add more. The intense fragrance of these resins is believed to purify the environment, creating a sacred space conducive to meditation.

Meditation and Ritual Use: As the smoke rises, focus on your intention or prayer. The sacred smoke is said to carry these to the divine, creating a bridge between the physical and spiritual realms. During meditation, the aromatic properties of Frankincense and Myrrh can aid in deepening your focus and enhancing your spiritual connection.

Safety and Considerations: Always use tongs or heat-resistant gloves when handling hot charcoal to avoid burns. Keep the burner on a heat-resistant surface to prevent damage to your furniture or altar. Never leave burning resins unattended, and ensure the charcoal is completely extinguished after use.

Storage of Resins: Keep your Frankincense and Myrrh resins in a cool, dry place, away from direct sunlight. An airtight container is ideal to preserve their fragrance and potency. Properly stored, these resins can last for years, retaining their spiritual and healing properties.

Holy Basil (Tulsi) for Divine Connection: Holy Basil, also known as Tulsi (Ocimum sanctum), is revered in many traditions for its protective and purifying qualities. To incorporate Holy Basil into your spiritual practices, you can create a simple tea or use the leaves and flowers in altar decorations. For a Tulsi tea, steep a teaspoon of dried Holy Basil leaves in boiling water for about 5-10 minutes. Strain and drink the tea as a daily ritual to invite divine protection, health, and clarity into your life. Holy Basil can also be grown in your home or garden, serving as a living embodiment of the sacred, purifying your space and offering daily reminders of your spiritual intentions.

Rose for Opening the Heart Chakra: The rose (Rosa spp.) has long been associated with the heart chakra and is used in rituals to promote love, healing, and emotional openness. To use roses in your spiritual practice, consider adding rose petals to your bath, creating a rose water spray for your space, or simply keeping fresh roses on your altar. Rose essential oil can also be used in diffusers or applied to the wrists and heart area (diluted with a carrier oil) to help open and balance the heart chakra, inviting love and compassion into your life.

CHAPTER 3: HERBS FOR SPIRITUAL GROWTH

Frankincense and Myrrh for Meditation

To effectively incorporate **Frankincense and Myrrh** into your meditation practice for enhanced focus and spiritual awareness, follow these detailed instructions:

Creating a Meditation Space: First, designate a quiet, comfortable area in your home where you can sit or lie down undisturbed. This space should be clean and arranged in a way that promotes relaxation and concentration. Consider adding elements that engage the senses, such as soft pillows, calming colors, and, most importantly, a small table or surface for your **Frankincense and Myrrh** burning setup.

Preparing the Resins: For meditation, you will need small, manageable pieces of **Frankincense (Boswellia sacra)** and **Myrrh (Commiphora myrrha)** resins. If your resins are in large chunks, gently crush them into smaller pieces with a mortar and pestle. This increases the surface area that will be exposed to heat, allowing for a more consistent release of smoke and aroma.

Setting Up for Burning: Place your heat-resistant burner or censer on the table or surface in your meditation space. Ensure it is stable and positioned on a heatproof mat to prevent any damage to your furniture. If using a charcoal burner, have a bowl of sand beneath it as an additional precaution against heat.

Lighting the Charcoal: Using a pair of metal tongs, hold a self-lighting charcoal disc and light it with a lighter or match. Wait until the charcoal is fully ignited, evident by a layer of gray ash covering its surface. This usually takes a few minutes. Carefully place the lit charcoal in your burner.

Burning the Resins: With a small spoon or tweezers, gently place a piece of **Frankincense** and a piece of **Myrrh** onto the hot charcoal. The resins will begin to melt and release their aromatic smoke. Adjust the amount based on your preference for the intensity of the fragrance. A balanced approach is to start with less and add more as needed.

Engaging in Meditation: As the sacred smoke begins to fill your space, sit comfortably in your designated meditation spot. Close your eyes and take several deep breaths, inhaling the aromatic compounds released by the **Frankincense and Myrrh**. These scents will aid in calming your mind, deepening your breath, and centering your focus.

Focusing Your Intentions: With each inhalation, envision the smoke carrying away any negative thoughts or distractions, leaving your mind clear and focused. With each exhalation, release any tension held within your body. Set an intention for your meditation session, whether it's seeking clarity on a specific issue, connecting with your spirituality, or simply achieving a state of deep relaxation.

Concluding Your Session: Once your meditation session is complete, take a moment to gradually bring your awareness back to your surroundings. Gently extinguish the charcoal if any remains lit, ensuring that it's completely cooled before disposal. Reflect on the sense of peace and clarity achieved during your session, carrying these feelings with you as you move forward in your day.

Cleaning and Storage: After the burner has cooled, clean any residue and store your **Frankincense and Myrrh** resins in airtight containers to maintain their potency. Keep your burner and other materials neatly stored in your meditation space, ready for your next session.

By following these steps, you can create a deeply enriching meditation experience, harnessing the ancient spiritual and focusing properties of **Frankincense and Myrrh**. This practice not only enhances your meditation sessions but also connects you to a long history of spiritual tradition.

Holy Basil for Divine Connection

Holy Basil, known scientifically as Ocimum sanctum, carries a profound spiritual significance across various cultures, particularly within the Indian subcontinent where it's revered as a manifestation of the goddess Tulsi. Integrating Holy Basil into daily spiritual practices can significantly enhance one's connection to the divine, fostering a harmonious balance between the physical, mental, and spiritual realms. To achieve this divine connection, it's essential to understand the multifaceted uses of Holy Basil, from its physical preparation to its incorporation into rituals that honor its sacredness.

For those seeking to cultivate a deeper spiritual connection through the use of Holy Basil, consider starting with the creation of a Tulsi sanctuary in your home. This can be as simple as dedicating a small altar or space where Holy Basil plants or leaves are kept. Ensure this space is positioned in an area that receives ample sunlight, ideally near a window facing east to catch the morning sun, symbolizing the new beginnings and purity that Tulsi brings into one's life. This sacred space not only serves as a focal point for daily meditation and prayer but also invites positive energy and purity into the home, aligning with Tulsi's protective and purifying nature.

Incorporating Holy Basil into daily meditation and prayer rituals can be profoundly impactful. Begin by lighting a candle or an oil lamp near the Tulsi plant each morning or evening as a symbolic offering, representing the light of consciousness illuminating the darkness of ignorance. As you light the candle, recite a simple mantra or prayer that resonates with your intention for divine connection, such as "May the sacred presence of Tulsi bring health, happiness, and spiritual awakening into my home and heart." This act of reverence acknowledges the sanctity of Holy Basil and its role as a bridge between the earthly and the divine.

Preparing and consuming Tulsi tea is another tangible way to internalize the sacred energy of Holy Basil. To prepare the tea, use fresh or dried Tulsi leaves. If using fresh leaves, gently wash a handful of leaves in cool water. If dried leaves are your choice, measure out approximately one teaspoon per cup of water. Bring water to a boil, then pour it over the leaves, allowing them to steep for about 5 to 10 minutes. As you sip the tea, visualize its healing and purifying properties circulating throughout your body, nourishing your soul, and connecting you to the divine essence of life.

For those who practice yoga or other forms of spiritual exercise, incorporating Tulsi leaves or essential oil into your practice can enhance the experience. Place Tulsi leaves or a few drops of the essential oil on your yoga mat or meditation cushion as a way to sanctify your practice space. The aroma of Holy Basil acts as a grounding and centering force, deepening your focus and elevating your spiritual practice by creating an atmosphere of sacredness and serenity.

Engaging with Holy Basil in these ways transforms it from a mere plant into a living symbol of divine connection, integrating its sacred presence into the fabric of daily life. Through the mindful use of Tulsi, one can cultivate a deeper sense of harmony, health, and holistic well-being, bridging the gap between the mundane and the spiritual.

Rose for Heart Chakra Healing

The rose, with its exquisite fragrance and delicate petals, has been a symbol of love and emotional healing across cultures for centuries. Its association with the heart chakra is profound, as it aids in opening, balancing, and healing this vital energy center. The heart chakra, located at the center of the chest, is the core of our emotional wellbeing, influencing our capacity for love, compassion, and connection. To utilize the rose for heart chakra healing and in love rituals, follow these detailed practices:

Creating a Rose Petal Bath: Begin by gathering fresh rose petals, preferably from organic roses to avoid pesticides. You will need about one to two cups of petals. Fill your bathtub with warm water and add the rose petals. As the water turns fragrant and takes on the essence of the roses, immerse yourself in the bath. While soaking, visualize the water infused with rose energy, enveloping your heart chakra in a healing and loving embrace. This ritual aids in releasing emotional blockages, fostering self-love, and preparing the heart for receiving and giving love.

Rose Quartz and Rose Petal Meditation: For this practice, you will need a rose quartz crystal, known for its heart-healing properties, and a handful of fresh or dried rose petals. Sit in a quiet space where you won't be disturbed. Hold the rose quartz in your left hand, the receiving hand, to welcome its energy into your heart space. Scatter the rose petals around you or place them on your heart center. Close your eyes, breathe deeply, and visualize a pink light emanating from the crystal, surrounded by the gentle essence of roses, filling your heart chakra with unconditional love and healing. Meditate in this space for about 10-15 minutes, allowing the combined energies of rose quartz and rose petals to work on your heart chakra.

Rose Essential Oil Anointing: Rose essential oil is a potent concentrate of the rose's healing properties. To use it for heart chakra work, dilute a few drops of rose essential oil with a carrier oil, such as jojoba or sweet almond oil, maintaining a ratio of 1:10. Gently anoint your heart chakra area with the oil, moving in a clockwise direction to open and activate this energy center. This practice can be done daily, especially during times of emotional distress or when working on enhancing your capacity for love and empathy.

Crafting a Rose Petal Love Sachet: This ritual involves creating a small sachet filled with dried rose petals, rose quartz chips, and a few drops of rose essential oil. Use a pink or green cloth to represent love and the heart chakra. Once filled, tie the sachet with a natural string and keep it under your pillow, in your purse, or anywhere close to you. The sachet serves as a talisman to attract love, promote emotional healing, and maintain an open, balanced heart chakra.

Rose Tea Ceremony for Self-Love: Brew a cup of rose tea using dried organic rose buds or petals. As you prepare the tea, set your intention for self-love and healing. With each sip, imagine yourself absorbing the rose's healing energy, filling your entire being with love and compassion for yourself. This ceremony can be a daily ritual to nurture your heart chakra and reinforce the practice of self-love.

BOOK 26: PREPARING FOR HERBAL EMERGENCIES

CHAPTER 1: HERBAL FIRST AID KIT

Essential Herbs for Cuts and Bruises

Arnica, calendula, and yarrow stand out as essential herbs for managing cuts, burns, and bruises, each bringing unique healing properties to the table. Starting with arnica, known for its potent anti-inflammatory and pain-relieving qualities, it's crucial to understand that it should never be applied to open wounds. Instead, arnica is most effective when used on bruises or areas of swelling that do not have broken skin. For optimal use, consider creating an arnica-infused oil by steeping dried arnica flowers in a carrier oil such as coconut or olive oil for several weeks, straining, and then applying topically to affected areas. This method helps to dilute arnica's potent compounds, making it safer for skin application.

Moving on to calendula, this herb is celebrated for its wound-healing abilities, thanks to its anti-inflammatory, antimicrobial, and astringent properties. Calendula can be applied directly to cuts and burns to promote faster healing and reduce the risk of infection. For a homemade calendula remedy, gently simmer dried calendula petals in a carrier oil for a few hours, strain, and store in a dark glass bottle. This infused oil can be applied directly to the skin or turned into a salve by mixing with beeswax, offering a soothing and protective barrier for damaged skin.

Yarrow, with its ability to stop bleeding and serve as a natural astringent, is invaluable for first aid. Fresh yarrow leaves can be crushed or chewed and applied directly to wounds to staunch bleeding. Alternatively, for a more convenient and hygienic application, dry yarrow leaves and flowers can be powdered and kept on hand to sprinkle on cuts and abrasions. Yarrow's antimicrobial properties also help prevent wound infection, making it a dual-action herb for emergency kits.

Each of these herbs can be grown in a home garden or sourced from reputable suppliers to ensure quality and potency. When preparing any herbal remedy, it's essential to use clean, sterilized containers and utensils to avoid contamination. Label each preparation with the date and contents to ensure safety and effectiveness. Remember, while these herbal remedies can provide immediate and effective care for minor injuries, they are not substitutes for professional medical treatment in the case of severe burns, deep cuts, or persistent wounds. Always consult with a healthcare provider for serious injuries or if there is any concern about the wound healing process.

Herbs for Common Ailments

For managing **headaches**, peppermint oil stands out due to its menthol content, which can help relax muscles and ease pain. To use, mix 2-3 drops of peppermint essential oil with a tablespoon of a carrier oil such as sweet almond or jojoba oil. Apply this blend to the temples and forehead, avoiding the eye area, for a cooling sensation that can alleviate headache symptoms. Additionally, drinking peppermint tea can also provide relief from tension headaches due to its muscle-relaxing properties.

For **nausea**, ginger is highly effective. Its compounds, such as gingerol, directly affect the digestive system and can help reduce feelings of nausea. To prepare a ginger remedy, peel and slice a 2-inch piece of fresh ginger root. Simmer it in 2 cups of water for about 10 minutes. Strain and drink the tea warm, optionally sweetening it with a teaspoon of honey. For convenience, ginger capsules containing 500-1000 mg of ginger powder can be taken as directed on the package, usually not exceeding 4 grams of ginger per day.

When addressing **minor infections**, echinacea is a powerful herb known for its immune-boosting properties. It can be particularly beneficial for respiratory tract infections. For a homemade echinacea tincture, fill a jar with dried echinacea flowers and leaves, then cover with vodka, ensuring the plant material is completely submerged. Seal the jar and store it in a cool, dark place for 4-6 weeks, shaking it every few days. Strain the mixture through a cheesecloth into a clean bottle. Take 1-2 teaspoons of this tincture up to three times a day at the first sign of an infection. Note: Echinacea should be used in cycles of 2-3 weeks on, followed by a one-week break.

For all remedies, ensure the ingredients are sourced from reputable suppliers to guarantee purity and potency. Always perform a patch test when applying oils topically for the first time to check for any allergic reactions. Pregnant or nursing women and individuals with pre-existing health conditions should consult a healthcare provider before incorporating these remedies into their regimen.

Portable Kits for Travel

Creating a portable herbal first aid kit for travel involves selecting compact, versatile items that can address a wide range of common ailments from digestive issues to minor cuts and bruises. Begin by choosing a small, durable container that can easily fit into a backpack or suitcase. A waterproof pouch or a hard-shell case with compartments is ideal to protect the contents from moisture and damage during travel.

For digestive discomforts, include **peppermint tea bags** and **ginger capsules**. Peppermint can alleviate symptoms of indigestion and nausea, while ginger is effective against motion sickness and stomach upset. Both are lightweight and take up minimal space.

For cuts, scrapes, and skin irritations, pack a small bottle of **calendula tincture** or a tube of **calendula cream**. Calendula is known for its soothing, antimicrobial properties that promote wound healing. Additionally, include a few **sterile gauze pads** and **adhesive bandages** to cover and protect minor wounds.

For headaches and muscle aches, a small vial of **lavender essential oil** can be both calming and pain-relieving when applied to the temples or sore muscles. Ensure the oil is stored in a leak-proof container to prevent spills.

For immune support, especially important in unfamiliar environments, bring along **elderberry capsules** or **echinacea tincture**. Both can be used at the first sign of a cold to boost the immune system. Remember to pack a small measuring dropper for tinctures to ensure proper dosage.

For insect bites and stings, include a small jar of **witch hazel extract** or **aloe vera gel**. Witch hazel can reduce itching and inflammation, while aloe vera soothes and heals the skin. If traveling to an area with mosquitoes, consider adding a **natural insect repellent** made from essential oils like citronella or lemon eucalyptus.

To address the risk of dehydration, especially during outdoor adventures or in hot climates, pack **electrolyte powder packets** that can be mixed with water. Dehydration can exacerbate many health issues, and maintaining electrolyte balance is crucial.

For organization within your kit, use small, labeled bags or containers to group items by their use – for example, digestive aids, wound care, and pain relief. This organization makes it easier to find what you need quickly in an emergency.

Lastly, include a compact reference guide or notes on the use and dosage of each item in your kit. Even if you are familiar with these remedies, having a reference can be invaluable in stressful situations or if someone else needs to use the kit.

Remember, while a travel herbal first aid kit can be a valuable resource for managing minor health issues on the go, it is not a substitute for professional medical care in the case of serious illness or injury. Always assess the situation carefully and seek medical attention when needed.

CHAPTER 2: EMERGENCY HERBAL PREPARATIONS

For **burns, aloe vera** is unparalleled in its soothing and healing properties. The gel inside the aloe vera leaf is rich in compounds that reduce inflammation and promote skin regeneration. To use, slice a leaf from an aloe vera plant, split it open, and apply the fresh gel directly to the burn. For more severe burns, the gel can be refrigerated before application for additional cooling relief. Ensure the burn is cleaned before applying aloe vera to prevent infection. For convenience, aloe vera gel can be pre-extracted and stored in the refrigerator in a sterile container for up to one week. When purchasing commercial aloe vera gel, opt for products with high aloe vera content and minimal additives.

Insect bites and stings can be effectively managed with **witch hazel** and **baking soda**. Witch hazel, applied with a cotton ball directly to the bite, offers immediate relief from itching and reduces inflammation due to its astringent properties. Baking soda can be made into a paste with water and applied to the bite to neutralize the acidic venom of insect stings, providing pain relief. For multiple bites, a bath with a cup of baking soda can offer widespread relief. Store witch hazel in a cool, dark place and ensure baking soda is kept moisture-free in an airtight container for longevity.

For **headache relief, peppermint and lavender essential oils** are highly effective. Peppermint oil, when diluted with a carrier oil like coconut or jojoba oil, can be massaged into the temples and back of the neck to relieve tension headaches. The cooling effect of menthol in peppermint oil eases pain and relaxes muscles. Lavender oil, known for its calming properties, can be inhaled or applied similarly to peppermint oil to reduce stress-related headaches. Always perform a patch test with essential oils to ensure no allergic reaction occurs. Essential oils should be stored in dark, glass bottles away from direct sunlight to preserve their potency.

Dehydration can be a concern in various emergency situations, making **oral rehydration salts (ORS)** a vital component of any herbal emergency kit. An ORS can be made by mixing 6 teaspoons of sugar and half a teaspoon of salt in 1 liter of purified water. This solution replenishes lost fluids and electrolytes quickly and efficiently. For taste, a squeeze of lemon juice or a small amount of orange juice can be added. Ensure the water used is clean and safe for consumption. Store sugar, salt, and citrus fruits in a cool, dry place to maintain their quality.

Diarrhea can lead to dehydration and nutrient loss, making **ginger tea** an effective remedy due to its anti-inflammatory and anti-microbial properties. To prepare, slice fresh ginger root and simmer in water for 10-15 minutes. Strain and drink the tea warm. Ginger powder can also be used in a pinch, with ¼ teaspoon mixed in hot water. Ginger aids in soothing the stomach and reducing intestinal inflammation. Store fresh ginger in the refrigerator and ginger powder in an airtight container in a cool, dark place.

For anxiety and stress, chamomile tea is a gentle, effective remedy. Chamomile has mild sedative properties that can calm the nervous system and promote relaxation. Steep dried chamomile flowers in hot water for 5-10 minutes, strain, and enjoy. For stronger effects, increase the steeping time. Chamomile can also be used in baths for a relaxing experience. Dried chamomile should be stored in an airtight container away from light and moisture to maintain its therapeutic properties.

When assembling an herbal emergency kit, consider the specific needs of those who may use it, including any allergies or sensitivities. Label all homemade preparations with their contents and the date of creation to ensure they are used while still effective. Always consult with a healthcare professional before using herbal remedies, especially in emergencies, to ensure they are appropriate for the situation and will not interfere with any medical conditions or medications.

CHAPTER 3: HERBAL REMEDIES FOR LONG-TERM CRISES

In long-term crises where access to conventional medical resources may be limited, establishing a reliable herbal medicine cabinet becomes essential. The focus here is on selecting herbs that are versatile, have a long shelf life, and can address a wide range of health concerns.

Aloe Vera is indispensable for skin health, offering soothing relief for burns, cuts, and other skin irritations. To prepare aloe vera for long-term storage, extract the gel from the leaf and blend it until smooth. This gel can be frozen in ice cube trays and then transferred to a freezer bag, ensuring you have a ready supply for topical applications.

Echinacea is renowned for its immune-boosting properties. For a long-lasting echinacea preparation, consider making a tincture. Fill a jar with dried echinacea plant parts, covering them with a high-proof alcohol like vodka to extract the active compounds. Store this mixture in a cool, dark place for up to six weeks, shaking it daily. After straining, the tincture can be stored in dark glass dropper bottles and kept in a cool, dark cabinet for several years.

Peppermint is a versatile herb for digestive issues, headaches, and respiratory problems. To preserve peppermint, dry the leaves and then store them in an airtight container away from light. For a peppermint oil infusion, submerge dried peppermint leaves in a carrier oil like almond or olive oil, and let the mixture sit in a sunny spot for about two weeks before straining. This oil can be applied topically for headaches or muscle pain, or a few drops can be added to tea for digestive relief.

Lavender is essential for stress, anxiety, and sleep disturbances. Lavender flowers can be dried and stored in sachets for use in drawers or under pillows to promote relaxation and sleep. Additionally, lavender oil can be made by infusing dried flowers in a carrier oil, similar to peppermint preparation, and used in baths or applied topically to calm nerves.

Ginger is crucial for nausea, digestive discomfort, and inflammation. Fresh ginger root can be sliced and dried for storage. To use, rehydrate the slices in hot water for tea. Ginger can also be powdered and stored in an airtight container for adding to food or making capsules for easy ingestion.

Turmeric, with its powerful anti-inflammatory properties, is another root that can be dried and powdered. Turmeric powder can be encapsulated or added to warm milk with a bit of black pepper to increase its bioavailability and effectiveness in reducing inflammation.

Garlic, known for its antimicrobial and immune-supporting qualities, can be stored in oil to create an infused garlic oil. Peel and lightly crush garlic cloves, then submerge them in olive oil in a sealed jar. Store this in the refrigerator and use it both for its health benefits and to add flavor to cooking.

Calendula, beneficial for skin health and wound healing, can be used to make a healing salve. Melt beeswax in a double boiler, then add infused calendula oil (prepared by steeping dried calendula petals in a carrier oil for several weeks). Pour this mixture into small jars or tins and allow it to cool and solidify.

For each of these preparations, it's critical to label containers with the date of preparation and the contents. Regularly check your supplies to ensure they remain potent and discard any that show signs of spoilage. By preparing and storing these herbal remedies, you can create a comprehensive herbal first aid kit that will serve you well in long-term crises, ensuring you have the means to support your health when traditional medical resources may not be readily available.

BOOK 27: SEASONAL HERBAL PRACTICES

CHAPTER 1: SPRING RENEWAL WITH HERBS

As spring arrives, it's an ideal time to rejuvenate your body and home with the power of herbs. This season, focus on **detoxification** and **cleansing** to shake off the sluggishness of winter. Begin by incorporating **dandelion** and **nettle** into your daily regimen. Dandelion, with its potent liver-supporting properties, can be used to make a detoxifying tea. Simply steep 1-2 teaspoons of dried dandelion root in boiling water for about 10 minutes. This tea aids in flushing out toxins and supports overall liver health. Nettle, known for its nutrient-rich profile, can be brewed similarly to dandelion. It's particularly effective in cleansing the blood and boosting energy levels as it's packed with vitamins A, C, and iron.

For your home, create a **spring renewal herbal spray** to purify the air and uplift the mood. Combine **lavender** and **rosemary** essential oils with distilled water in a spray bottle. Lavender brings a sense of calm and relaxation, while rosemary's invigorating scent helps to clear the mind and enhance concentration. Use about 10 drops of each essential oil per 1 cup of water. Shake well before each use and spray around your living spaces to refresh and energize your home environment.

To support your body's natural detoxification processes, add **burdock root** to your diet. Its blood-cleansing abilities make it a valuable herb for spring cleansing. Prepare a simple decoction by simmering 1 tablespoon of dried burdock root in 2 cups of water for about 15 minutes. Strain and drink the tea once cool. Burdock root not only supports liver and kidney function but also aids in clearing the skin of blemishes and toxins.

Lastly, embrace the practice of dry brushing before your morning shower. Use a brush made from natural fibers and gently brush your skin in a circular motion towards the heart. This exfoliates dead skin cells, stimulates the lymphatic system, and encourages new cell growth. Following dry brushing, shower as usual and consider applying an oil infused with **calendula** or **chamomile** to nourish and soothe the skin. These herbs are excellent for calming inflammation and promoting skin regeneration, making them perfect for a springtime skincare routine.

CHAPTER 2: SUMMER COOLING AND PROTECTION

Cooling Teas for Heat Relief Provides recipes using peppermint and hibiscus to beat the heat.

Beneficial effects
Cooling Teas for Heat Relief combines the refreshing qualities of peppermint and the tart, fruity essence of hibiscus to create a beverage that not only cools the body on hot summer days but also offers health benefits. Peppermint is known for its ability to soothe stomach issues and improve digestion, while hibiscus has been shown to lower blood pressure and support liver health. Together, they make a hydrating drink that helps beat the heat while promoting overall wellness.

Portions
4 servings

Preparation time
10 minutes

Cooking time
5 minutes to boil water, then allow to cool or chill

Ingredients
- 4 cups of water
- 1/4 cup dried peppermint leaves
- 1/4 cup dried hibiscus flowers
- Honey or stevia to taste (optional)
- Ice cubes for serving
- Lemon slices for garnish (optional)

Instructions
1. Bring 4 cups of water to a boil in a large pot.

2. Once the water is boiling, remove it from the heat and add 1/4 cup of dried peppermint leaves and 1/4 cup of dried hibiscus flowers to the pot.

3. Cover the pot with a lid and let the mixture steep for about 15-20 minutes. The longer it steeps, the stronger the flavors will be.

4. After steeping, strain the tea through a fine mesh sieve into a large pitcher, pressing on the leaves and flowers to extract as much liquid as possible. Discard the used peppermint leaves and hibiscus flowers.

5. If desired, sweeten the tea with honey or stevia according to taste. Stir well until the sweetener is fully dissolved.

6. Allow the tea to cool to room temperature. For a quicker cooling process, place the pitcher in the refrigerator until chilled.

7. Serve the tea over ice cubes in individual glasses. Garnish each glass with a lemon slice for an added touch of flavor and visual appeal.

Variations
- For a sparkling version, mix half of the cooled tea with an equal amount of sparkling water just before serving.

- Add a few fresh mint leaves or hibiscus petals to each glass for a more decorative presentation and a burst of fresh flavor.
- Incorporate a splash of lime juice for a tangy twist that complements the flavors of peppermint and hibiscus.

Storage tips

Store any leftover tea in a sealed pitcher or bottle in the refrigerator for up to 3 days. It's best enjoyed cold, so keep it chilled until ready to serve.

Tips for allergens

For those with sensitivities to honey, stevia serves as a natural, low-calorie sweetener alternative that won't spike blood sugar levels. If using stevia, start with a small amount and adjust according to taste, as it is much sweeter than honey.

Scientific references

- "Hibiscus sabdariffa L. in the treatment of hypertension and hyperlipidemia: A comprehensive review of animal and human studies," published in Fitoterapia, highlights the blood pressure-lowering effects of hibiscus.
- "Peppermint and its functionality: A review," published in the Journal of Food Science, discusses the digestive benefits of peppermint and its potential for improving gastrointestinal health.

Bug Repellent Sprays and Balms

Creating bug repellent sprays and balms with citronella as the primary ingredient offers a natural and effective way to deter pests during the summer months. Citronella, known for its distinctive lemony scent, is a potent essential oil derived from the leaves and stems of different species of Cymbopogon (lemongrass). The process of crafting these products involves careful selection of complementary ingredients to enhance the repellent properties and ensure skin safety.

For a citronella bug repellent spray, begin by gathering a clean spray bottle, preferably made of glass to preserve the integrity of essential oils. You will need distilled water as the base of your spray, witch hazel to help disperse the oil evenly throughout the water, and citronella essential oil. To make a 4-ounce batch, mix approximately 2 ounces of distilled water with 1.5 ounces of witch hazel. Add 50-60 drops of citronella essential oil. For added efficacy, consider incorporating other essential oils known for their repellent properties, such as eucalyptus, lavender, or tea tree oil, limiting the total number of drops to 70 to ensure skin safety. Shake the mixture well before each use, and apply liberally to exposed skin, avoiding the eyes and mouth.

For a citronella bug repellent balm, which offers a more concentrated and portable option, you will need beeswax, coconut oil, shea butter, and citronella essential oil. Start by melting 2 tablespoons of beeswax over a double boiler. Once melted, add 2 tablespoons of coconut oil and 1 tablespoon of shea butter, stirring until the mixture is well combined and smooth. Remove from heat and let it cool slightly before adding 30-40 drops of citronella essential oil. Pour the mixture into small tins or lip balm tubes and allow it to solidify. This balm can be applied directly to the skin, focusing on pulse points where the body heat will help to diffuse the scent more effectively.

When working with essential oils, it's crucial to ensure the correct dilution to prevent skin irritation. Always perform a patch test on a small skin area before widespread use, especially for individuals with sensitive skin or allergies. Additionally, while citronella is safe for most adults and children, it's advisable to consult a healthcare provider before using on young children or if you are pregnant.

Storing your citronella bug repellent products properly will extend their shelf life. Keep sprays and balms in a cool, dark place away from direct sunlight. The spray should be used within 3-6 months, while the balm, thanks to the stabilizing properties of beeswax and coconut oil, can last up to a year. Always label your homemade products with the date of creation to keep track of their freshness.

CHAPTER 3: AUTUMN AND WINTER WELLNESS

Immune Support with Elderberry & Echinacea

To bolster immune support during the colder seasons, incorporating **elderberry** and **echinacea** into your wellness routine can be highly beneficial. These herbs have been revered for centuries for their ability to enhance the body's resistance to infections. Here, we will detail how to prepare effective remedies from these powerful plants.

Elderberry Syrup Preparation:

1. **Ingredients**:
   - 1/2 cup dried elderberries (Sambucus nigra)
   - 2 cups water
   - 1 cup raw honey
   - Optional: 1 cinnamon stick, 3 cloves, and a piece of fresh ginger for additional flavor and benefits

2. **Instructions**:
   - Combine the elderberries and water in a saucepan. If you're using the optional ingredients, add them now.
   - Bring the mixture to a boil, then reduce the heat and simmer for about 20-30 minutes, or until the liquid has reduced by half.
   - Remove from heat and let the mixture cool to a manageable temperature. Then, mash the berries using a spoon or masher to release any remaining juice.
   - Strain the mixture through a fine mesh strainer or cheesecloth into a bowl, pressing on the solids to extract as much liquid as possible.
   - Once the liquid has cooled to lukewarm, stir in the raw honey until well combined. The honey not only sweetens the syrup but also adds its own antimicrobial properties.
   - Transfer the syrup to a sterilized glass bottle. Store in the refrigerator for up to two months.

Echinacea Tincture Preparation:

1. **Ingredients**:
   - 1/4 cup dried echinacea root (Echinacea purpurea or Echinacea angustifolia)
   - 1/2 liter vodka or brandy (at least 40% alcohol by volume)

2. **Instructions**:
   - Place the dried echinacea root in a clean glass jar.
   - Pour the vodka or brandy over the roots, ensuring they are completely submerged. If they float to the top, you can weigh them down with a clean stone or similar object.
   - Seal the jar tightly and label it with the date and contents.
   - Store the jar in a cool, dark place for 4-6 weeks, shaking it gently every few days to help the extraction process.
   - After the infusion period, strain the tincture through a fine mesh strainer or cheesecloth into another clean glass jar or bottle. Squeeze or press the soaked echinacea to extract as much liquid as possible.
   - Store the tincture in a cool, dark place. It will remain potent for several years.

Usage Guidelines:

- **Elderberry Syrup**: For immune support during the cold seasons, adults can take 1 tablespoon daily, and children (over one year old) can take 1-2 teaspoons daily. If you're already experiencing cold or flu symptoms, the dosage can be increased to 4 times a day.
- **Echinacea Tincture**: Adults can take 1-2 ml, 3 times a day at the first sign of cold or flu symptoms. For children, consult a healthcare provider for the appropriate dosage, as alcohol-based tinctures may not be suitable for young children.

Important Considerations:

- Always source your herbs from reputable suppliers to ensure they are free from contaminants and have been correctly identified.
- Pregnant or breastfeeding women should consult with a healthcare provider before using these remedies.
- Individuals with autoimmune diseases should also seek medical advice before using echinacea due to its immune-stimulating properties.
- Label your homemade remedies with the date of preparation to keep track of their shelf life.

Warming Herbal Teas and Tonics

To craft a **warming herbal tea** that not only soothes the soul but also supports circulation during the colder months, one can turn to the potent duo of **cinnamon** and **ginger**. These spices, revered for their warming properties and health benefits, make an excellent base for a tonic that can help fend off the chill of autumn and winter.

Ingredients:

- 1 tablespoon of freshly grated **ginger root** (Zingiber officinale) – known for its ability to boost circulation and immune function.
- 1 cinnamon stick (Cinnamomum verum) – chosen for its warming effects and ability to regulate blood sugar levels.
- 4 cups of water – serves as the base of your tea, allowing the flavors and properties of the herbs to infuse.
- Optional: Honey or maple syrup to taste – natural sweeteners that can add a soothing texture and flavor.
- Optional: A slice of lemon – adds a vitamin C boost and a refreshing tang.

Preparation:

1. Begin by bringing the 4 cups of water to a boil in a medium-sized pot.
2. Once boiling, reduce the heat to a simmer and add the grated ginger root and cinnamon stick.
3. Allow the mixture to simmer gently for 15-20 minutes. This slow simmering process helps to extract the active compounds from the ginger and cinnamon, ensuring their therapeutic benefits are imparted into the tea.
4. After simmering, remove the pot from the heat and strain the tea into a large pitcher or directly into serving cups, discarding the ginger and cinnamon remnants.
5. If desired, sweeten each cup with honey or maple syrup to taste and add a slice of lemon for an extra boost of flavor and vitamin C.

Serving:

Serve the tea warm, ideally soon after preparation to enjoy its maximum warming effects. This tea can be consumed 2-3 times a day, especially during cold mornings or evenings, to help maintain warmth and circulation.

Storage:

Any leftover tea can be stored in the refrigerator for up to 2 days. Reheat gently on the stove or enjoy cold for a refreshing twist.

Benefits:

- **Ginger** is a powerful anti-inflammatory that can help reduce soreness and inflammation in the body. Its warming effect is also beneficial for stimulating circulation, making it an ideal remedy for cold hands and feet during the winter months.

- **Cinnamon** not only adds a delightful flavor but also contributes to the health of the circulatory system. It's been studied for its effects on blood sugar regulation, which is crucial for maintaining energy levels and overall wellness.

Additional Tips:

- For a stronger tea, allow the ginger and cinnamon to simmer for up to 30 minutes.

- To enhance the tea's circulatory benefits, consider adding a pinch of cayenne pepper. Start with a small amount, as cayenne is very spicy.

- For those interested in exploring the synergistic effects of herbs, adding a cardamom pod to the simmering process can introduce additional digestive and respiratory benefits.

This warming herbal tea blend offers a comforting, flavorful way to support the body during the colder seasons, leveraging the ancient wisdom of cinnamon and ginger to promote warmth and wellness from within.

BOOK 28: HERBAL APPLICATIONS IN COOKING

CHAPTER 1: CULINARY HERBS FOR EVERYDAY HEALTH

Culinary herbs not only add flavor to our meals but also offer a range of health benefits that can enhance everyday wellness. Incorporating these herbs into your cooking is a simple and effective way to boost nutrition and support overall health. Here are some key culinary herbs and their health benefits:

- **Basil**: Known for its sweet and peppery flavor, basil is rich in antioxidants, particularly flavonoids, which protect the body's cells from damage. It also has anti-inflammatory and antibacterial properties. Fresh basil leaves can be added to salads, soups, and pasta dishes.

- **Rosemary**: This aromatic herb is not only a memory enhancer but also contains compounds that offer anti-inflammatory, antioxidant, and antimicrobial benefits. Rosemary can be used to season meats, soups, and bread.

- **Thyme**: Thyme is packed with vitamin C and is also a good source of vitamin A. It's known for its ability to support respiratory health, making it a great addition to teas and dishes during cold and flu season. Thyme can be used fresh or dried in sauces, stews, and marinades.

- **Oregano**: Often used in Italian and Mediterranean cuisines, oregano is known for its potent antioxidant properties, thanks to the compound carvacrol. It can help fight bacteria and has been linked to reducing viral infection. Oregano can be sprinkled on pizzas, into sauces, and over grilled vegetables.

- **Mint**: Mint is not just for freshening breath; it also has digestive benefits, helping to ease indigestion and symptoms of IBS. Fresh mint leaves can be used in teas, cocktails, and salads.

- **Cilantro**: Also known as coriander, cilantro is rich in immune-boosting antioxidants. It's known to help lower blood sugar levels and fight inflammation. Cilantro can be used in salsa, guacamole, and as a garnish for a variety of dishes.

- **Parsley**: This herb is a nutritional powerhouse, packed with vitamins A, C, and K. It can help with bone health and immune function. Parsley can be used in soups, salads, and as a garnish.

Incorporating these herbs into your diet can be as simple as sprinkling them over your favorite dishes before serving. Not only will they enhance the flavor of your meals, but they'll also provide a nutritional boost.

CHAPTER 2: HERBAL INFUSIONS FOR BEVERAGES

Moving forward from the foundational understanding of culinary herbs, let's delve into the art of crafting herbal infusions for beverages, a method that not only elevates the sensory experience of drinking but also imbues our bodies with the myriad health benefits these plants offer. Herbal infusions, commonly known as herbal teas, are an accessible and enjoyable way to incorporate the healing properties of herbs into your daily routine. Here, we will explore several recipes that harness the flavors and benefits of various herbs, providing detailed instructions to ensure you can recreate these healthful drinks at home.

Lemon Verbena and Mint Iced Tea

Ingredients:

- 1/4 cup fresh lemon verbena leaves
- 1/4 cup fresh mint leaves
- 4 cups boiling water
- Honey or maple syrup to taste
- Ice cubes
- Lemon slices for garnish

Instructions:

1. Place the lemon verbena and mint leaves in a large heatproof pitcher.
2. Pour the boiling water over the herbs and let steep for 15-20 minutes, depending on your desired strength.
3. Strain the mixture, removing the leaves, and sweeten with honey or maple syrup to taste.
4. Allow the tea to cool to room temperature, then refrigerate until chilled.
5. Serve over ice cubes, garnished with lemon slices.

Hibiscus and Rosehip Refreshing Cooler

Ingredients:

- 1/4 cup dried hibiscus flowers
- 1/4 cup dried rosehips
- 4 cups boiling water
- Honey or maple syrup to taste
- Ice cubes
- Orange slices for garnish

Instructions:

1. Combine the hibiscus flowers and rosehips in a heatproof pitcher.
2. Add the boiling water and let steep for 20 minutes for a deep, rich flavor.
3. Strain the infusion, discarding the solids, and sweeten as desired with honey or maple syrup.
4. Cool to room temperature, then refrigerate until thoroughly chilled.
5. Serve over ice, garnished with orange slices for a citrusy note.

Lavender and Lemon Zest Herbal Water

Ingredients:

- 2 tablespoons dried lavender flowers

- The zest of 1 lemon, avoiding the white pith
- 4 cups cold water
- Honey or maple syrup to taste (optional)

Instructions:

1. In a large jar, combine the lavender flowers and lemon zest with cold water.
2. Cover and refrigerate for at least 4 hours, or overnight for a stronger infusion.
3. Strain the water to remove the lavender and lemon zest. Sweeten if desired.
4. Serve chilled for a refreshing and calming beverage.

Each of these recipes showcases the versatility of herbal infusions, offering options for both hot and cold preparations. When selecting herbs for your infusions, always ensure they are of the highest quality, preferably organic, to avoid the ingestion of pesticides and other chemicals. Additionally, while these beverages provide health benefits, it's important to consume them in moderation as part of a balanced diet. Remember, the key to enjoying herbal infusions is experimentation; feel free to adjust the quantities of herbs or mix and match different herbs according to your taste preferences and health needs.

Teas for Digestion and Relaxation Provides recipes using chamomile, mint, and fennel.

Beneficial effects

Combining chamomile, mint, and fennel into a tea creates a soothing blend that can aid digestion, reduce stress, and promote relaxation. Chamomile is known for its calming properties, helping to ease the mind and reduce anxiety. Mint stimulates digestion and can relieve symptoms of irritable bowel syndrome, such as bloating and indigestion. fennel is traditionally used to treat various digestive ailments, including heartburn, gas, and bloating. Together, these herbs offer a natural way to support digestive health while also providing a calming effect on the body and mind.

Portions

2 servings

Preparation time

5 minutes

Cooking time

10 minutes

Ingredients

- 2 cups of water
- 1 tablespoon dried chamomile flowers
- 1 tablespoon dried mint leaves
- 1 teaspoon fennel seeds
- Honey or lemon slices (optional, for flavor)

Instructions

1. Begin by bringing 2 cups of water to a boil in a medium saucepan.
2. While the water is heating, place 1 tablespoon of dried chamomile flowers, 1 tablespoon of dried mint leaves, and 1 teaspoon of fennel seeds into a tea infuser or directly into the saucepan.
3. Once the water reaches a rolling boil, reduce the heat to low and submerge the tea infuser with the herbs into the water. If the herbs are directly in the pan, ensure they are fully immersed.

4. Cover the saucepan with a lid and allow the mixture to simmer gently for 10 minutes. This slow simmering process helps to extract the flavors and beneficial properties from the herbs.

5. After 10 minutes, remove the saucepan from the heat. If using a tea infuser, carefully remove it from the water. If the herbs are loose, strain the tea through a fine mesh sieve into a pitcher or directly into serving cups.

6. For added flavor, sweeten the tea with honey to taste or garnish with a slice of lemon in each cup.

7. Serve the tea warm, encouraging slow sipping to fully enjoy its therapeutic benefits.

Variations

- For a cooler, refreshing version, allow the tea to cool to room temperature, then refrigerate until chilled. Serve over ice for a soothing summer beverage.

- Add a slice of fresh ginger to the saucepan along with the other herbs for an extra digestive boost and a spicy flavor note.

- For a caffeine kick, include a bag of green tea during the simmering process, removing it after 3 minutes to prevent bitterness.

Storage tips

This tea is best enjoyed fresh but can be stored in a sealed container in the refrigerator for up to 2 days. Reheat gently on the stove or enjoy chilled. Stir well before serving as natural sediments may settle at the bottom.

Tips for allergens

Individuals with allergies to pollen or specific herbs should proceed with caution and may need to substitute or omit certain ingredients. For those sensitive to honey, stevia or maple syrup can serve as alternative sweeteners.

Herbal Tonics and Cordials

Creating herbal tonics and cordials with elderberry and lemon balm begins with understanding the unique properties and flavors of these herbs. Elderberry, known for its immune-boosting qualities, offers a rich, fruity flavor that pairs well with the calming, citrusy notes of lemon balm. To harness these benefits, one must carefully select high-quality, organic elderberries and fresh lemon balm leaves, ensuring the potency and purity of the ingredients.

The process of making an elderberry and lemon balm tonic starts with preparing a decoction of elderberries. This involves adding one cup of dried elderberries to four cups of water in a heavy-bottomed saucepan. The mixture should be brought to a boil, then simmered on low heat for 45 minutes to an hour, reducing the liquid by half to concentrate the flavors and active compounds. It's crucial to maintain a gentle simmer and avoid boiling vigorously to preserve the delicate nutrients in the elderberries.

While the elderberry decoction simmers, a lemon balm infusion can be prepared by steeping a generous handful of fresh lemon balm leaves in two cups of boiling water. This should be covered and allowed to infuse for about 15 to 20 minutes. The lemon balm infusion brings a refreshing, aromatic quality to the tonic, complementing the deep, berry flavors of the elderberry.

After both the elderberry decoction and lemon balm infusion have been prepared, they should be strained to remove the solids. The liquids are then combined in a clean saucepan, and the mixture is gently warmed. At this stage, sweeteners such as raw honey or maple syrup can be added to taste, typically starting with a quarter cup and adjusting according to preference. The addition of sweetener not only enhances the flavor but also acts as a preservative for the tonic.

To further preserve the tonic and add complexity to its flavor profile, a small amount of alcohol, such as brandy or vodka, can be mixed in. This step is optional but recommended if the tonic is intended for long-term storage. Approximately one-quarter cup of alcohol per pint of tonic will suffice. The alcohol acts as a solvent, extracting additional beneficial compounds from the herbs and extending the shelf life of the tonic.

Once the tonic is fully blended, it should be transferred to sterilized glass bottles, sealed tightly, and stored in a cool, dark place. The tonic will be ready to use immediately but will continue to mature and develop in flavor over several weeks. For daily immune support, a tablespoon of the tonic can be taken directly or diluted in water or tea.

Creating a lemon balm and elderberry cordial involves a similar process, with an emphasis on achieving a sweeter, more syrup-like consistency suitable for use in beverages or as a dessert topping. The primary difference lies in the ratio of water to elderberries and the amount of sweetener used. For a cordial, the elderberry decoction should be made more concentrated by using half the amount of water. After combining with the lemon balm infusion and sweetener, the mixture should be simmered until it thickens slightly to a syrupy consistency.

In crafting these herbal tonics and cordials, attention to detail, from the selection of ingredients to the precision of the cooking process, ensures a final product that is not only beneficial for health but also a pleasure to consume. The rich, comforting flavors of elderberry and the soothing, aromatic qualities of lemon balm come together to create beverages that soothe the body and delight the senses.

Infused Waters for Everyday Hydration

Infused waters offer a refreshing and hydrating way to enjoy the benefits of herbs daily. To create infused waters for everyday hydration using **rosemary** and **basil**, begin by selecting fresh, organic herbs. Freshness is key to ensuring the water is infused with the full flavor and benefits of the herbs.

For **rosemary-infused water**, start by washing a sprig of rosemary under cold water to remove any dirt or impurities. Lightly bruise the leaves by rolling them between your fingers to release the essential oils. Fill a pitcher with about 32 ounces of cold or room temperature filtered water. Add the bruised rosemary sprig to the pitcher. For a more pronounced flavor, you can chop the rosemary leaves before adding them to the water. Cover the pitcher and refrigerate for at least 4 hours, or overnight for a stronger infusion. The longer it infuses, the more pronounced the flavor will be. Before serving, consider adding a few slices of lemon or cucumber for an extra refreshing taste.

For **basil-infused water**, begin by gently rinsing about 10-12 fresh basil leaves. Similar to the rosemary, bruise the basil leaves to release their aromatic oils. Place the leaves into a 32-ounce pitcher of cold or room temperature filtered water. To enhance the flavor profile, add slices of fresh strawberries or raspberries to the pitcher along with the basil. This combination creates a sweet and herbaceous beverage. Cover and refrigerate for 4 hours to overnight, allowing the flavors to meld. The resulting water will have a subtle basil flavor with hints of the added fruit.

When preparing infused waters, always use a clean pitcher and utensils to prevent contamination. Glass pitchers are preferred as they do not impart any unwanted flavors into the water. Infused waters should be consumed within 24 to 48 hours for best quality and freshness. Discard any remaining water after this period, especially if the herbs begin to look wilted or the water appears cloudy.

Lemon Verbena and Mint Iced Tea

Beneficial effects

Lemon Verbena and Mint Iced Tea offers a refreshing and soothing beverage, perfect for hot summer days. Lemon Verbena is known for its calming effects and ability to aid digestion, while mint provides a cooling sensation and helps to relieve symptoms of indigestion and inflammation.

Together, they create a delicious drink that not only quenches thirst but also promotes relaxation and digestive health.

Portions
4 servings

Preparation time
15 minutes

Cooking time
5 minutes to boil water, then allow to cool or chill

Ingredients
- 4 cups of water
- 1/4 cup fresh lemon verbena leaves
- 1/4 cup fresh mint leaves
- 2 tablespoons honey (optional)
- Ice cubes
- Lemon slices for garnish

Instructions
1. Bring 4 cups of water to a boil in a large pot.
2. Once the water is boiling, remove it from the heat. Add 1/4 cup of fresh lemon verbena leaves and 1/4 cup of fresh mint leaves to the hot water.
3. Cover the pot with a lid and allow the herbs to steep for about 10 minutes. This duration ensures that the water becomes well-infused with the flavors and therapeutic properties of the herbs.
4. After steeping, strain the tea through a fine mesh sieve into a large pitcher, pressing on the leaves to extract as much flavor as possible. Discard the leaves.
5. If desired, stir in 2 tablespoons of honey while the tea is still warm. This will help the honey dissolve more effectively, sweetening the tea.
6. Allow the tea to cool to room temperature. For a quicker cooling process, place the pitcher in the refrigerator until chilled.
7. To serve, fill glasses with ice cubes and pour the chilled tea over the ice. Garnish each glass with a slice of lemon for an added touch of flavor and visual appeal.

Variations
- For a sparkling twist, replace 1 cup of water with 1 cup of sparkling water, adding it to the tea after it has cooled to room temperature.
- Add a few slices of cucumber to the pitcher before chilling for a refreshing and hydrating variation.
- For an herbal boost, include a few sprigs of fresh lavender or rosemary during the steeping process for additional flavor and potential stress-relieving benefits.

Storage tips
Store any leftover Lemon Verbena and Mint Iced Tea in a sealed pitcher or bottle in the refrigerator for up to 3 days. It's best enjoyed cold, so keep it chilled until ready to serve.

Tips for allergens
For those with allergies or sensitivities to honey, stevia or agave syrup can serve as a natural, low-calorie sweetener alternative that won't spike blood sugar levels. If using stevia, start with a small amount and adjust according to taste, as it is much sweeter than honey.

Scientific references

- "A Review of the Bioactivity and Potential Health Benefits of Peppermint Tea (Mentha piperita L.)", published in Phytotherapy Research, highlights the digestive and anti-inflammatory benefits of mint.
- "Lemon Verbena: A Lemonscented Herb From South America", published in Nutrition Today, discusses the calming effects and digestive health benefits of lemon verbena.

Hibiscus and Rosehip Refreshing Cooler

Beneficial effects

The Hibiscus and Rosehip Refreshing Cooler combines the tart, cranberry-like flavor of hibiscus with the sweet, tangy essence of rosehips, creating a delicious and revitalizing beverage. Hibiscus is rich in vitamin C and antioxidants, which can help to lower blood pressure, support liver health, and offer anti-inflammatory benefits. Rosehips, the fruit of the rose plant, are also packed with vitamin C, aiding in immune system support and skin health. This cooler is not only a delightful way to stay hydrated but also provides a natural boost to your body's defenses and overall wellness.

Portions

4 servings

Preparation time

15 minutes

Cooking time

5 minutes to boil water, then allow to cool or chill

Ingredients

- 4 cups of water
- 1/4 cup dried hibiscus flowers
- 1/4 cup dried rosehips
- 2 tablespoons honey or to taste (optional)
- Ice cubes for serving
- Lemon slices for garnish (optional)

Instructions

1. Bring 4 cups of water to a boil in a large pot.
2. Once boiling, remove the pot from heat and add 1/4 cup of dried hibiscus flowers and 1/4 cup of dried rosehips to the hot water.
3. Cover the pot and allow the mixture to steep for 10 minutes. The steeping time extracts the flavors and beneficial properties from the hibiscus and rosehips, creating a richly colored and flavorful base for the cooler.
4. Strain the mixture through a fine mesh sieve into a large pitcher, pressing on the flowers and rosehips to extract as much liquid as possible. Discard the solids.
5. Stir in 2 tablespoons of honey to the strained liquid while it's still warm, adjusting the amount according to your sweetness preference. The honey will dissolve more easily in warm liquid.
6. Allow the cooler to come to room temperature, then refrigerate until chilled. This process can take about 1-2 hours.
7. To serve, fill glasses with ice cubes and pour the Hibiscus and Rosehip Cooler over the ice. Garnish each glass with a slice of lemon for an extra touch of freshness and vitamin C.

Variations
- For a sparkling Hibiscus and Rosehip Cooler, replace 1 cup of water with sparkling water. Add the sparkling water after the mixture has cooled to maintain its fizz.
- Enhance the flavor with fresh mint leaves by adding them to the pot during the steeping process.
- Create an adult version of the cooler by adding a splash of rum or vodka to each glass before serving.

Storage tips
The Hibiscus and Rosehip Cooler can be stored in the refrigerator in a sealed pitcher or bottle for up to 3 days. It's best enjoyed cold, so keep it chilled until ready to serve. Stir or shake well before serving as natural sediments may settle at the bottom.

Tips for allergens
For those with allergies or sensitivities to honey, stevia or maple syrup can be used as alternative sweeteners. Always ensure that the dried hibiscus flowers and rosehips are sourced from reputable suppliers to avoid cross-contamination with allergens.

Lavender and Lemon Zest Herbal Water

Beneficial effects
Lavender and Lemon Zest Herbal Water offers a refreshing and calming beverage that harnesses the soothing properties of lavender, known for its ability to reduce anxiety, promote relaxation, and support sleep. The addition of lemon zest not only adds a vibrant, uplifting flavor but also provides vitamin C and antioxidants, which can boost the immune system and improve skin health. This herbal water is a delightful way to hydrate while also enjoying the therapeutic benefits of its natural ingredients.

Portions
4 servings

Preparation time
10 minutes

Cooking time
N/A

Ingredients
- 4 cups of filtered water
- 2 tablespoons of dried lavender flowers
- Zest of 1 lemon, ensuring to avoid the white pith as it can be bitter
- Honey or stevia to taste (optional)

Instructions
1. Begin by bringing 4 cups of filtered water to a near boil in a medium saucepan or kettle.
2. While the water is heating, thoroughly wash the lemon. Use a zester or a fine grater to zest the lemon, taking care to only remove the outer colored part of the peel.
3. Place the dried lavender flowers and lemon zest in a large pitcher or jar.
4. Once the water is heated but not boiling, pour it over the lavender and lemon zest in the pitcher.
5. Allow the mixture to steep for about 5 minutes. For a stronger flavor and more pronounced benefits, you can steep for up to 10 minutes.
6. Strain the herbal water through a fine mesh sieve to remove the lavender flowers and lemon zest, pressing gently to extract maximum flavor.

7. If desired, sweeten the herbal water with honey or stevia according to taste. Stir well until fully dissolved.

8. Serve the Lavender and Lemon Zest Herbal Water immediately over ice for a refreshing drink, or allow it to cool and then refrigerate to serve chilled.

Variations

- For a sparkling variation, replace 1 cup of filtered water with 1 cup of sparkling water, adding it after the mixture has been steeped and cooled.
- Add a few fresh mint leaves to the pitcher before pouring in the hot water for an extra refreshing twist.
- Incorporate a few slices of fresh cucumber for a spa-like beverage that's perfect for relaxation and hydration.

Storage tips

Store any leftover Lavender and Lemon Zest Herbal Water in a sealed glass container in the refrigerator for up to 2 days. For best flavor, consume within 24 hours.

Tips for allergens

For those with sensitivities or allergies to honey, stevia serves as a natural, low-calorie sweetener alternative that doesn't affect blood sugar levels. Always ensure that the lavender used is culinary grade to avoid the ingestion of any harmful pesticides or chemicals.

BOOK 29: HERBS FOR GLOBAL HEALING

CHAPTER 1: AFRICAN AND NATIVE HERBAL WISDOM

In African and Native American traditions, herbs are not just for physical healing but also for spiritual wellness and connecting with nature. **Baobab** is revered in many African cultures for its ability to store water and sustain life. Its leaves, rich in vitamin C, are used to boost immunity and energy levels. To prepare a baobab leaf infusion, dry the leaves thoroughly under the sun until they are crisp. Crush the dried leaves into a fine powder using a mortar and pestle. Steep one teaspoon of this powder in boiling water for 10 minutes, strain, and enjoy the drink once a day for immune support.

Moringa, another powerhouse, is known as the "miracle tree" for its nutrient-rich leaves. To harness its benefits, harvest fresh moringa leaves and wash them in clean water. Pat the leaves dry and remove them from the stems. Lay the leaves out on a clean cloth in a well-ventilated area away from direct sunlight, allowing them to dry for a few days until crisp. Once dry, grind the leaves into a fine powder using a food processor. Store the powder in an airtight container. Add half a teaspoon to smoothies or soups daily to increase energy and nutrient intake.

In Native American healing, **White Sage** is used for purification and cleansing ceremonies. To create a white sage smudge stick, gather fresh white sage leaves and tie them into a bundle using natural cotton string. Start at the base, wrapping the string tightly around the bundle, and work your way to the top before securing the end. Allow the bundle to dry in a cool, dark place for at least a week. Once dried, it can be lit and used to cleanse spaces of negative energy.

Echinacea is widely used to strengthen the immune system. For an echinacea tincture, fill a jar with dried echinacea flowers and leaves, then cover with vodka, ensuring the plant material is completely submerged. Seal the jar and store it in a cool, dark place, shaking it daily for four to six weeks. Strain the mixture through a fine mesh sieve, and store the liquid in dark dropper bottles. Use 20-30 drops in water up to three times daily at the first sign of a cold.

These practices highlight the deep connection between these cultures and their environment, utilizing the natural world to promote physical and spiritual well-being.

CHAPTER 2: ASIAN AND EUROPEAN HERBAL PRACTICES

In the realm of Asian herbal practices, **Ginseng** stands as a cornerstone for its remarkable energy-boosting and revitalizing properties. To harness the full potential of Ginseng, it's essential to select the highest quality roots, preferably those that have been aged for at least six years, as they contain the highest concentration of active compounds. Begin by slicing the Ginseng root thinly, which increases the surface area for extraction. For a simple Ginseng tea, steep about 5 grams of sliced Ginseng in 250 ml of boiling water for 15 to 20 minutes. This method allows the water to become infused with Ginseng's therapeutic properties, creating a potent tonic that can help enhance physical stamina and mental alertness. For those looking to incorporate Ginseng into their daily regimen, consider taking this tea in the morning to kickstart the day with an energy boost.

Transitioning to European herbal traditions, **Lavender** is celebrated for its calming and soothing effects, particularly beneficial for those struggling with stress and sleep disturbances. To create a Lavender infusion that promotes relaxation and a peaceful night's sleep, begin with dried Lavender flowers, ensuring they are organically sourced to avoid any chemical contaminants. Use approximately one tablespoon of dried Lavender per cup of boiling water. Cover and steep for 5 to 10 minutes. This steeping time allows the essential oils and active ingredients to be released into the water, creating a fragrant and therapeutic tea. For enhanced benefits, enjoy a cup of Lavender tea approximately one hour before bedtime to help ease into a state of relaxation and prepare for restful sleep.

Both of these practices, from Asia and Europe, reflect the deep-rooted belief in the power of nature to heal and nurture the body and mind. By integrating these ancient remedies into modern wellness routines, individuals can tap into the timeless wisdom that has supported human health for centuries. Whether seeking to boost energy levels with Ginseng or to find tranquility through Lavender, these herbal traditions offer natural pathways to achieving balanced health and wellbeing.

CHAPTER 3: INTEGRATING GLOBAL PRACTICES

Integrating global practices into a holistic health regimen involves a thoughtful blend of traditions, respecting the origins and wisdom of each. To effectively incorporate these diverse healing modalities, one must first understand the principles behind each practice and how they can complement modern wellness approaches. For instance, the adaptogenic properties of **Ashwagandha** from Ayurvedic medicine can be combined with the calming effects of **Lavender** from European herbalism to create a comprehensive stress-relief protocol. This requires sourcing high-quality, organic Ashwagandha root powder and Lavender flowers, ensuring the purity and potency of these herbs.

To prepare an **Ashwagandha and Lavender stress-relief tea**, measure one teaspoon of Ashwagandha powder and add it to a tea infuser along with a tablespoon of dried Lavender flowers. Place the infuser in a cup of boiling water and steep for 10 minutes. This allows the water to extract the active compounds from the herbs, creating a potent therapeutic beverage. The Ashwagandha provides a grounding, restorative effect, while the Lavender offers a soothing, aromatic quality, addressing both the physical and emotional aspects of stress.

For those seeking to enhance cognitive function, combining **Ginkgo Biloba** from traditional Chinese medicine with **Rosemary** from Mediterranean herbal practices offers a synergistic approach. Ginkgo Biloba leaves should be sourced in their dried form, ideally from a reputable supplier that verifies the absence of contaminants. Rosemary, known for its memory-enhancing properties, should be used fresh for maximum efficacy. To create a **Ginkgo and Rosemary cognitive tonic**, simmer one tablespoon of dried Ginkgo leaves and a sprig of fresh Rosemary in two cups of water for 20 minutes. This slow simmering process extracts the flavonoids and terpenes from the herbs, which are believed to support blood circulation to the brain and improve concentration. Strain the tonic and consume it in the morning to kickstart mental clarity and focus for the day.

In addressing digestive health, the carminative effects of **Ginger** from Asian herbalism can be paired with the soothing properties of **Peppermint** from Western herbal traditions. To harness these benefits, fresh Ginger root and dried Peppermint leaves are ideal. Begin by grating one tablespoon of fresh Ginger root into a pot with four cups of water, bringing it to a boil. Add two tablespoons of dried Peppermint leaves, reduce the heat, and simmer for 15 minutes. This combination works to ease digestive discomfort, with Ginger stimulating digestion and Peppermint relaxing the digestive tract muscles. Strain the mixture and drink warm after meals to aid digestion and alleviate symptoms like bloating and gas.

Integrating these global practices requires not only an understanding of the individual herbs but also knowledge of how to combine them effectively. Each blend should be tailored to the individual's needs, considering factors such as existing health conditions, allergies, and personal preferences. Documentation of the effects, both positive and negative, is crucial in refining the approach and achieving the desired health outcomes. By embracing the diversity of global herbal traditions, individuals can create a personalized, holistic health regimen that draws on the collective wisdom of cultures around the world.

BOOK 30: SUSTAINING HERBAL KNOWLEDGE

CHAPTER 1: TEACHING HERBAL WISDOM

To effectively teach herbal wisdom, it's crucial to start by identifying the foundational herbs that have been universally recognized for their medicinal properties. These include **Echinacea** for immune support, **Ginger** for digestive health, and **Lavender** for stress relief. Each herb comes with its unique set of benefits, preparation methods, and safety considerations. For instance, when discussing **Echinacea**, emphasize its role in enhancing the immune system, but also caution against its use in autoimmune diseases due to its stimulating effects on the immune response.

When introducing these herbs, use clear, accessible language to explain how to identify high-quality herbs. This involves checking for vibrant colors, potent aromas, and, when possible, sourcing from organic growers to avoid pesticide exposure. For **Ginger**, highlight the importance of a fresh, spicy aroma as an indicator of its potency, and for **Lavender**, point out the deep purple color and sweet floral scent as signs of a high-quality herb.

Preparation techniques form the next critical part of teaching herbal wisdom. This includes demonstrating how to create simple **infusions** and **decoctions**, which are the backbone of herbal medicine. For an **infusion**, use **Lavender** as an example: explain that steeping the flowers in hot water for 5-10 minutes will create a calming tea, perfect for reducing anxiety or aiding sleep. For a **decoction**, use **Ginger** to illustrate how simmering the root in water for 20-30 minutes can extract a higher concentration of its digestive-aiding compounds.

Safety is paramount in herbal medicine, so it's essential to teach how to recognize and avoid toxic plants. Incorporate visual aids, like photographs or live samples, to help students distinguish between safe herbs and their dangerous look-alikes. For example, differentiate between **Echinacea** and other coneflowers that might not offer the same immune-boosting benefits and could potentially be harmful.

Finally, encourage hands-on learning by organizing workshops where students can practice making their herbal remedies under guidance. This could involve preparing a simple **Lavender** oil for stress relief by infusing dried lavender in a carrier oil like almond or olive oil for several weeks. Or, creating a **Ginger** tincture by soaking the root in alcohol to extract its active compounds, which can then be used in small doses to aid digestion.

By breaking down each concept with detailed explanations and practical demonstrations, students will gain a comprehensive understanding of herbal wisdom. This approach ensures they not only learn about the various herbs and their uses but also how to safely and effectively incorporate them into daily life for improved health and wellness.

CHAPTER 2: BUILDING A LEGACY OF HERBAL PRACTICES

To build a legacy of herbal practices, it's essential to document and share your knowledge and experiences. Start by creating a detailed journal or digital archive where you record every herb you work with, including its **Latin name, common name, harvesting locations**, **harvesting times**, and **specific uses**. For each herb, note down the **soil type** it thrives in, **sunlight requirements, watering frequency**, and any **companion plants** that support its growth. This documentation becomes invaluable not only for your reference but as a guide for future generations interested in herbalism.

When harvesting herbs, always use clean, sharp tools to ensure a clean cut that will heal quickly, minimizing damage to the plant. For roots, use a garden fork to gently lift the soil around the plant before easing the root out. Leaves should be picked in the morning after the dew has evaporated but before the sun is too high, to ensure they retain their essential oils. Flowers are best harvested just as they open, using scissors or your fingers to snip them gently. Always leave enough of the plant behind to ensure its continued growth and health.

Drying herbs requires a well-ventilated, dark, and dry space. Tie herbs in small bundles and hang them upside down, or lay them out on a mesh screen. Some herbs, like basil and mint, have high moisture content and may mold if not dried quickly; for these, consider using a dehydrator set at a low temperature. Once dried, store the herbs in airtight containers, away from light and heat, to preserve their potency. Label each container with the herb's name, harvest date, and any specific notes about its properties or intended use.

Creating tinctures and infusions is another key aspect of preserving herbal knowledge. For tinctures, finely chop or grind the dried herb and cover it with a solvent like alcohol or vinegar in a glass jar, ensuring the herb is completely submerged. Seal the jar tightly and store it in a cool, dark place, shaking it daily for four to six weeks. After this period, strain the liquid through a fine mesh sieve or cheesecloth into a clean, dark glass bottle. Label the bottle with the herb's name, the type of solvent used, and the date of preparation.

Teaching others is a crucial step in building a legacy. Host workshops or create online tutorials demonstrating how to identify, harvest, dry, and prepare herbs. Cover the basics of making teas, tinctures, salves, and oils, emphasizing the importance of respecting the plants and their habitats. Encourage participants to start their own herbal journals, documenting their learning process and any recipes they create.

Finally, engage with the community by participating in local farmers' markets, offering consultations, or starting an herbal blog. Share your knowledge freely but also encourage feedback and discussions. This not only enriches your understanding but fosters a community of like-minded individuals passionate about herbalism. Building a legacy is not about hoarding knowledge but about sharing and growing it collectively.

CHAPTER 3: PRESERVING HERBAL TRADITIONS

In the modern world, preserving herbal traditions extends beyond personal practice into the digital realm, ensuring that the wealth of knowledge accumulated over centuries remains accessible and relevant. The first step in this preservation effort is to digitize herbal knowledge. This involves creating comprehensive online databases that catalog herbs, their uses, preparation methods, and any cultural or historical significance. Each entry should include high-resolution images of the herb, detailed descriptions of its appearance, optimal growing conditions, and step-by-step guides for harvesting and preparation. For example, a digital entry for **Lavender** would not only describe its calming properties but also offer video tutorials on creating lavender-infused oils, drying techniques for long-term storage, and recipes for teas or baths.

Another crucial aspect is the development of mobile applications focused on herbal education. These apps can offer features like plant identification through photo recognition, personalized remedy recommendations based on symptoms or desired outcomes, and interactive forums where users can share experiences, ask questions, and connect with experienced herbalists. For instance, a user could upload a photo of **Echinacea** and receive information on its immune-boosting properties, along with user-submitted reviews on its effectiveness in cold prevention.

Social media platforms play a significant role in preserving and disseminating herbal traditions. Creating content that educates and engages, such as short-form videos demonstrating herb harvesting or preparation of simple remedies, can reach a broad audience and inspire interest in herbalism. A series of Instagram posts could detail the process of making a **Ginger** tincture, from selecting the right type of ginger to the final bottling, each accompanied by tips on usage and storage.

Online courses and webinars offer structured learning opportunities for those interested in deepening their herbal knowledge. These can range from beginner-friendly introductions to specific topics like medicinal mushrooms or advanced courses on creating complex herbal formulations. A webinar might cover the safe use of **Adaptogens**, including **Ashwagandha** and **Rhodiola Rosea**, explaining how to incorporate them into daily routines for stress management.

Preserving herbal traditions also involves advocacy and community engagement. This could mean partnering with local schools to introduce herbal education programs, organizing community herb gardens to foster hands-on learning, or lobbying for the inclusion of herbal medicine in public health discussions. A community project might involve planting a public medicinal herb garden with informational plaques next to each plant, such as **Calendula** for skin health, explaining its uses and benefits.

Finally, the preservation of herbal traditions in a modern world requires a commitment to sustainability. This means promoting ethical wildcrafting practices, supporting organic and biodynamic farming, and advocating for the conservation of indigenous plants and their habitats. An online campaign could focus on the importance of preserving **Wild Ginseng**, highlighting its medicinal value and the threats to its natural habitats.

By leveraging technology, engaging with communities, and advocating for sustainability, we can ensure that herbal traditions are not only preserved but continue to flourish in the modern world. Through these efforts, the ancient wisdom of herbalism becomes a living, evolving practice that enriches our lives and connects us more deeply to the natural world.

Made in the USA
Middletown, DE
13 December 2024